CONTENTS

Introduction 4

Breakfasts 8

Snacks 40

Soups, Salads & Sides 78

Lunches 142

Dinners 208

Desserts 302

Baked 348

Drinks 370

Index 376

INTRODUCTION

Every parent wants to give their child the best nutritional start in life and to cook healthy meals that the whole family can enjoy. *The Big Book of Quick, Easy Family Recipes* features 500 recipes that are packed with nutrients for a healthy diet, showing you how to create tasty, wholesome meals without spending a lot of money, time or effort. All the recipes have been devised with simplicity and speed in mind, so that even the most hectic of family lives need not be a barrier to eating well.

ABOUT THIS BOOK

The main aim of this book is to inspire. The majority of the recipes are quick and easy to prepare; others take a little forethought and preparation but can be made in bulk and frozen for future use. Many of the recipes will also keep for a few days in the fridge, allowing you to plan ahead.

The emphasis is on good-quality, nutritious fresh food without being too worthy. There are some recipes for sweet desserts and treats, although many are fruit-based and refined sugars have been kept to a minimum. It's just a case of learning to be sparing with treats – if you cut them out completely, they become more tempting. A balanced diet can handle an indulgence every now and then.

The recipes have been created to appeal to both adults and children from the age of three. Try to enjoy these recipes as a family and eat together as often as you can. As for portion sizes, these are averages only, as the size of meals you need to make will obviously differ widely depending on whether you have a picky five-year-old or a ravenous teenager.

SPECIAL DIETS

With a few simple substitutions many of the recipes in this book that contain meat or dairy can be adjusted to suit a vegetarian or vegan diet. Tofu and tempeh make great alternatives to meat, cow's milk can easily be swapped for a dairy-free alternative, and butter can be replaced with vegetable spread.

If your child or another family member is a vegetarian or vegan, has an allergy to nuts or an intolerance of dairy products, eggs, wheat or gluten, you will need to take more care when preparing their meals.

The symbols shown below are used throughout the book to indicate which recipes are safe for particular diets.

KEY TO SYMBOLS

 Vegetarian
Gluten-free
 Wheat-free
 Dairy-free

The BIG BOOK of QUICK, EASY FAMILY RECIPES

500 SIMPLE, HEALTHY IDEAS YOU & YOUR KIDS CAN ENJOY

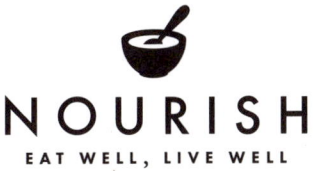

NOURISH
EAT WELL, LIVE WELL

THE BIG BOOK OF QUICK, EASY FAMILY RECIPES

Gemini Adams, Christine Bailey, Nicola Graimes and Charlotte Watts

First published in the UK and USA in 2019 by
Nourish, an imprint of Watkins Media Limited
Unit 11, Shepperton House, 83-93 Shepperton Road
London N1 3DF

enquiries@nourishbooks.com

Recipes in this book have been previously published in the following volumes:

The Top 100 Recipes for Brainy Kids
    by Christine Bailey
The Top 100 Recipes for Happy Kids
    by Charlotte Watts and Gemini Adams
The Top 100 Recipes for a Healthy Lunchbox
    by Nicola Graimes
The Big Book of Quick and Easy Family Recipes
    by Kirsten Hartvig

Copyright © Watkins Media Limited 2019
Text copyright © Gemini Adams, Christine Bailey, Nicola Graimes, Kirsten Hartvig and Charlotte Watts 2019
Photography copyright © Watkins Media Limited

The right of Gemini Adams, Christine Bailey, Nicola Graimes, Kirsten Hartvig and Charlotte Watts to be identified as the Authors of this text has been asserted in accordance with the Copyright, Designs and Patents Act of 1988.

All rights reserved. No part of this book may be reproduced in any form or by any electronic or mechanical means, including information storage and retrieval systems, without permission in writing from the publisher, except by a reviewer who may quote brief passages in a review.

A CIP record for this book is available from the British Library

ISBN: 978-1-84899-359-4

10 9 8 7 6 5 4 3 2 1

Commissioning Editor: Kate Fox
Managing Editor: Daniel Hurst
Head of Design: Georgina Hewitt
Production: Uzma Taj

Typeset in Estilo
Colour reproduction by XY Digital
Printed in China

Publisher's note

While every care has been taken in compiling the recipes for this book, Watkins Media Limited, or any other persons who have been involved in working on this publication, cannot accept responsibility for any errors or omissions, inadvertent or not, that may be found in the recipes or text, nor for any problems that may arise as a result of preparing one of these recipes. If you are pregnant or breastfeeding or have any special dietary requirements or medical conditions, it is advisable to consult a medical professional before following any of the recipes contained in this book.

Notes on the recipes

Unless otherwise stated:
Use medium fruit and vegetables
Use medium (US large) organic or free-range eggs
Use granulated sugar
Do not mix metric, imperial and US cup measurements:
    1 tsp = 5ml 1 tbsp = 15ml 1 cup = 240ml

nourishbooks.com

NUTRITION

RECOGNIZING THE RIGHT FOODS

Use natural, whole foods, comprising fresh produce as much as possible. Whole foods are those that by and large do not come from a packet, but are natural, fresh and preferably organic. Where possible, always choose organic, especially meat and dairy, to expose your family to fewer hormones and antibiotics. Wash all fruit and vegetables before preparing them.

Avoid processed foods, which often have added preservatives and colours, many of which can be harmful to children's developing bodies. Of course, it is pretty challenging to avoid such products altogether, so try introducing an 80:20 ratio. Aim to use 80 per cent whole foods in your family's diet, allowing 20 per cent for occasional convenience foods.

TIPS FOR A HEALTHY BALANCED DIET

- Make breakfast a priority – a proper mealtime rather than a rushed snack. Protein (from eggs, nuts, seeds, yogurt and whole grains) is especially important at breakfast, as it helps to create all the chemicals the body needs to function throughout the day and slows down the release of sugars.

- At lunch and dinner, eat plenty of vegetables, fruits, beans and pulses, seeds, nuts and whole grains, such as oats, whole wheat, brown rice, rye and millet.

- Eat a good mix of dietary protein, including fish, chicken, turkey, bananas, yogurt, eggs, beans, nuts (especially almonds), seeds, quinoa, cottage cheese, avocados and wholegrain crackers.

- Eat oily fish two or three times a week – the essential fatty acids, known as omega-3 oils, that they contain are crucial for children's brain development and function.

- Change refined "white" sources of bread, rice and pasta to wholegrain or "brown" versions, which have their fibre left intact.

- Don't have sweets, chocolate, cakes, biscuits and pastries as snacks, but save them for rare treats. Instead, try flapjacks, fruit, savoury snacks, and healthy nut-and-seed bars, which cause fewer energy highs and lows.

- Drink plenty of fluids every day, but reduce sugary drinks and sodas. Try diluted fruit juices, natural smoothies or, preferably, water.

- Keep desserts free from added sugar and eat slow sugar-release fruits – peaches, blackberries, blueberries, raspberries, plums, strawberries, apricots (fresh and dried), figs, apples, pineapple (fresh), cherries, oranges, melon and watermelon.

A BALANCED PLATE

A nutritionally balanced meal should feature one or more items from each of the following food groups.

FRUIT AND VEG
The more colouful and varied, the better.

DAIRY
Good sources of calcium are vital, but can be high in saturated fat, so use in moderation. Choose from: cheeses (lower-fat cream or hard cheeses, Quark, mozarella, feta); yogurt (plain or fromage frais); milk or milk alternatives.

PROTEIN
Lean, cooked chicken, turkey or beef; fish and seafood (especially oily fish such as herring, salmon, trout and mackerel); eggs; nuts, nut butters and seeds; beans, pulses and hummus; vegetarian sausages and nut cutlets; tofu.

STARCHY CARBS
Wholegrain bread, rice, pasta and noodles; potatoes; grains (quinoa or bulgur wheat).

FATS
Small amounts of healthier oils (such as olive oil) and unsaturated fats should be used for cooking and in dressings or spreads.

SHOPPING AND PLANNING AHEAD
A little forethought makes preparing meals so much easier. Not only does it relieve the daily panic of what to serve, but it also makes the weekly shop more straightforward. Write down a daily menu for the week ahead – it can be made up of fresh fruit and vegetables, freshly prepared foods, and some pre-prepared and frozen dishes, as well as those invaluable leftovers. Use the menu to write a shopping list and try to stick to the list when you go shopping!

FRESH FRUIT AND VEG
Buy as fresh as possible and only as much as you need for the week. If you can, opt for organic, seasonal varieties. Make the most of local farmer's markets and delivery boxes.

CHILLED FOODS
Most chilled foods have a very limited shelf life, so buy regularly in small amounts.

STORECUPBOARD
Most of these foods will keep for weeks or months, so it's a good idea to keep a varied selection. Keep an eye on best-before and use-by dates and note that some products require chilling after opening.

BREADS
Bread is most nutritious when made with wholemeal flour and also contains a higher amount of fibre. Store a supply of bread in the freezer to avoid running out.

FROZEN FOODS
Freeze homemade soups and other prepared foods in single portions. Frozen fruits and vegetables make a convenient standby and are often more nutritious than fresh, having been frozen soon after picking. Purées, compotes and sauces all freeze well.

A HEALTHY ATTITUDE TO FOOD

The whole family can eat and enjoy the recipes in this book. Sitting down for meals as a family is a vital part of a child's relationship with food. Even if there are just two of you, eating the same foods at the table together can encourage an open-minded attitude to food. This will give your child an appreciation of healthy foods that hopefully will last them a lifetime, and will undoubtedly encourage them to experiment with foods that they have never seen before or have previously been unwilling to try.

MAKING FOOD FUN

- Introduce games about food – who can guess where in the world a food comes from, how it's grown, and so on.

- Encourage your child to grow his or her own food, even if it is just a pot of herbs on a windowsill. A child is more likely to enjoy what they are eating if they have grown and cared for it themselves, giving them a great sense of achievement.

- Encourage your child to join you in the kitchen. Ask them to help you prepare foods; open their appreciation of flavours and seasoning by inviting them to enjoy and participate in all stages of the cooking process.

INTRODUCING NEW FOODS

A child's development goes through many stages, and that applies to learning to appreciate new foods as much as it does to walking and talking. Here are some ideas to make introducing new foods easier:

- Give unfamiliar foods in small amounts on the side of the plate with little fuss and no insistence that your child eats them. Even if your child leaves them the first few times, after seeing them for the fifth time, he or she may just make that decision to try.

- Mix new foods with old favourites: try adding a new vegetable to a pizza or in a soup or stir-fry; or simply hide new foods in wraps, mashed in with others, and in stews.

- Eat the food yourself in front of your child for a few days before offering it to them – you may find that your child even asks to try it.

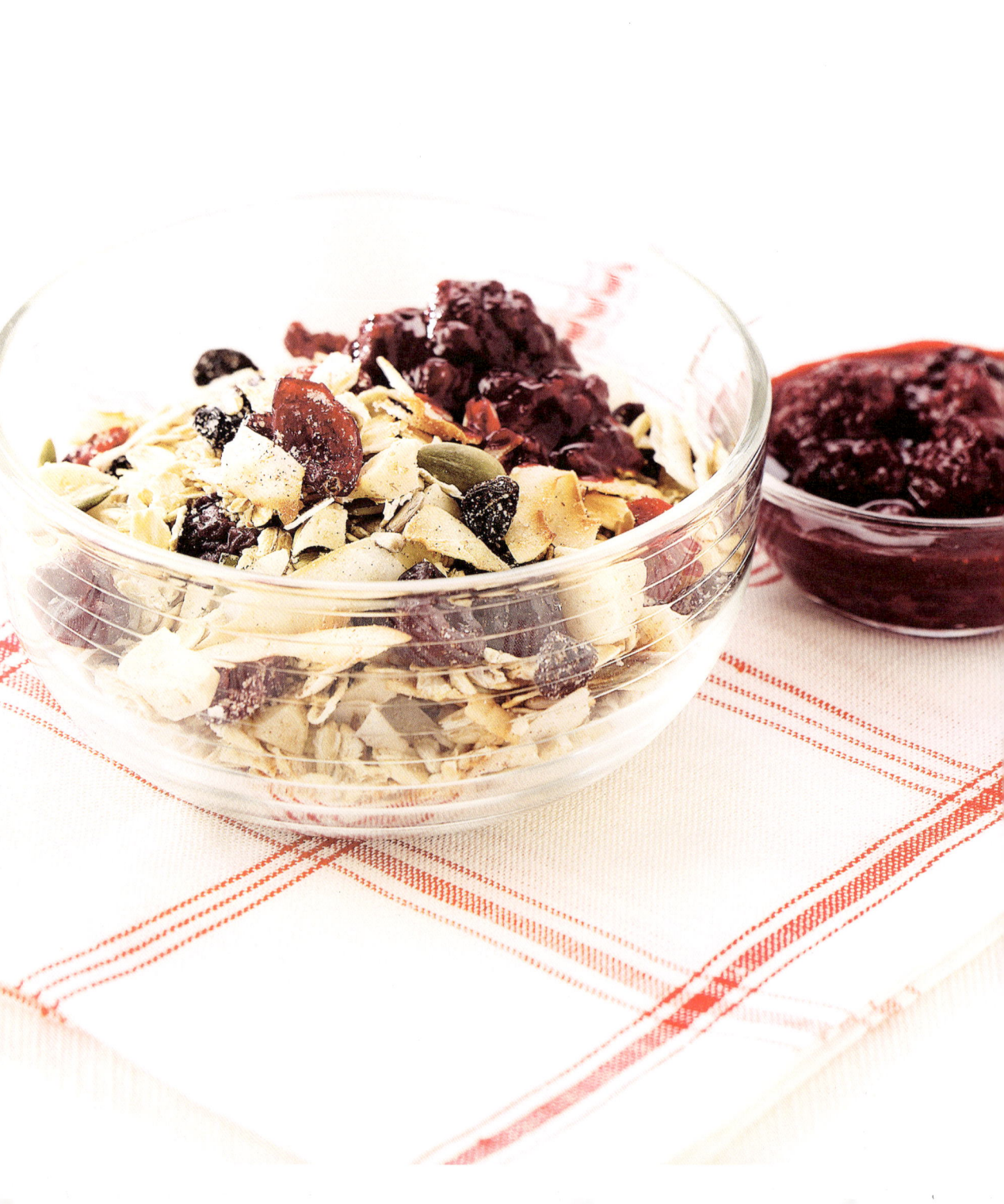

Breakfasts

Breakfast is one of the most important meals of the day – a good healthy breakfast helps us to concentrate, feel alert and perform at our best during the day, whether at school or work. So, for an early energy boost and to maintain a steady blood-sugar level throughout the morning, try some of these mouthwatering recipes designed to tempt even the most reluctant breakfast eater.

Kickstart your day with delicious Fruit and Seed Granola (see page 11) or Tropical Yogurt Pots (see page 18); for something on-the-go choose the oaty Breakfast Bars (see page 20) or Blueberry and Apple Muffins (see page 25); or for a really substantial and sustaining meal, try Banana and Buckwheat Pancakes (see page 26) or the Baked Bean Melt (see page 34).

001 BERRY MUSELI

SERVES 4
PREPARATION
10 minutes
COOKING
10 minutes

STORAGE
The muesli will keep in an airtight container for up to 2 weeks. The compote will keep in the fridge for up to 2 days.

175g/6oz/2 cups porridge (rolled) oats
4 tbsp unsweetened coconut flakes
4 tbsp roughly chopped macadamia nuts
4 tbsp ground almonds
3 tbsp pumpkin seeds
3 tbsp sunflower seeds
1 tsp ground cinnamon
75g/3oz/½ cup mixed dried berries, such as cranberries, blueberries and cherries
milk, to serve

BERRY COMPOTE:
250g/9oz/1 cup mixed berries, fresh or frozen
3 tbsp apple juice

1. Put the oats, coconut and macadamia nuts in a non-stick frying pan (skillet) and cook over a gentle heat, stirring frequently, for 2–3 minutes until lightly browned. Remove from the heat and leave to cool.

2. Put the oat mixture in a bowl and stir in the almonds, pumpkin and sunflower seeds, cinnamon and dried berries.

3. To make the berry compote, put the berries in a pan with the apple juice. Heat gently until just boiling, then simmer for 5 minutes, or until the berries are soft. Set aside to cool.

4. Spoon the muesli into four bowls and add milk to taste. Serve topped with the berry compote.

BREAKFAST | 11

002 MILLET AND APPLE PORRIDGE

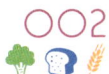

SERVES 4
PREPARATION
10 minutes
COOKING
35 minutes

STORAGE
Leftovers will keep
in the fridge for up
to 2 days.

125g/4½oz/¾ cup millet
2 small eating apples, peeled, cored and diced
150ml/5fl oz/scant ⅔ cup milk
50g/1¾oz/⅓ cup cashew nuts
4 dried apricots
1 tsp ground cinnamon
1 tbsp honey or agave nectar
1 tbsp ground flaxseeds

1. Put the millet in a pan, pour in 750ml/26fl oz/3 cups water and bring to a boil. Reduce the heat, and simmer, covered, for 15 minutes.

2. Stir in the apples and continue simmering for a further 15 minutes until almost all the water has been absorbed. Remove from the heat and set aside.

3. Blend the milk, nuts, apricots, cinnamon, honey or agave nectar and flaxseeds in a blender or food processor until smooth.

4. Stir the nut mixture into the millet and serve hot or cold.

003 FRUIT AND SEED GRANOLA

SERVES 4-6
PREPARATION
10 minutes
COOKING
35 minutes

STORAGE
Store in an airtight
container for up to
2 weeks.

250g/9oz/2¾ cups porridge (rolled) oats
60g/2¼oz/½ cup flaked almonds
60g/2¼oz/½ cup pecans, roughly chopped
60g/2¼oz/½ cup sunflower seeds
60g/2¼oz/½ cup pumpkin seeds
4 tbsp sesame seeds
3 tbsp light olive or vegetable oil
200ml/7fl oz/scant 1 cup apple juice
75g/2½oz/½ cup dried apricots, roughly chopped
75g/2½oz/½ cup dried mixed berries or cherries

1. Preheat the oven to 180°C/350°F/gas mark 4.

2. Put the oats, nuts and seeds into a large bowl. Mix the oil with the apple juice and stir it into the dry ingredients.

3. Spread out the mixture on a large baking sheet and bake for 30 minutes, or until golden, stirring halfway through cooking. Stir in the dried apricots and berries and bake for a further 5 minutes.

4. Leave to cool before serving or storing.

004 SWEET QUINOA

SERVES 4
PREPARATION 2 minutes
COOKING 18 minutes

STORAGE
Keep in the fridge for 24 hours and reheat in the microwave.

700ml/24fl oz/3 cups water
230g/8oz/2 cups quinoa
250ml/9fl oz/1 cup milk
2 tsp ground cinnamon

1. Pour the water into a small saucepan, add the quinoa and simmer over a low heat for 15 minutes, stirring occasionally.

2. When the mixture has thickened, add the milk and stir over a low heat for a further 2 minutes.

3. Remove from the heat, add the cinnamon and stir. Pour into bowls. Add extra milk to cool, or brown sugar to sweeten, if absolutely necessary.

005 GRILLED PEACHES with MACADAMIA CREAM

SERVES 4
PREPARATION 10 minutes
COOKING 15 minutes

STORAGE
The cream will keep in the fridge for up to 3 days. The cooked peaches will keep in the fridge for up to 1 day.

olive oil, for greasing
4 peaches, halved and pitted
3 tbsp honey or agave nectar
2 tsp dairy-free margarine
100g/3½oz/scant 1 cup macadamia nuts
juice of 2 oranges
1–2 drops vanilla extract

1. Preheat the oven to 180°C/350°F/gas mark 4 and grease a baking dish with oil.

2. Put the peaches in the dish, cut-side up, drizzle over half the honey or agave nectar and dot with the margarine. Bake for 10–15 minutes until slightly softened.

3. Blend the remaining honey or agave and the rest of the ingredients in a blender until smooth. Serve the peaches warm with the macadamia cream.

BREAKFAST | 13

006 MORNING MUESLI

SERVES 4
PREPARATION
5 minutes

STORAGE
You can store the muesli in an airtight container for up to 1 month.

110g/4oz/²/₃ cup dried apricots
110g/4oz/²/₃ cup dried prunes
110g/4oz/²/₃ cup hazelnuts
50g/2oz/²/₃ cup pumpkin seeds
230g/8oz/2 cups granola
230g/8oz/2 cups porridge (rolled) oats

1. Roughly chop the apricots and prunes.

2. Place in a large mixing bowl and add all the other ingredients.

3. Mix well, then serve in smaller bowls, adding milk as required.

007 CRUNCHY PORRIDGE
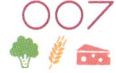

SERVES 4
PREPARATION
2 minutes
COOKING
10 minutes

STORAGE
Keep in the fridge for up to 6 hours and reheat in the microwave.

230g/8oz/2 cups porridge (rolled) oats
600ml/21fl oz/2½ cups soya milk
2 tbsp molasses or brown sugar
4 tbsp sunflower seeds
4 tbsp pumpkin seeds

1. Pour the oats and soya milk into a saucepan and warm over a medium heat. Alternatively, pour the milk and oats into a bowl and cook for 3 minutes in the microwave.

2. Bring to the boil, stirring regularly. Alternatively, remove from the microwave after 3 minutes, stir and return to the microwave for a further 2–4 minutes.

3. When the mixture has thickened slightly, add the molasses or brown sugar and stir. Remove from the heat and serve in individual bowls with the seeds scattered on top.

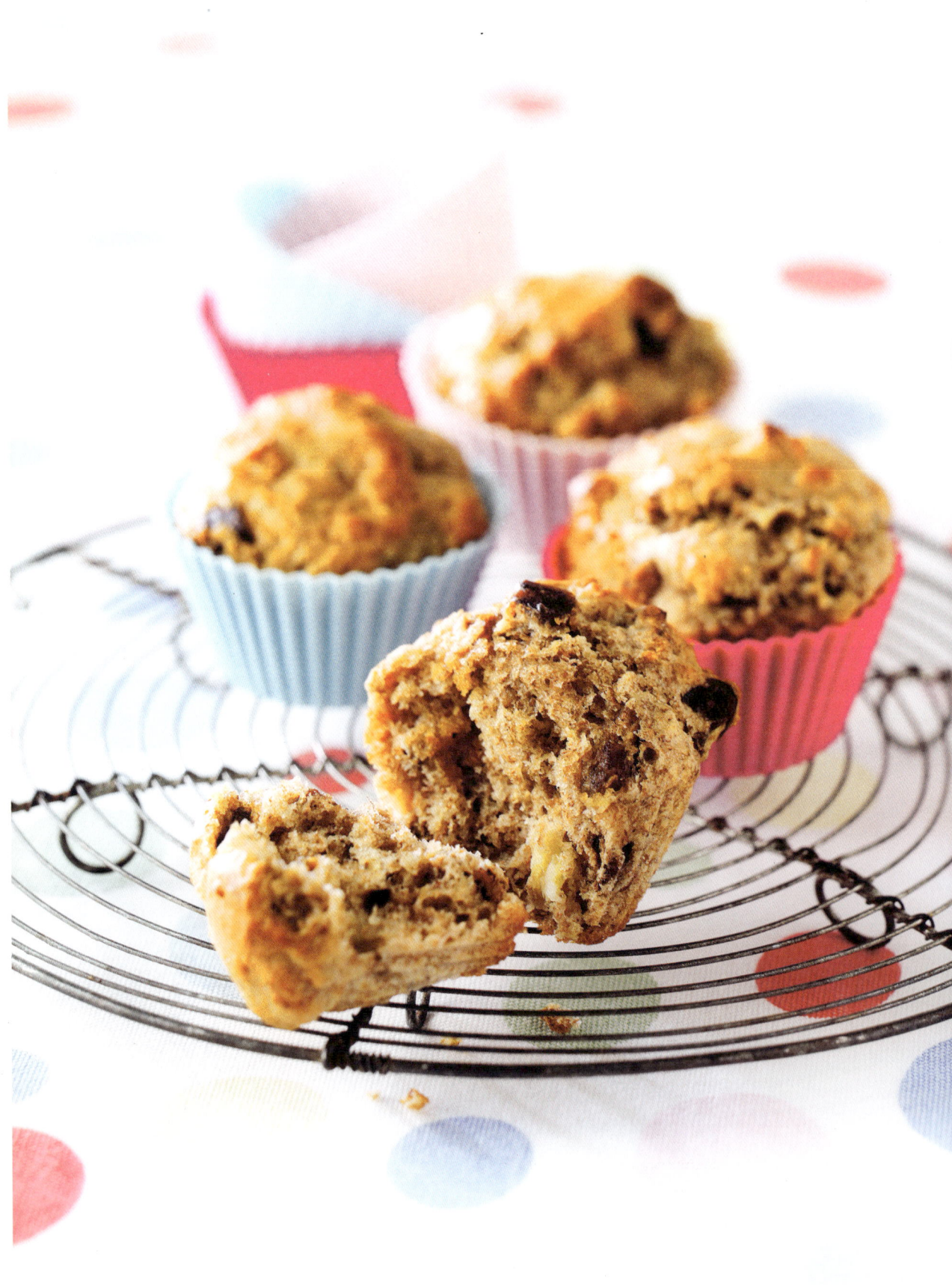

008 DATE and WALNUT MUFFINS

MAKES 12
PREPARATION
5 minutes
COOKING
25 minutes

STORAGE
Store in an airtight container in the fridge for up to 3 days or in the freezer for up to 3 months.

- 300g/10½ oz/2¼ cups wholemeal (wholewheat) flour
- 2 tsp baking powder
- 1 tsp bicarbonate of soda (baking soda)
- 50g/2oz/¼ cup caster (superfine) sugar
- 100g/3½oz/heaped ¾ cup walnuts, chopped
- 100g/3½oz/¾ cup dates, chopped
- 2 large ripe bananas
- 300ml/10½fl oz/1¼ cups plain yogurt
- 5 tbsp light olive oil
- 1 egg, beaten

1. Preheat the oven to 180°C/350°F/gas mark 4 and line a 12-hole muffin tin (pan) with muffin cases.

2. Mix the flour, baking powder, bicarbonate of soda (baking soda), sugar, walnuts and dates in a large bowl.

3. Mash the bananas in a separate bowl, then stir in the yogurt, oil and egg. Make a well in the middle of the dry ingredients, pour in the yogurt mixture and fold both mixtures together until just combined.

4. Spoon the mixture into the muffin cases. Bake for 20–25 minutes until well risen, golden brown, set and springy to the touch. Leave to cool slightly before serving.

009 BERRY SALAD

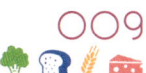

SERVES 4
PREPARATION
5 minutes

STORAGE
Best eaten immediately.

- 200g/7oz/2 cups strawberries, hulled and sliced
- 100g/3½oz/⅔ cup each of raspberries, blackberries and blackcurrants
- 200g/7oz/1 cup cherries, halved and pitted
- 2 tbsp almond butter
- 4 apricots, pitted and chopped

1. Mix the berries and cherries in a glass bowl.

2. Blend the almond butter and the apricots with enough water to make a thick cream.

3. Add the cream to the mixed berries and gently coat. Serve immediately.

010 RAISIN FRENCH TOAST

SERVES 4
PREPARATION
10 minutes
COOKING
8 minutes

STORAGE
Best eaten immediately.

3 eggs, beaten
4 tbsp low-fat crème fraîche
1 tsp ground cinnamon
2 ripe peaches, pitted
25g/1oz/¼ cup raisins
8 slices of wholemeal bread
1 tbsp butter
1 tbsp olive oil

1. In a large bowl, whisk the eggs with the crème fraîche and cinnamon until frothy.

2. Purée the peaches in a blender and mix in the raisins. Spread the purée on half the bread slices and top with the remaining slices to make sandwiches.

3. Melt the butter with the olive oil in a large frying pan (skillet). Dip a sandwich into the egg mixture, turn it a couple of times to make sure it is well soaked, then fry for 1–2 minutes on each side until golden and crisp. Repeat with the remaining sandwiches. Cut into triangles and serve immediately.

011 DRIED FRUIT with FRESH STRAWBERRIES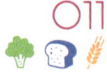

SERVES 4
PREPARATION
10 minutes

STORAGE
Best eaten immediately.

4 dried bananas, chopped
8 dates, pitted and chopped
8 dried figs, chopped
2 handfuls raisins
2 pears, cored and chopped
2 apples, cored and chopped
40 strawberries, halved
plain yogurt or soya yogurt, to serve

1. Place all the fruit (except for the strawberries) in a bowl and gently mix.

2. Spoon the mixed fruit onto plates, garnish with strawberries and serve with yogurt.

012 HOT WAFFLES with FRESH FRUIT

SERVES 4
PREPARATION
10 minutes

STORAGE
Best eaten immediately.

8 small Belgian waffles
4 mandarins, peeled and chopped
2 bananas, peeled and sliced
2 pears, halved, cored and sliced
2 tbsp chopped walnuts
4 tbsp maple syrup

1. Toast the waffles and place them on serving plates.

2. Pile the fruit on top, sprinkle with walnuts, drizzle over the maple syrup, and serve immediately.

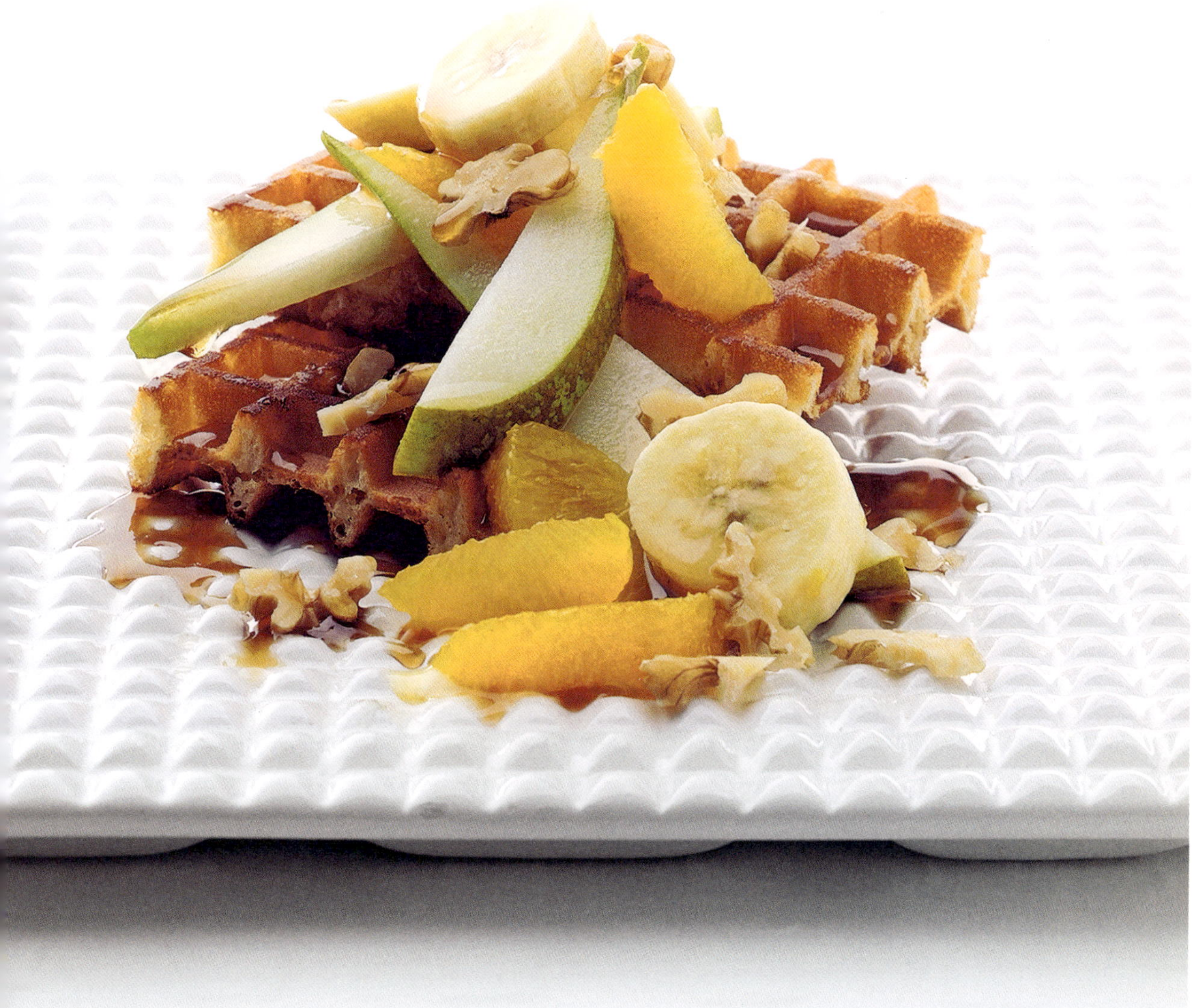

013 TROPICAL YOGURT POTS

SERVES 4
PREPARATION
10 minutes
COOKING
2 minutes

STORAGE
Prepare in advance and store in the fridge for up to 1 day. Store the nut-and-seed topping in an airtight container for up to 2 days.

- 25g/1oz/¼ cup desiccated (dried shredded) coconut
- 40g/1½oz/¼ cup macadamia nuts
- 3 tbsp cashew nuts
- 3 tbsp pumpkin seeds
- 1 tbsp ground flaxseeds
- 4 sharon fruit, halved
- juice of 1 orange
- 250ml/9fl oz/1 cup plain yogurt
- 2 passionfruit, pulp strained to remove seeds

1. Lightly toast the coconut and nuts in a non-stick frying pan (skillet) for 1–2 minutes, stirring frequently until they are golden brown.

2. Place the coconut and nuts in a blender with the pumpkin seeds and pulse to chop the mixture finely. Transfer to a bowl and stir in the flaxseeds.

3. Put the sharon fruit, orange juice and yogurt in the blender and blend until smooth.

4. Divide the yogurt mixture among four glasses or bowls and swirl in the passionfruit pulp. Top with the nut and seed mixture and serve.

014 LAYERED FRUIT AND NUT SALAD

SERVES 4
PREPARATION
10 minutes

STORAGE
Best eaten immediately.

- 2 mangoes, peeled and sliced
- 2 bananas, peeled and sliced lengthways
- 8 plums, pitted and sliced
- 200g/7oz/1½ cups raspberries
- 2 papaya, peeled, deseeded and diced
- 4 tbsp cashew nuts
- 2 tbsp maple syrup
- 200ml/7fl oz/scant 1 cup plain or soya yogurt

1. Arrange the mango, banana, plums and raspberries in layers in a serving dish.

2. Blend the papaya with the cashew nuts, maple syrup and yogurt. Pour the sauce over the fruit layers and serve.

015 CITRUS FRUIT SALAD

SERVES 4
PREPARATION 10 minutes

STORAGE Best eaten immediately.

2 oranges, peeled and sliced
2 pink grapefruits, peeled and sliced
2 clementines, peeled and sliced
maple syrup to taste

1. Place the fruit in a glass serving bowl. Drizzle with the maple syrup and serve.

016 MELLOW MELON

SERVES 4
PREPARATION 10 minutes

STORAGE Best eaten immediately.

1 cantaloupe melon, peeled, deseeded and diced
1 large bunch green grapes, halved
2 oranges, peeled, halved and sliced
4 ripe green figs, quartered
2 bananas, peeled and sliced
2 large fresh dates, pitted
2 tsp maple syrup

1. Mix the melon, grapes, orange and figs in a bowl.
2. Blend the banana with the dates, maple syrup and enough water to make a thick, smooth sauce.
3. Pour the sauce over the fruit and serve.

017 BREAKFAST BARS

MAKES 12–16
PREPARATION 15 minutes
COOKING 30 minutes

STORAGE
Store in an airtight container in the fridge for up to 3 days or freeze for up to 3 months.

olive oil, for greasing
425g/15oz/3$^{2}/_{3}$ cups dates
200ml/7fl oz/scant 1 cup apple juice
100g/3$^{1}/_{2}$oz/$^{1}/_{2}$ cup peanut butter
225g/8oz/2$^{1}/_{2}$ cups porridge (rolled) oats
150g/5$^{1}/_{2}$ oz/1$^{1}/_{2}$ cups wholemeal (wholewheat) flour
2 tbsp ground flaxseeds
1 tsp baking powder
1 tsp ground cinnamon

1. Preheat the oven to 190°C/375°F/gas mark 5 and grease a shallow 20 x 26cm/ 8 x 10in baking tin (pan) with oil.

2. Put the dates and apple juice in a saucepan and bring to a boil, then reduce to a simmer for 2 minutes.

3. Cool slightly, then purée in a food processor. Set aside just over half the purée in a bowl. Add the peanut butter to the remaining purée and process again to form a thick paste.

4. Mix the oats, flour, flaxseeds, baking powder and cinnamon in a bowl. Stir in the peanut butter mixture to form a sticky dough. Press half the dough into the tin (pan) and spread the date purée on top. Scatter over lumps of the remaining dough and press down to cover the date layer.

5. Bake for 20–25 minutes until golden brown. Cool in the tin (pan) for 10–15 minutes before turning out. Cut into small bars and cool completely, then serve.

018 PRUNE AND APRICOT YOGURT

SERVES 4
PREPARATION 5 minutes

STORAGE
Keep in the fridge for up to 2 days.

110g/4oz/$^{2}/_{3}$ cup dried prunes
110g/4oz/$^{2}/_{3}$ cup dried apricots
230g/8oz/1$^{1}/_{2}$ cups granola
350g/12oz/1$^{1}/_{2}$ cups plain yogurt
4 tbsp sunflower seeds

1. Roughly chop the prunes and apricots.

2. Mix the prunes, apricots, granola and yogurt in a large bowl. Divide between serving dishes and sprinkle with the sunflower seeds.

019 NUT AND CHERRY OAT BARS

MAKES 12–14
PREPARATION
15 minutes
COOKING
30 minutes

STORAGE
Store in an airtight container for up to 3 days.

olive oil, for greasing
150g/5½oz/1¼cups dates
150g/5½oz/1 cup cashew nuts, soaked in water overnight and drained
185ml/6fl oz/¾ cup apple juice
3 tbsp honey or agave nectar
225g/8oz/2½ cups porridge (rolled) oats
3 tbsp sesame seeds
3 tbsp sunflower seeds
3 tbsp ground flaxseeds
90g/3¼oz/⅔ cup dried cherries

1. Preheat the oven to 180°C/350°F/gas mark 4 and grease a shallow 20 x 33cm/8 x 13in baking tin (pan) with oil.

2. Process the dates, cashews, apple juice and honey or agave nectar in a food processor or blender to form a smooth purée.

3. Put the porridge oats, seeds and dried cherries in a large bowl. Add the purée and stir to combine thoroughly. Spread the mixture in the prepared tin (pan).

4. Bake for 25–30 minutes until golden brown. Leave to cool for 10 minutes, then cut into 12–14 bars while still warm. Leave in the tin until completely cool, then serve.

020 APRICOT AND TOFU SMOOTHIE

SERVES 4
PREPARATION
5 minutes

STORAGE
Best drunk immediately, but it will keep for 3–4 hours in the fridge.

3 apricots, pitted
3 ready-to-eat dried apricots
1 small peach, pitted
150ml/5fl oz/scant ⅔ cup pineapple juice
250g/9oz silken tofu

1. Blend all the ingredients in a blender until smooth and creamy.

2. Divide the drink among four glasses and serve.

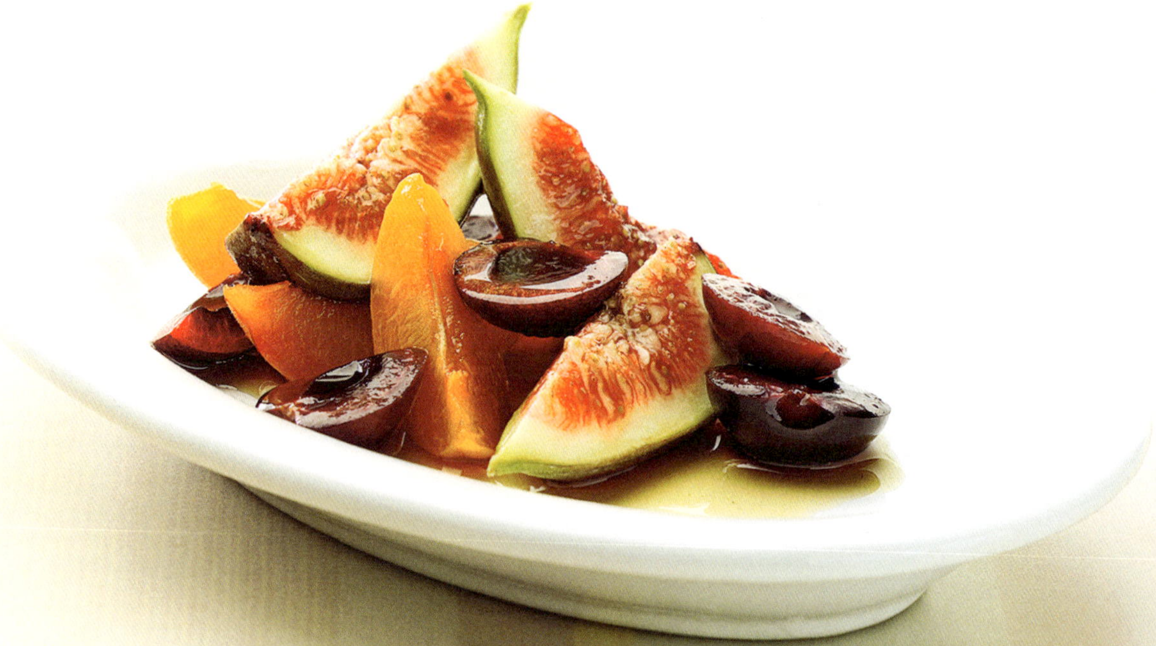

021 POACHED FIGS, APRICOTS AND CHERRIES

SERVES 4
PREPARATION
5 minutes
COOKING
15 minutes

STORAGE
Leftovers will keep in the fridge for up to 2 days.

300ml/10½fl oz/1¼ cups apple juice
2 tsp maple syrup
8 fresh figs, quartered
8 apricots, quartered and pitted
16 cherries, halved and pitted
4 tbsp orange juice

1. Heat the apple juice in a large heavy saucepan with the maple syrup. Add the figs, apricots and cherries. Bring to the boil, cover and gently simmer for 5 minutes.

2. Lift out the fruit with a slotted spoon and transfer to a serving bowl. Bring the juice back to the boil and reduce to a thick syrup.

3. Pour the syrup over the fruit, add the fresh orange juice and serve with crème fraîche or soya cream.

022 ZESTY CITRUS PANCAKES

MAKES 6–8
PREPARATION 10 minutes
COOKING 20 minutes

STORAGE
Leftovers will keep in the fridge for up to 2 days.

50g/1¾ oz/scant ½ cup plain (all-purpose) flour
25g/1oz/scant ¼ cup wholemeal (wholewheat) flour
25g/1oz/scant ¼ cup ground flaxseeds
grated zest of 1 orange
2 eggs, beaten
250ml/9fl oz/1 cup milk
2 tbsp olive oil
1 orange, peeled and segmented

CREAMY CITRUS SAUCE
juice and grated zest of 4 oranges
2 tbsp honey or agave nectar
250g/9oz mascarpone cheese

1. Sift the flours into a bowl. Stir in the flaxseeds and orange zest, then make a well in the middle and add the eggs. Whisk in the milk until a smooth batter forms.

2. Heat a little of the oil in a frying pan (skillet). Add about 2–3 tablespoons of batter, tilting the pan to form a pancake. Cook for 1 minute, or until set and brown underneath, then flip the pancake and cook the other side for 10–20 seconds. Transfer to a warm plate. Repeat with the remaining batter.

3. To make the sauce, simmer the orange juice, zest and honey or agave nectar for 2 minutes until slightly thickened. Put the mascarpone in a bowl and whisk in the orange mixture.

4. Top the pancakes with the sauce and orange segments and serve.

023 FRUITY PANCAKES

SERVES 4
PREPARATION
10 minutes
COOKING
20 minutes

STORAGE
Best eaten immediately.

PANCAKE BATTER
250g/9oz/2 cups plain (all-purpose) flour
4 eggs, beaten
250ml/9fl oz/1 cup milk
2 tbsp vegetable oil or butter
large pinch of sea salt

FILLING
2 bananas, peeled and thinly sliced
2 nectarines, quartered and sliced
16 gooseberries, halved
6 plums, quartered
oil, for frying
¼ tsp ground cinnamon
4 tbsp hazelnuts, chopped

1. Mix the batter ingredients with 250ml/9fl oz/1 cup of water and set aside.

2. Combine the fruit in a bowl.

3. Heat a little oil in a frying pan (skillet) and add a small ladleful of batter to the pan, swirling the batter so that it fills the pan. Fry each pancake for 2 minutes on each side, then keep warm while you cook the remainder. Fill each pancake with 2 tablespoons of fruit and sprinkle with a little cinnamon and a few hazelnuts. Serve immediately, with lemon wedges and maple syrup.

024 BLUEBERRY AND APPLE MUFFINS

MAKES 12
PREPARATION 10 minutes
COOKING 30 minutes
STORAGE You can keep the cooked muffins for up to 1 week in an airtight container.

115g/4oz butter
55g/2oz/¼ cup brown sugar
2 eggs
½ tsp ground cinnamon
2 tbsp marmalade
zest of 1 orange
115g/4oz/1 cup self-raising (self-rising) flour
115g/4oz/1 cup porridge (rolled) oats
1 apple, cored and grated
115g/4oz/1 cup blueberries

1. Preheat the oven to 200°C/400°F/gas mark 6. Cream together the butter and sugar. Stir in the eggs, cinnamon, marmalade and orange zest.

2. Add the flour and oats, beating together until smooth. Gently stir in the apple and blueberries.

3. Divide the mixture between 12 muffin cases. Bake in the oven for 20–30 minutes or until golden.

4. Transfer to a wire rack and leave to cool.

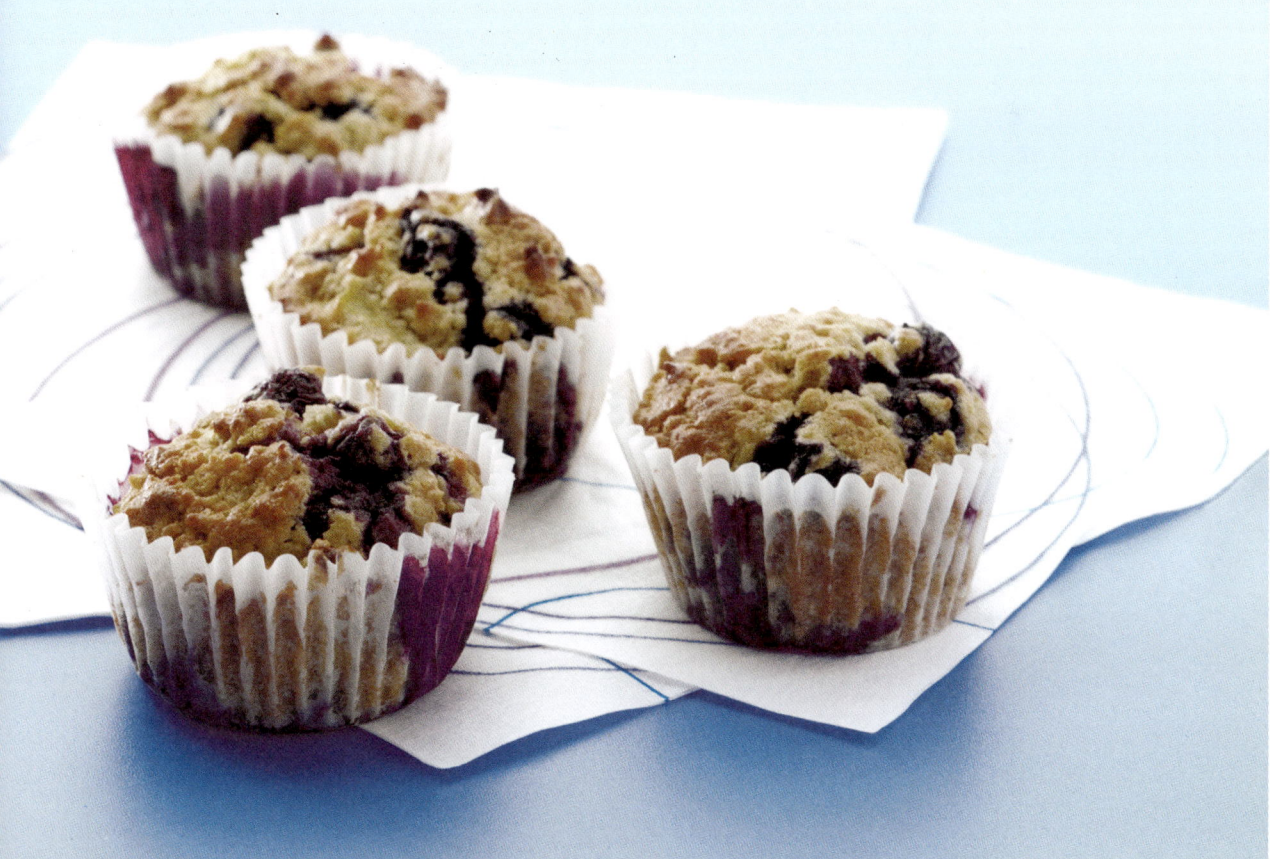

025 BANANA and BUCKWHEAT PANCAKES

MAKES 6-10 PANCAKES
PREPARATION 35 minutes
COOKING 10 minutes
STORAGE You can refrigerate the pancake mixture for up to 3 days.

175g/6oz/1½ cups buckwheat flour
2 eggs
375ml/13fl oz/1½ cups milk
oil, for frying
2 large bananas, cut into slices
55g/2oz/⅓ cup flaked (slivered) almonds
maple syrup, to serve

1. Sift the flour into a mixing bowl. Add the eggs and milk and whisk together until smooth. Leave in the fridge for 30 minutes.

2. Wipe a large frying pan (skillet) with oil, and heat. When hot, pour in 2 tablespoons of the batter and tip the frying pan so that the mixture covers the base of the pan. Cook the pancake on both sides until lightly browned. Repeat until all the batter is used up.

3. Serve each pancake with the banana slices, a sprinkle of almonds and a drizzle of maple syrup.

026 OATMEAL PANCAKES with SALMON

MAKES 12 PANCAKES
PREPARATION 10 minutes
COOKING 15 minutes
STORAGE Leftovers will keep in the fridge for up to 2 days.

75g/2½oz/⅔ cup fine oatmeal
75g/2½oz/⅔ cup plain (all-purpose) flour
1 tsp baking powder
1 egg, beaten
125ml/4fl oz/½ cup milk
1 tbsp olive oil
200g/7oz hot-smoked salmon
5 tbsp crème fraîche
1 tbsp chopped dill
grated zest of 1 lemon

1. Put the oatmeal in a food processor and pulse to break down. Add the flour and baking powder and pulse to mix. Add the egg and, with the processor running, pour in the milk to make a smooth, thick batter.

2. Heat the oil in a frying pan (skillet). Drop 4 spoonfuls of batter into the pan to make small pancakes, spacing them apart. Cook for 3 minutes, or until just set on top and golden underneath, then turn and cook the other side for 1–2 minutes until brown underneath. Repeat with the remaining batter.

3. Flake the salmon into a bowl. Mix in the crème fraîche, dill and lemon zest. Top the pancakes with the salmon mixture and serve.

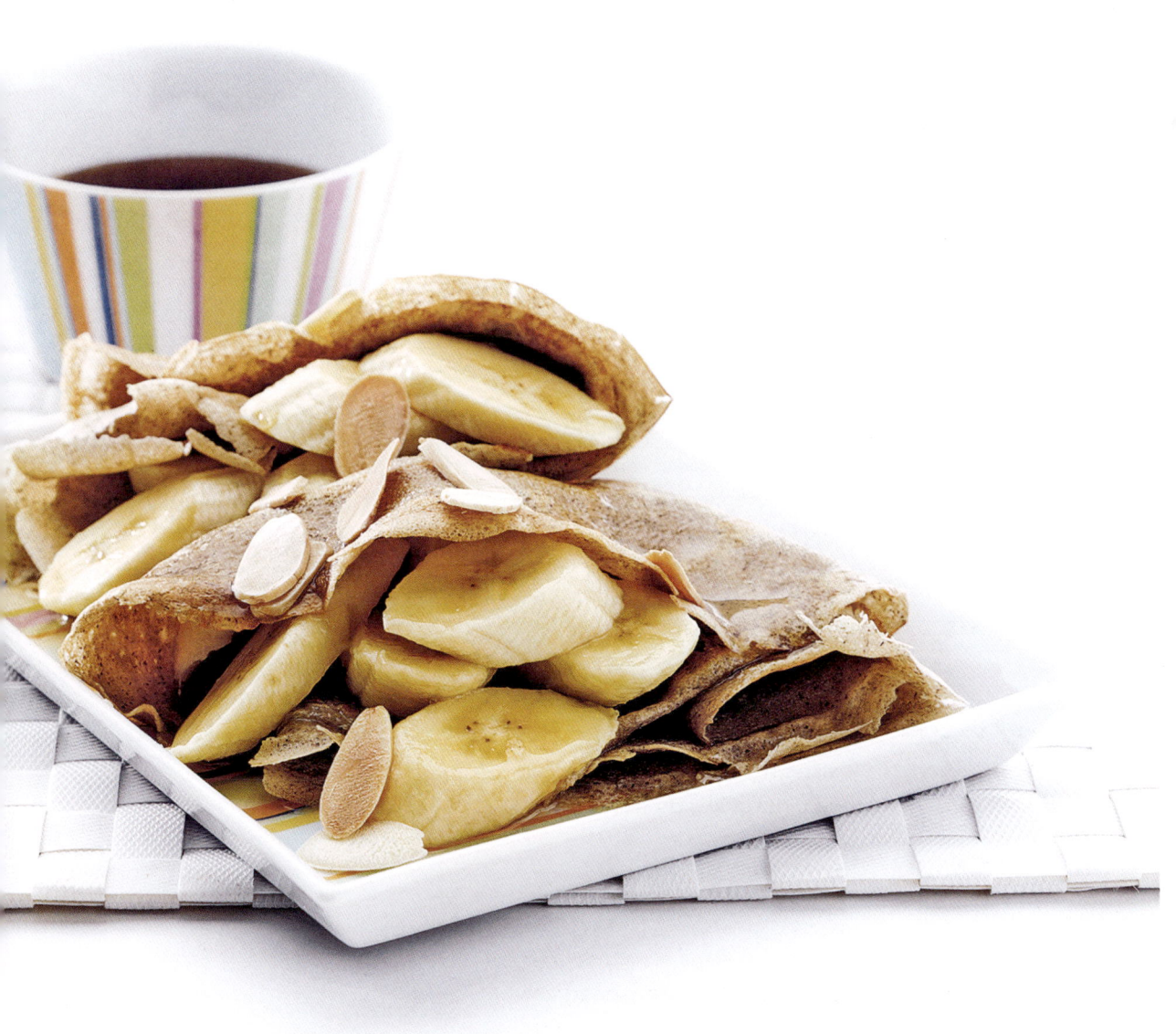

027 BUCKWHEAT GALETTES with VEGETABLES

SERVES 4
PREPARATION 10 minutes
COOKING 30 minutes

GALETTES
250g/9oz/2 cups buckwheat flour
large pinch of salt
2 eggs
4 tsp baking powder
4 tbsp vegetable oil
600ml/21fl oz/2½ cups milk
oil, for frying

FILLING
2 shallots, finely chopped
2 bay leaves
large pinch of mace
2 cloves garlic, crushed
500g/18oz mushrooms, chopped
400ml/14floz/1²⁄₃ cups vegetable stock
2 tsp cornflour (cornstarch), dissolved in a little cold water
250g/9oz cooked green beans, finely chopped
250g/9oz/generous 2 cups cooked sweetcorn kernels

1. Mix the flour, salt and egg or baking powder in a bowl. Add the oil and the milk, little by little, until you get a smooth batter. Set aside.

2. Fry the shallots in a large pan with a little oil for 3 minutes. Add the bay leaves, mace and garlic. Heat through, add the mushrooms and stir-fry for 2 minutes, then add the stock. Leave to simmer.

3. Meanwhile, fry the galettes one at a time in a frying pan (skillet) with a little oil. Keep warm while you finish the sauce.

4. Add the cornflour (cornstarch) to the mushroom sauce and cook until it thickens.

5. Fill the galettes with a spoonful each of the mushroom sauce and the cooked green beans and sweetcorn mixture, and serve.

028 MEDITERRANEAN MELTS

SERVES 4
PREPARATION 5 minutes
COOKING 10 minutes

STORAGE
Keep in the fridge for 1 day.

4 slices rye bread
200g/7oz goat's cheese
16 cherry tomatoes
50g/2oz/²⁄₃ cup chopped basil leaves

1. Preheat the grill (broiler) to medium. Spread the slices of rye bread with the goat's cheese. Chop the cherry tomatoes in half and arrange them evenly over the top

2. Place under the grill (broiler) for 5-10 minutes until the cheese has melted.

3. Sprinkle with the chopped basil before serving.

029 PIPÉRADE PITTA

SERVES 4
PREPARATION
10 minutes
COOKING
4 minutes

STORAGE
Make on the day.

4 tbsp olive oil
1 red (bell) pepper, diced
4 tomatoes, halved, deseeded and diced
4 spring onions (scallions), finely chopped
4 tbsp milk
8 free-range eggs, lightly beaten
salt and freshly ground black pepper
4 wholemeal pittas

(1) Heat the oil in a frying pan (skillet) and fry the (bell) pepper gently for 1 minute, then add the tomatoes and spring onions (scallions) and cook for one minute more.

(2) Mix the milk into the beaten eggs, season, and add to the pan. Cook until the egg is scrambled (about 2 minutes), stirring constantly with a wooden spoon to stop it sticking.

(3) Warm the pittas slightly to make opening them easier. Cut in half crossways then spoon the pipérade inside. Leave to cool before wrapping or serve hot.

030 CREAMED SALMON RICE CAKES

SERVES 4
PREPARATION
10 minutes

STORAGE
You can keep the topping mix in the fridge for up to 2 days.

2 avocados
50g/2oz/1/2 cup spinach, chopped
50g/2oz/2/3 cup chopped coriander (cilantro)
110g/4oz smoked salmon, chopped
4 tbsp cream cheese
freshly ground black pepper
juice of 1/2 lemon
8 plain rice cakes (no salt added)
8 sprigs parsley

(1) Scoop out the avocado flesh into a small mixing bowl. Add the chopped spinach, coriander (cilantro) and salmon and then stir in the cream cheese.

(2) Add some black pepper and squeeze in the lemon juice. Stir the mixture well until creamy in texture.

(3) Spread each rice cake equally with the mixture, garnish with parsley and serve.

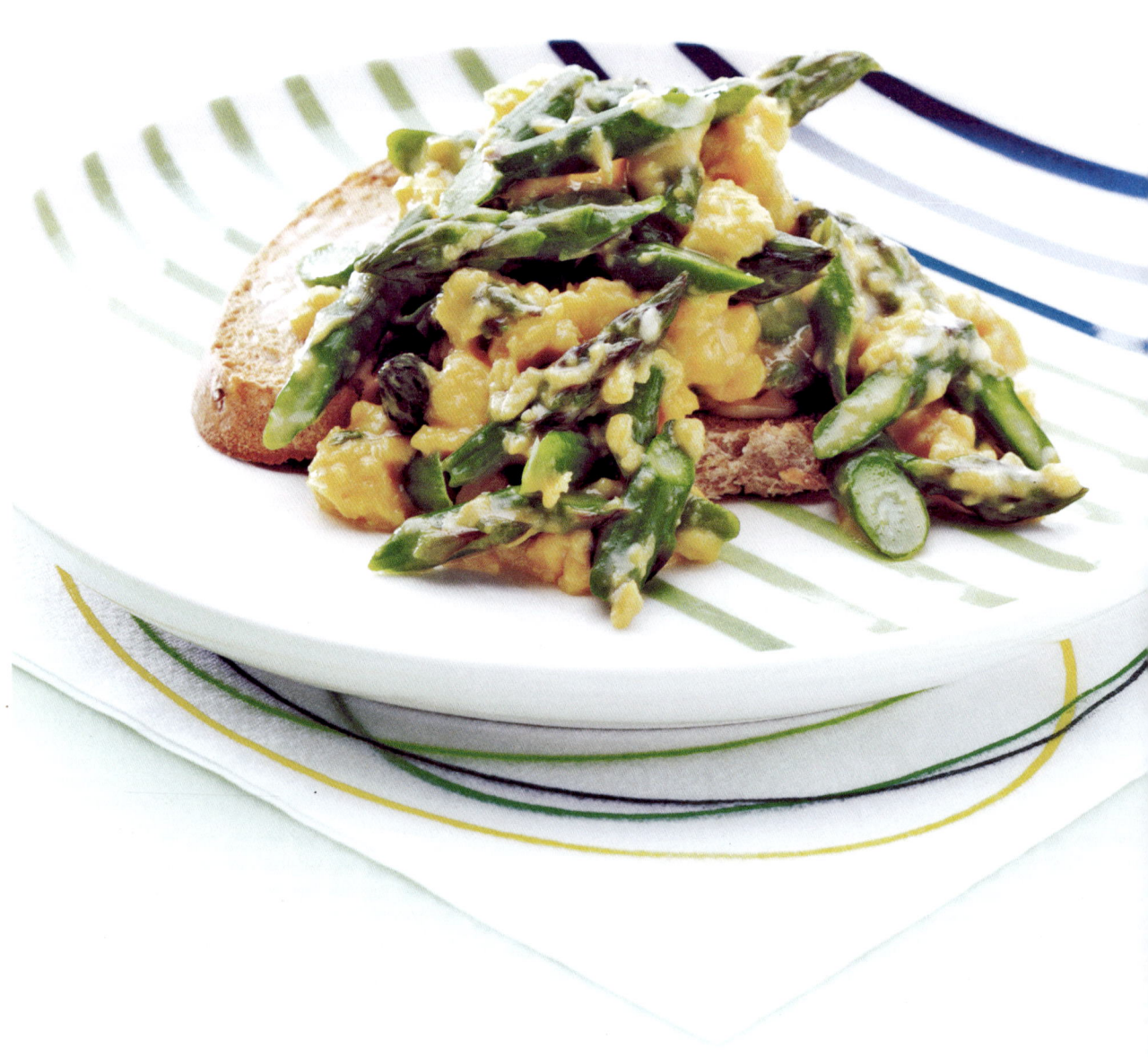

031 ASPARAGUS EGG SCRAMBLE

SERVES 4
PREPARATION 5 minutes
COOKING 10 minutes
STORAGE You can refrigerate for a few hours and serve cold.

4 tbsp olive oil
400g/14oz asparagus, finely chopped
8 eggs
120ml/4fl oz/½ cup milk
½ tsp celery salt
50g/2oz butter, plus extra for spreading
8 slices rye bread

1. Heat the olive oil in a non-stick saucepan. Add the asparagus and stir-fry gently for 3-4 minutes.

2. Crack the eggs into a jug, add the milk, celery salt and butter and beat with a fork.

3. Gently heat a non-stick pan and pour in the egg mixture. Stir continuously over a gentle heat until the liquid begins to congeal and then add the asparagus.

4. Meanwhile, toast the rye bread and spread with a little butter. Serve the asparagus scramble over the rye bread.

032 POPEYE BAKED EGGS

SERVES 4
PREPARATION 5 minutes
COOKING 15 minutes
STORAGE Best eaten immediately.

1 tbsp butter, plus extra for greasing
400g/14oz baby spinach leaves, washed
freshly ground black pepper
4 eggs
185ml/6fl oz/¾ cup crème fraîche
freshly grated nutmeg
75g/2½ oz Cheddar cheese, grated

1. Preheat the oven to 200°C/400°F/gas mark 6 and grease four individual shallow baking dishes with butter.

2. Melt the butter in a saucepan over a low heat and add the spinach. Cover and cook for 20 seconds, until wilted. Divide the spinach among the prepared dishes and season with black pepper.

3. Make a slight indentation in the middle of each portion of spinach and crack 1 egg into each. Carefully spoon the crème fraîche around the eggs. Season with a little nutmeg and sprinkle the grated Cheddar over the eggs.

4. Bake for 10-12 minutes until the eggs are just set. Serve immediately.

033 EGGLESS TOFU AND HERB OMELETTES

SERVES 2
PREPARATION
10 minutes
COOKING
5 minutes

STORAGE
Best eaten immediately.

250g/9oz tofu, crumbled
200ml/7fl oz/scant 1 cup cup soya or rice milk
2 tbsp wheat flour
2 tsp baking powder
sea salt and black pepper to taste
1 tbsp each finely chopped chives, parsley and chervil or tarragon
oil, for frying

1. Blend the tofu with the milk in a blender or food processor. Transfer to a mixing bowl, add the flour and the baking powder and season. Add the herbs and mix again.

2. Heat a little oil in a frying pan (skillet). Pour in half of the tofu batter and spread it evenly over the pan. Turn down the heat and gently cook until the topside is firm. Sprinkle with oil, turn and cook the other side. Remove from the heat and serve.

3. Repeat with the remaining batter to make a second omelette.

034 EGGLESS SPRING OMELETTES

SERVES 4
PREPARATION
10 minutes
COOKING
5 minutes

STORAGE
Best eaten immediately.

200g/7oz/1½ cups wheat flour
1 tsp sea salt
2 tsp baking powder
large pinch of saffron
400ml/14fl oz/1⅔ cups water
black pepper to taste
oil, for frying
40g/1½oz/¼ cup fresh green peas, blanched
2 tbsp fresh mint, finely chopped

1. Mix the flour, salt, baking powder and saffron in a bowl. Add the water, whisk to a smooth batter and season.

2. Heat a little oil in a frying pan (skillet). Pour in half of the batter and spread it evenly to form a thin pancake. Turn down the heat and cook slowly until the topside begins to firm. Spread half of the peas and mint over half of the omelette, fold and fry on each side for 30 seconds. Remove from the heat and serve.

3. Repeat with the remaining batter to make a second omelette.

035 MUSHROOM OMELETTES

SERVES 4
PREPARATION 5 minutes
COOKING 15 minutes
STORAGE Best eaten immediately.

8 eggs
1 tsp freshly ground black pepper
½ tsp celery salt
2 tsp dried oregano
160ml/5fl oz/⅔ cup milk
2 tbsp olive oil
1 large red onion, peeled and diced
230g/8oz/2 cups mushrooms, sliced
150g/6oz/1 cup goat's cheese
50g/2oz/⅔ cup chopped parsley

1. Put the eggs into a bowl and beat with a fork. Add the pepper, salt, oregano and milk, stirring together well.

2. Heat half the oil in a small frying pan (skillet), add the onions and mushrooms, and sauté until softened.

3. Remove from the heat and drain off any excess oil. Add the onion and mushroom mix to the beaten eggs and stir well. Heat the remaining oil in the frying pan (skillet), add a quarter of the mixture and cook the omelette for 3–4 minutes.

4. Crumble a quarter of the goat's cheese on top, then turn the omelette and cook the other side. Repeat with the remaining ingredients until you have four individual omelettes. Serve, garnished with chopped parsley.

036 BREAKFAST KEBABS

SERVES 4
PREPARATION
5 minutes
COOKING
10 minutes

STORAGE
Best eaten immediately.

32 cherry tomatoes
32 button mushrooms
8 eggs
50g/2oz/⅔ cup chopped parsley

1. Skewer 4 tomatoes and 4 mushrooms alternately onto a skewer, and repeat until you have used all the tomatoes and mushrooms (making 8 skewers).

2. Place the kebabs under a grill (broiler) and cook for 10 minutes, until lightly browned.

3. Crack the eggs into a poacher and cook for 4–6 minutes. Serve the kebabs alongside the poached eggs, garnished with chopped parsley.

037 BAKED BEAN MELT

SERVES 4
PREPARATION
10 minutes
COOKING
30 minutes

STORAGE
Store any leftover baked beans in the fridge for up to 3 days.

160ml/5fl oz/⅔ cup vegetable oil
1 large onion, peeled and diced
6 cloves garlic, crushed
2 red (bell) peppers, deseeded and chopped
500ml/17fl oz/2 cups water
500ml/17fl oz/2 cups maple syrup
400g/14oz/2 cups tomato purée (paste)
4 tbsp blackstrap molasses
4 tbsp apple cider vinegar
2 tsp Dijon mustard
1 tsp freshly ground black pepper
4 x 400-g/14-oz cans cooked pinto beans, drained
8 soda bread farls
300g/10½oz/2 cups Cheddar cheese

1. Preheat the oven to 170°C/325°F/gas mark 3. Heat the oil in a large pan. Add the onion, garlic and red pepper and sauté for several minutes, then set aside.

2. In a large bowl, whisk together the water, maple syrup, tomato purée (paste), molasses, vinegar, mustard and black pepper. Then add the beans and vegetable mixture and stir together. Pour into a large casserole dish, cover and bake for 30 minutes, adding more water if necessary.

3. Lightly toast the soda bread farls and grate the cheese. When the beans are cooked, remove and serve over the soda farls with the grated cheese sprinkled over the top.

038 EGGLESS PANCAKES with SPINACH FILLING

SERVES 4
PREPARATION
10 minutes
COOKING
20 minutes

STORAGE
Best eaten immediately.

BATTER
250g/9oz/2 cups plain (all-purpose) flour
2 tsp baking powder
large pinch of salt
200ml/7fl oz/scant 1 cup milk or soya milk
200ml/7fl oz/scant 1 cup water
4 tbsp vegetable oil

FILLING
400g/14oz fresh spinach
2 tbsp plain (all-purpose) flour
200ml/7fl oz/scant 1 cup crème fraîche
large pinch of nutmeg and sea salt to taste
oil, for frying
Gruyère cheese (optional)

1. Mix the batter ingredients and set aside. Preheat the oven to 230°C/450°F/gas mark 8 or heat a grill (broiler).

2. Gently cook the spinach in a saucepan with a little water until soft. Add the flour and stir for 30 seconds, then add the crème fraîche, heat through and season with nutmeg and salt.

3. Heat a little oil in a frying pan (skillet), pour in the batter and fry the pancakes for 2 minutes on each side. Top with 1 tablespoon of filling, roll up and place in an ovenproof dish. Sprinkle with Gruyère cheese and grill (broil) or bake for a few minutes until the cheese melts. Serve hot.

039 VEGETABLE RÖSTIS with POACHED EGGS

SERVES 4
PREPARATION
15 minutes
COOKING
35 minutes

STORAGE
Make the röstis in advance and reheat in a warm oven while cooking the eggs. Leftovers will keep in the fridge for up to 1 day.

olive oil, for greasing
200g/7oz sweet potatoes, peeled and grated
100g/3½oz parsnips, peeled and grated
6 eggs
2 spring onions (scallions), chopped
75g/2¾oz goat's cheese, crumbled
freshly ground black pepper

1. Preheat the oven to 200°C/400°F/gas mark 6 and grease a large baking sheet with oil. Mix the sweet potatoes and parsnips in a bowl and season with pepper.

2. Put 2 of the eggs in a blender or food processor. Add the spring onions (scallions) and cheese and blend until smooth. Pour the mixture into the grated vegetables and mix well.

3. Using a spoon, shape the mixture into 8 equal patties and put them on the baking sheet. Bake for 30–35 minutes until the patties are golden brown and crisp.

4. Meanwhile, bring a large pan of water to the boil. Break 1 egg into a cup and then gently slide it into the water. Repeat with the remaining eggs and poach for 3–4 minutes, or until cooked to taste. Using a slotted spoon, remove the eggs from the pan and drain on paper towels.

5. Put the röstis on plates and top with the eggs. Serve immediately.

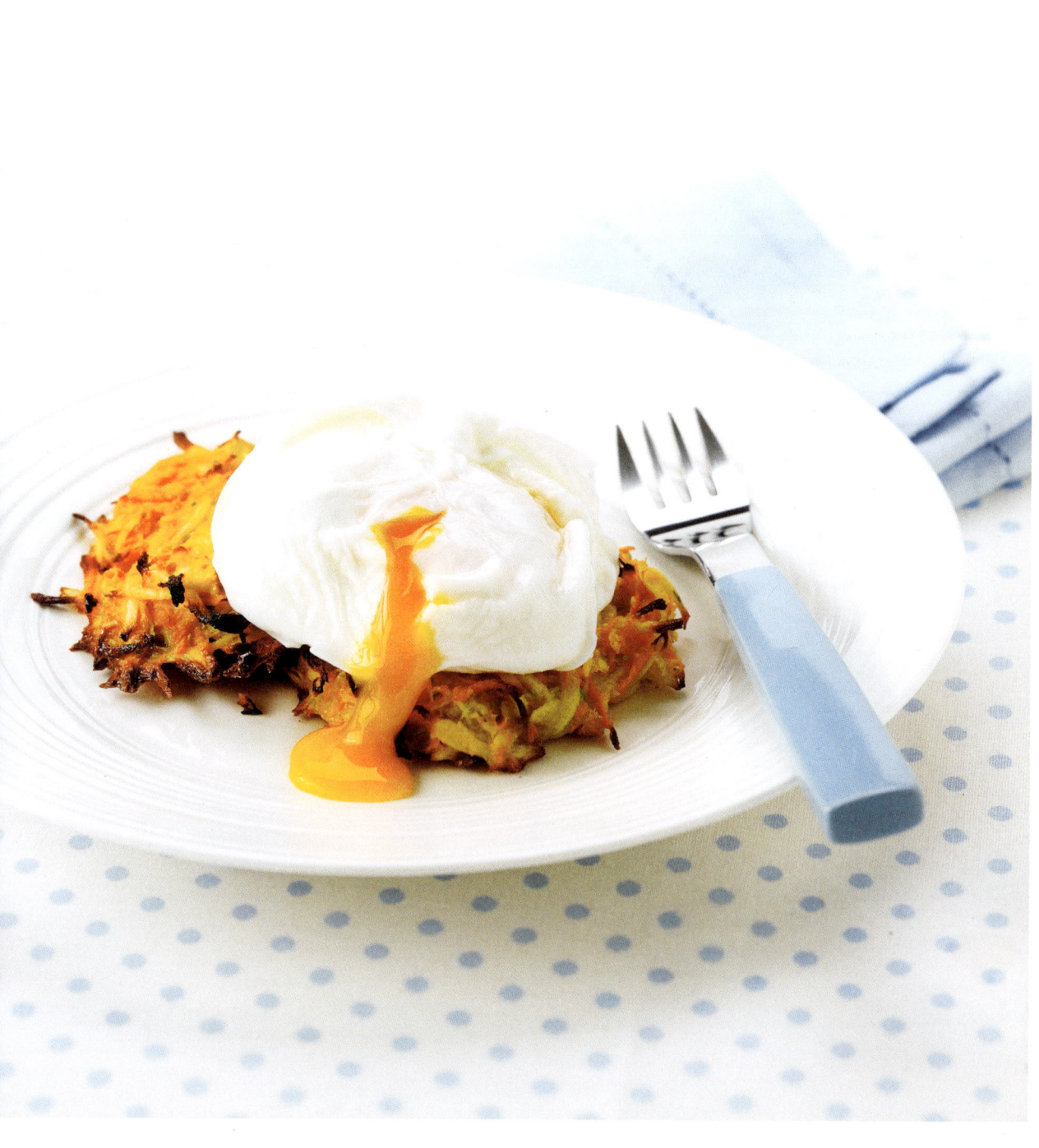

040 EGG AND TOMATO CUPS

SERVES 4
PREPARATION
15 minutes
COOKING
25 minutes

STORAGE
Best eaten immediately.

olive oil, for greasing
4 large tomatoes
1 slice lean ham, about 25g/1oz, diced
4 tbsp crème fraîche
1 tbsp finely chopped parsley leaves
few drops of Tabasco sauce
4 eggs
freshly ground black pepper

1. Preheat the oven to 200°C/400°F/gas mark 6 and lightly grease a shallow baking dish with oil. Slice the top off each tomato and use a spoon to scoop out and discard the seeds and juice. Place, cut-sides down, on paper towels to drain.

2. In a bowl, mix together the ham, crème fraîche and parsley and season with the Tabasco. Put the tomatoes in the dish, cut-sides up, and fill with the ham mixture.

3. Carefully crack 1 egg into each tomato and season with black pepper. Bake for 20–25 minutes until the eggs are just set. Serve immediately.

041 GIANT BAKED BEANS ON TOASTED RYE

SERVES 4
PREPARATION
5 minutes
COOKING
10 minutes

STORAGE
Leftovers will keep in the fridge for up to 2 days.

1 tbsp olive oil
1 small red onion, chopped
2 x 400-g (14-oz) cans butterbeans (lima beans), drained and rinsed
1 x 400-g (14-oz) can chopped tomatoes
3 tbsp tomato purée (paste)
pinch of ground allspice
pinch of ground cinnamon
3 tbsp apple juice
1 tbsp tamari
2 tsp cider vinegar
4 slices rye bread
1 tbsp chopped parsley

1. Heat the oil in a saucepan. Add the onion and cook for 2–3 minutes until softened.

2. Stir in the butterbeans (lima beans), tomatoes, tomato purée (paste), spices, apple juice, tamari and vinegar. Bring to the boil, reduce the heat and simmer gently for 5 minutes, or until heated through and thickened slightly.

3. Lightly toast the rye bread. Spoon the beans onto the bread and sprinkle with the parsley. Serve immediately.

042 BRUNCH BONANZA

SERVES 4
PREPARATION
10 minutes
COOKING
30 minutes

STORAGE
Best eaten immediately.

- 115g/4oz/1 cup mushrooms, peeled and sliced
- 16 cherry tomatoes, cut in half
- 1 onion, peeled and diced
- 2 cloves garlic, peeled and finely sliced
- 2 leeks, trimmed and sliced
- 2 sweet potatoes, peeled and chopped
- 8 sausages, sliced
- 3–4 tbsp olive oil
- 25g/1oz/$\frac{1}{3}$ cup chopped parsley

1. Preheat the oven to 190°C/375°F/gas mark 5. Scatter the mushrooms and cherry tomatoes into a medium-sized ovenproof dish. Add the onion, garlic, leek, sweet potato and sausages.

2. Drizzle the olive oil on top and sprinkle on the parsley. Bake in the oven for 20–30 minutes until the sweet potato is soft. Remove from the oven and serve.

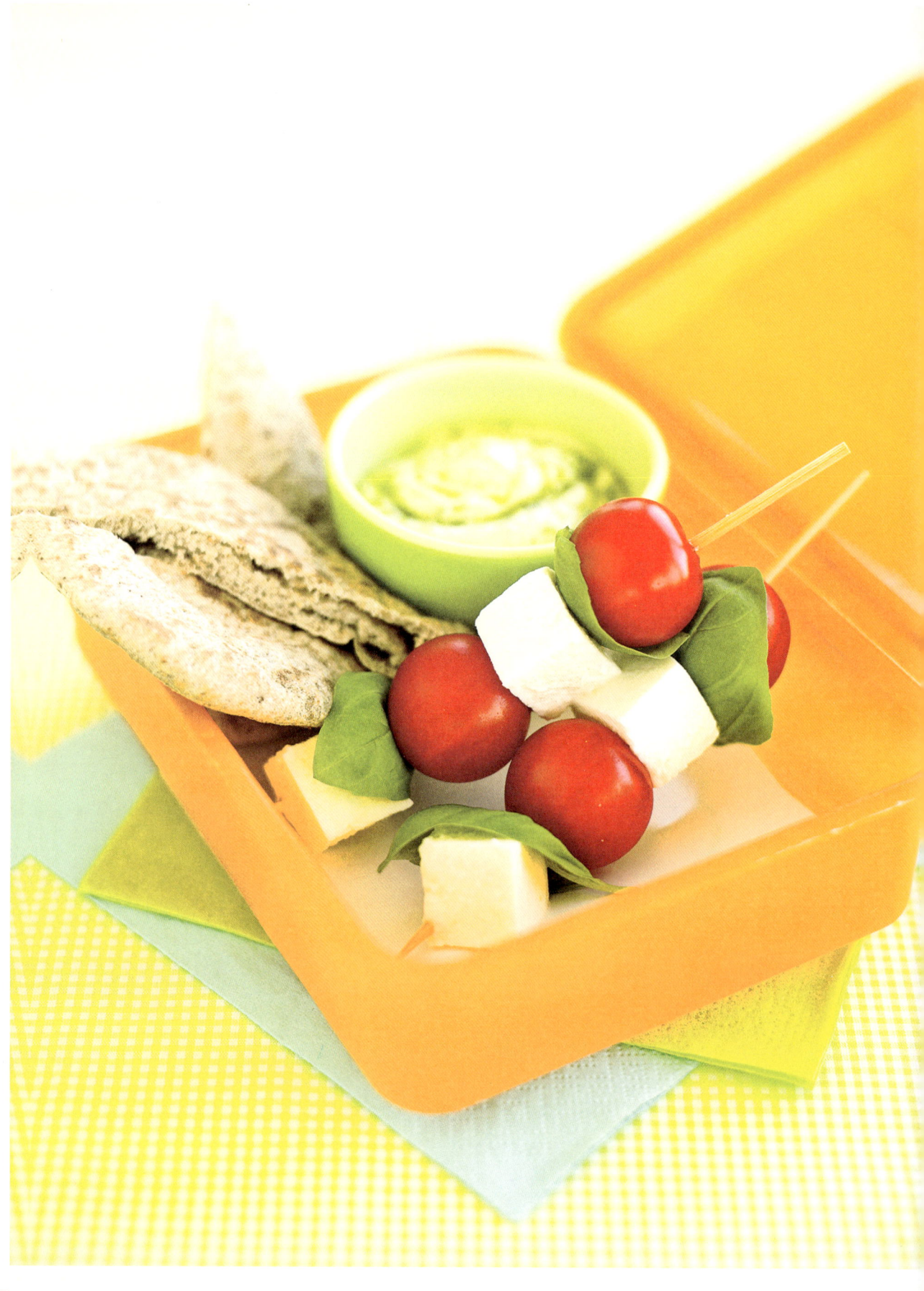

Snacks

Mealtimes are only half the story. When you or your kids are peckish between lunch and dinner, the next meal can seem a lifetime away. It can be all too tempting to reach for that packet of crisps or cookies, but shop-bought snacks can be high in saturated fats and sugars, with very little long-term nutritional benefit.

This chapter is packed with healthy, home-made treats that all the family will enjoy, and which avoid the sugar highs and energy slumps that processed snacks give. Whether it's colourful Tortilla Dippers with Tomato Salsa (see page 68) or refreshing Pineapple and Mint Frozen Yogurt (see page 77), these nutritionally balanced snacks will set you up for the rest of the day.

043 MOZZARELLA, CHERRY TOMATO AND BASIL STICKS

MAKES 4 STICKS

PREPARATION
10 minutes

STORAGE
Make the dip in advance and keep in the fridge for up to 1 week. Assemble the sticks on the day.

8 cherry tomatoes
8 basil leaves
8 x 1cm/½in cubes mozzarella cheese

PESTO DIP
60ml/2fl oz/¼ cup low-fat plain yogurt
1 tbsp green pesto

1. To make the dip, mix together the yogurt and pesto, then spoon into a small lidded pot.

2. Thread a cherry tomato on to a cocktail stick (toothpick), followed by a basil leaf and a cube of mozzarella. Add a second tomato, basil leaf and cube of mozzarella.

3. Assemble the remaining sticks in the same way. Serve the sticks with the pesto dip.

044 SALAMI, CHEESE and PINEAPPLE STICKS

MAKES 4 STICKS
PREPARATION
5 minutes

STORAGE
Make the day before and keep in the fridge overnight. Keep chilled until ready to eat.

4 thin slices salami
4 chunks pineapple
4 large bite-sized cubes Cheddar or other hard cheese

1. Fold a slice of salami in half then half again and thread on to a cocktail stick (toothpick), followed by a chunk of pineapple, then a chunk of Cheddar.

2. Repeat to make four sticks.

045 HAM ROLL-UPS

SERVES 1
PREPARATION
10 minutes

STORAGE
Make the day before and keep in the fridge overnight. Keep chilled until ready to serve.

2 thin slices square granary bread
a little butter
½ tsp mild mustard or chutney of choice
2 slices good-quality cooked ham, roughly the same size as the bread
2 long, thin sticks cucumber (the same length as each slice of bread), seeded

1. Remove the crusts from each slice of bread, then flatten them slightly by pressing down with your fingers. Mix the butter and mustard or chutney together in a bowl, then spread over the bread.

2. Lay a slice of ham on each slice of bread and place the cucumber diagonally across the ham.

3. Starting from one corner, roll each slice up tightly and place seam-side down on a board. Cut each roll-up in half at an angle, then wrap in clingfilm (plastic wrap) to keep their shape.

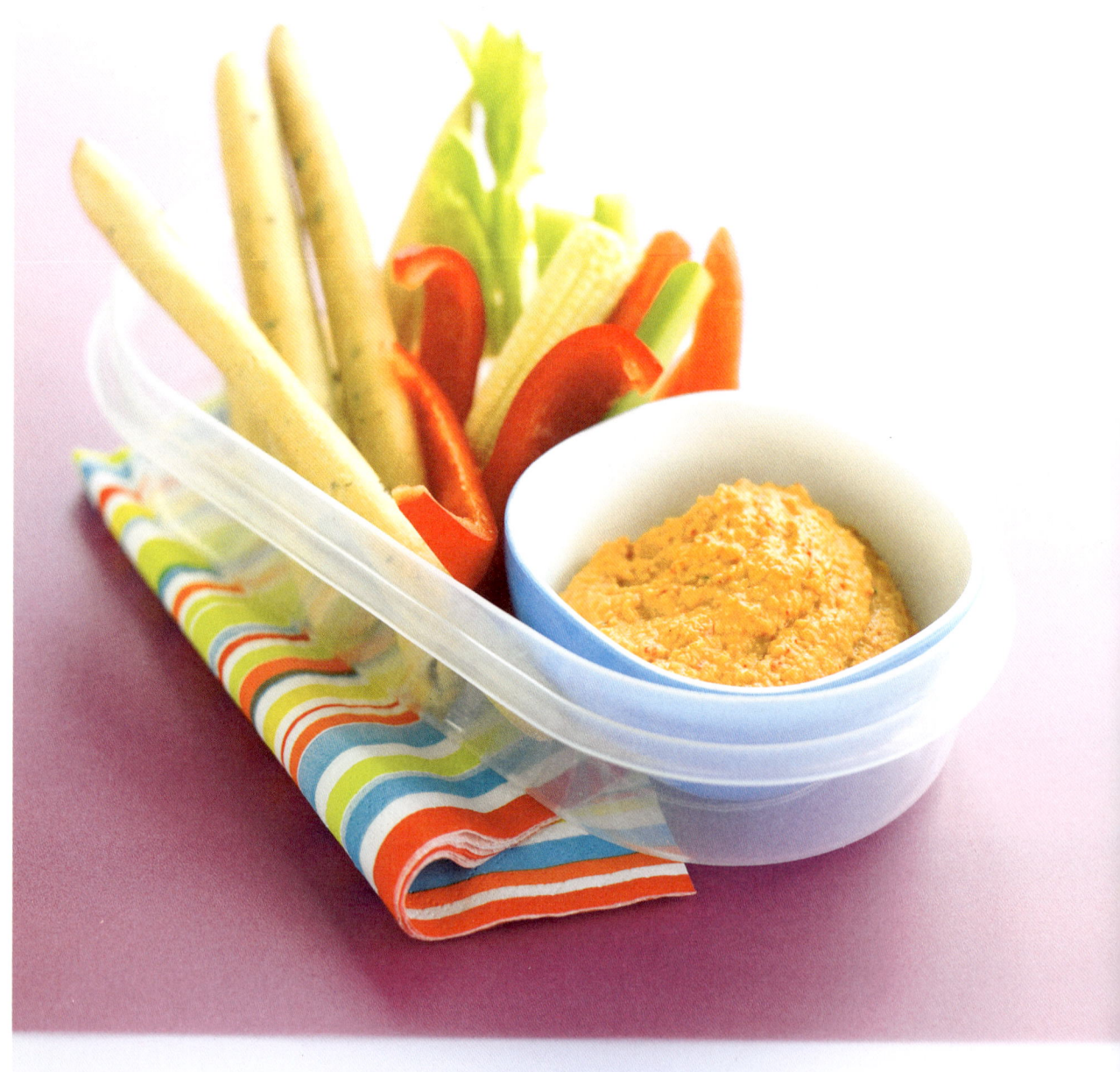

046 ROASTED RED PEPPER HUMMUS

SERVES 6
PREPARATION
15 minutes
COOKING
30 minutes

STORAGE
Make in advance and keep in the fridge for up to 1 week.

1 red (bell) pepper, deseeded and quartered
3 tbsp extra-virgin olive oil, plus extra for drizzling
235g/8½oz/heaped 1½ cups canned chickpeas (garbanzo beans), drained and rinsed
2 cloves garlic, halved
1 heaped tbsp tahini (sesame paste)
juice of ½ lemon
salt and freshly ground black pepper

1. Preheat the oven to 200°C/400°F/gas mark 6. Put the (bell) pepper quarters in a roasting tin (pan) with 1 tbsp of the oil. Toss the pepper in the oil until coated, then roast for 25–30 minutes, turning once, until the skin begins to blister and blacken.

2. Remove the pepper from the oven and leave until cool enough to handle, then peel off the skin.

3. Put the pepper in a food processor or blender with the chickpeas (garbanzo beans), garlic, tahini (sesame paste), lemon juice, 2 tablespoons water and the rest of the oil. Blend until the mixture forms a chunky, creamy purée, occasionally scraping the mixture down the sides of the processor or blender.

4. Transfer the hummus to a lidded pot. Season to taste and drizzle a little extra olive oil over the top.

047 HUMMUS AND RYE TOASTS

SERVES 2
PREPARATION
5 minutes

STORAGE
You can refrigerate overnight and eat the following morning.

4 slices rye bread
4 tbsp hummus
2 handfuls alfalfa sprouts
1 red (bell) pepper, deseeded and finely sliced

1. Toast the slices of rye bread for 1–2 minutes on each side. Spread each slice liberally with the hummus.

2. Sprinkle half a handful of alfalfa sprouts on top of each slice.

3. Garnish the slices with the red (bell) peppers.

048 HONEY-SESAME SAUSAGES

SERVES 2–4
PREPARATION
5 minutes
COOKING
15 minutes

STORAGE
Make in advance and keep in the fridge for up to 3 days. Keep chilled until ready to eat.

2 tsp olive oil
1 tbsp clear honey
1 tsp Dijon mustard
12 good-quality cocktail sausages
1 tsp sesame seeds (optional)

1. Preheat the oven to 180°C/350°F/gas mark 4. Mix together the oil, honey and mustard in a bowl. Add the sausages and turn to coat them in the mixture.

2. Arrange the sausages in a non-stick roasting tin (pan) and cook in the oven for about 12–14 minutes, turning occasionally, until almost cooked. Sprinkle the sesame seeds over, if using, and cook for another minute until the sausages are golden and cooked through. Leave to cool.

049 PEAR AND HAM BUNDLES

SERVES 1
PREPARATION
5 minutes

STORAGE
Make on the day. Keep chilled until ready to eat.

1 ripe (but not too soft) pear, quartered and cored
squeeze of lemon juice
2 slices Parma ham, halved

1. Place the pear quarters on a plate, squeeze the lemon juice over them and turn until they are coated – this will help to prevent them browning.

2. Wrap one strip of Parma ham around each pear quarter.

050 HERRINGS ON RYE

SERVES 1
PREPARATION
5 minutes

STORAGE
Make on the day. Keep chilled until ready to eat.

low-fat cream cheese, for spreading
2 slices rye bread
6 slices marinated herring (you choose the marinade)

1) Spread the cream cheese over each slice of rye bread and sandwich with the cheesy sides in the middle.

2) Put the herrings in a pot with a lid. To eat, fork the herrings on to the bread or eat them separately straight from the pot, if that is easier.

051 SMOKED SALMON SPIRALS

SERVES 1
PREPARATION
10 minutes

STORAGE
Make the day before and keep in the fridge overnight. Slice on the day. Keep chilled until ready to eat.

1 tbsp low-fat cream cheese
squeeze of lemon juice
1 slice wholemeal bread
1 slice white bread
slices of smoked salmon or trout
freshly ground black pepper

1) Mix the cream cheese with the lemon juice and season with black pepper.

2) Cut the crusts off both slices of bread and spread the lemon cream cheese over one slice. Arrange a layer of fish on the bread and top with the remaining slice of bread.

3) Press down on the sandwich to flatten it slightly, then roll it up tightly into a cylinder shape. Wrap in clingfilm (plastic wrap) until ready to slice. Cut the bread into 1cm/½in slices.

052 TUNA QUESADILLA

SERVES 1
PREPARATION
5 minutes
COOKING
3 minutes

STORAGE
Make on the day. Keep chilled until ready to eat.

2 slices mozzarella cheese
1 small soft flour tortilla
3–4 tbsp canned tuna, drained
2 slices tomato
olive oil, for brushing
freshly ground black pepper

1. Place the mozzarella in the centre of the tortilla. Top with the tuna and tomato, season, then fold in the sides of the tortilla to make a square parcel.

2. Brush a frying pan (skillet) with olive oil. Place the parcel seam-side down in the pan and fry over a low heat for about 3 minutes, turning once, until golden. Leave to cool before wrapping.

3. Alternatively, sandwich the filling between two tortillas, cook on both sides in a lightly oiled frying pan (skillet) until the cheese melts and the tortillas are slightly golden and crisp, then cut into wedges.

053 FISH PÂTÉ

SERVES 1–2
PREPARATION
10 minutes

STORAGE
You can refrigerate the fish pâté for up to 3 days, or freeze it for up to a month.

250g/9oz de-boned mackerel fillets, cooked
150g/5½oz/⅔ cup cream cheese
1 tbsp lemon juice
25g/1oz/⅓ cup chopped parsley
2 wholemeal brown bread rolls
butter, for spreading
55g/2oz/⅔ cup rocket (arugula)

1. Break up the mackerel fillets into a blender or food processor. Add the cream cheese and process until smooth. Squeeze in the lemon juice, add the chopped parsley and stir together.

2. Cut the bread rolls in half and butter the top side. Spread the fish pâté liberally on the bottom halves of the rolls, add half the rocket (arugula) to each one and then close the tops. (Put an extra lemon wedge into your child's lunchbox – if they smear the juice over their fingers after they've eaten, it will remove the fishy smell!)

054 HUMMUS and SEEDED CRACKERS

SERVES 6
PREPARATION 10 minutes
COOKING 10 minutes

STORAGE
The hummus will keep in the fridge for up to 4 days or in the freezer for up to 1 month. Store the crackers in an airtight container for up to 2 days.

1 x 400-g/14-oz can chickpeas (garbanzo beans), drained and rinsed
2 sun-dried tomatoes in oil, drained
1 tbsp lemon juice
2 cloves garlic, crushed
1 tbsp tahini (sesame paste)
3 tbsp flaxseed or hemp-seed oil
pinch of paprika

SEEDED CRACKERS
3 wholemeal pitta breads, halved lengthways
2 tbsp olive oil
3 tbsp sesame seeds
pinch of paprika
2 tbsp Parmesan cheese

1. Preheat the oven to 200°C/400°F/gas mark 6. To make the crackers, brush the pittas with the oil and cut them into small triangles. Put on a baking sheet, sprinkle with the seeds, paprika and Parmesan. Bake for 5–10 minutes, or until golden brown and crisp. Cool on a rack for 2–3 minutes.

2. Process the chickpeas (garbanzo beans), tomatoes, lemon juice, garlic and tahini (sesame paste) in a food processor or blender to form a thick purée. Add the oil and process until smooth and creamy.

3. Spoon the hummus into a bowl and sprinkle with the paprika. Serve with the seeded crackers.

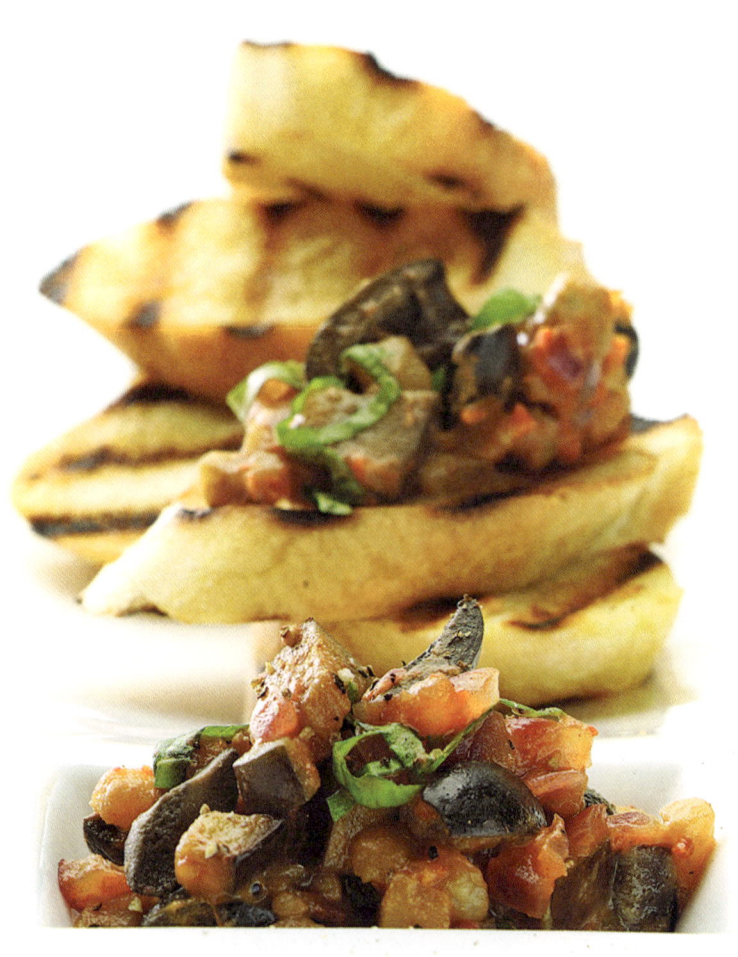

055 AUBERGINE (EGGPLANT) AND OLIVE PÂTÉ

SERVES 4–6
PREPARATION 10 minutes
COOKING 20 minutes
STORAGE Make in advance and keep in the fridge for up to 5 days.

2 tbsp olive oil
1 large red onion, finely chopped
2 medium aubergines (eggplant), diced
4 cloves garlic, crushed
4 tsp tamari
250g/9oz/1½ cups cherry tomatoes, blended
2 handfuls fresh basil
2 tsp Dijon mustard
20 black olives, pitted and chopped
sea salt and freshly ground black pepper to taste

1. Heat the oil in a frying pan (skillet) and sweat the onion until soft. Turn up the heat, add the aubergine (eggplant) and stir-fry until soft, about 10 minutes. Lower the heat, add the garlic, tamari (wheat-free soy sauce) and blended tomatoes, followed by the basil, mustard and olives. Very gently stir-fry for a further 5 minutes.

2. Season and serve on toasted bread with plenty of crispy green lettuce.

056 ROASTED AUBERGINE (EGGPLANT) DIP

SERVES 4
PREPARATION 15 minutes
COOKING 40 minutes
STORAGE Make in advance and keep in the fridge for up to 5 days.

1 large aubergine (eggplant)
2 cloves garlic
1 tbsp tahini (sesame paste)
1 tsp ground cumin
1 tsp ground coriander
2 tbsp extra-virgin olive oil
juice of ½ lemon
sea salt and freshly ground black pepper to taste

1. Preheat the oven to 200°C/400°F/gas mark 6. Prick the aubergine (eggplant) all over with a fork, then place in a roasting tin (pan). Roast for about 40 minutes, until the inside of the aubergine (eggplant) is very soft.

2. Leave to cool slightly, then halve the aubergine (eggplant) lengthways and scoop out the flesh with a spoon into a food processor or blender. Add the garlic, tahini (sesame paste), spices, olive oil and lemon juice. Process until smooth and creamy. Season to taste and serve with breadsticks or pitta bread slices.

057 BABA GANOUSH WITH AVOCADO AND FENNEL SALAD

SERVES 2–4
PREPARATION 20 minutes
COOKING 20 minutes

STORAGE
The salad is best eaten immediately. The baba ganoush will keep in the fridge for up to 5 days.

1 medium aubergine (eggplant)
2 tbsp lemon juice
1 tbsp tahini (sesame paste)
1 avocado, quartered and pitted
1 carrot, cut into peelings with a vegetable peeler
1 large tomato, chopped
1 small fennel bulb, finely chopped
1 bunch watercress, chopped
1 tbsp balsamic vinegar
2 tbsp walnut oil
sea salt and black pepper to taste

1. Prick the skin of the aubergine with a fork and grill (broil) it on all sides until it is soft and the skin charred, about 20 minutes. Cool under running water, halve and scoop out the flesh with a spoon into a food processor or blender. Blend the flesh with the lemon juice, tahini (sesame paste) and a pinch of salt.

2. Peel and slice the avocado and mix with the carrot, tomato, fennel and watercress in a salad bowl.

3. Make a dressing by whisking the balsamic vinegar and walnut oil with salt and pepper, pour over the salad and gently toss. Serve immediately with the baba ganoush and warm pitta bread.

058 HUMMUS RICE SNACKS

SERVES 2
PREPARATION 5 minutes

STORAGE
Store in a dry place for up to 4 hours.

4 rice cakes
115g/4oz/½ cup hummus
1 red (bell) pepper, deseeded and sliced lengthways
8 black olives, pitted and halved
4 sprigs basil

1. Spread each rice cake liberally with hummus and lay 3–4 strips of red (bell) pepper over each one.

2. Decorate with two olives and a sprig of basil and serve immediately.

059 SMASHED BEAN AND CARROT SPREAD

SERVES 4–6
PREPARATION
10 minutes
COOKING
5 minutes

STORAGE
Make in advance and keep in the fridge for up to 5 days.

1 carrot, sliced
2 tbsp extra-virgin olive oil
2 cloves garlic, crushed
1 tsp ground cumin
¼ tsp ground cinnamon
1 tsp ground coriander
2 pinches of chilli powder
200g/7oz/1½ cups canned butter (lima) beans, drained and rinsed
juice of 1 lemon
salt and freshly ground black pepper to taste

1. Steam the carrot until tender. Meanwhile, heat the oil in a saucepan and fry the garlic and spices for 1 minute. Add the beans, lemon juice and 2–3 tablespoons of water, then heat gently, stirring.

2. Put the carrot in a food processor or blender with the bean mixture. Process until smooth, adding a little extra water if necessary, then season to taste.

060 CREAMY GUACAMOLE

SERVES 2–4
PREPARATION
10 minutes

STORAGE
Make the day before and keep in the fridge overnight, or make on the day.

1 ripe avocado, halved and pitted
1 clove garlic, crushed
juice of ½ small lemon or juice of 1 lime
1 tbsp mayonnaise
1 tbsp finely chopped fresh coriander (cilantro) (optional)
salt and freshly ground black pepper to taste

1. Use a spoon to scoop the avocado out of its skin into a bowl. Stir in the garlic, lemon or lime juice and mayonnaise and mash using a fork to achieve the consistency you want.

2. Stir in the coriander (cilantro), if using, and season to taste.

061 PERUVIAN POLENTA CAKES

SERVES 4
PREPARATION
40 minutes
COOKING
20 minutes

STORAGE
Store leftovers in an airtight container in the fridge for up to 5 days.

600g/21oz/4 cups pre-cooked polenta (cornmeal)
2 fresh red chillies, finely chopped
4 tbsp fresh coriander (cilantro), finely chopped
1 tsp sea salt
about 500ml/17fl oz/2 cups boiling water
corn oil, for frying
2 large tomatoes, diced
1 large cucumber, grated
2 red (bell) peppers, quartered and sliced
4 tbsp lemon juice
2 tsp raw cane sugar
sea salt to taste

1. Place the cooked polenta (cornmeal) in a bowl, add the chilli, coriander (cilantro) and salt and mix well. Gradually pour in the boiling water and stir to a thick consistency. Leave to stand for 5 minutes, then mould the mixture with wet hands to make 24 round patties, about 5cm/2in in diameter by 1cm/$\frac{1}{2}$in thick.

2. Fry the cakes with a little corn oil in a frying pan (skillet) over a medium heat until golden, turning them frequently to prevent sticking.

3. Make a relish by mixing the tomato, cucumber, red (bell) pepper, lemon juice, sugar and salt. Serve the cakes hot with the relish on the side.

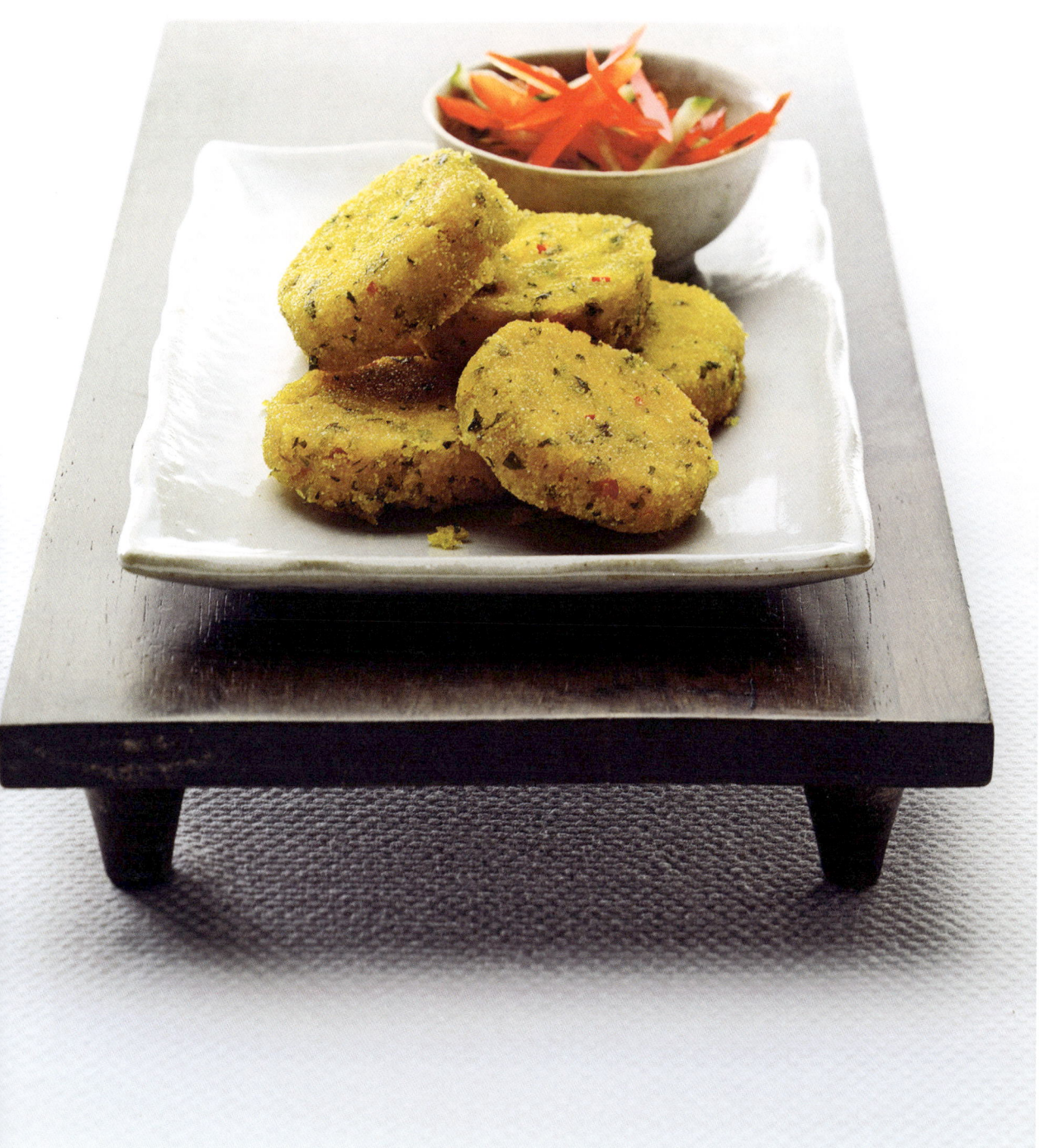

062 TZATZIKI

SERVES 4
PREPARATION
10 minutes

STORAGE
Make in advance and keep in the fridge for up to 3 days.

100g/3½oz/½ cup low-fat plain yogurt
10-cm/4-in piece courgette (zucchini), finely grated
2 small cloves garlic, crushed
4 tbsp finely chopped mint
salt and freshly ground black pepper to taste

1. Mix together the yogurt, courgette (zucchini), garlic and mint in a lidded pot or bowl.

2. Season to taste and serve with falafel or pitta bread.

063 PECAN PÂTÉ

SERVES 4
PREPARATION
5 minutes

STORAGE
Refrigerate for up to 5 days.

350g/12oz/2 cups pecans
4 carrots, peeled and grated
230g/8oz/1 cup alfalfa sprouts
2 tbsp olive oil
1 tsp celery salt
110g/4oz/1 cup chopped parsley

1. Put the pecans into a blender and process until they have become crumb-like. Add the carrots and alfalfa sprouts. Process for another minute, then add the olive oil, celery salt and parsley. Blend together into a smooth pâté, adding a little more olive oil if necessary.

064 SMOKED TOFU SALAD

SERVES 2-4

PREPARATION
15 minutes

STORAGE
The smoked tofu will keep for up to 2 days in the fridge. You can store the salad for up to 24 hours in the fridge.

250g/9oz smoked tofu, crumbled
4 tbsp lemon juice
2 tsp grated lemon zest
6 tbsp water
2 small shallots, finely chopped
2 cloves garlic, finely chopped
4 tbsp breadcrumbs
2 tbsp tomato ketchup (optional)
sea salt and black pepper to taste

SALAD
1 lettuce, shredded
2 carrots, grated or cut into peelings
2 large ripe tomatoes, sliced
2 tbsp capers
large handful Greek olives, pitted
4 tbsp fresh parsley, chopped

1. Blend the smoked tofu with the lemon juice, lemon rind and water. Add the shallot, garlic, breadcrumbs and tomato ketchup (if using). Season and keep in the fridge until needed.

2. Place the lettuce in a salad bowl and top with the carrot, tomato, capers, olives and parsley. Serve with the smoked tofu and warm pitta bread.

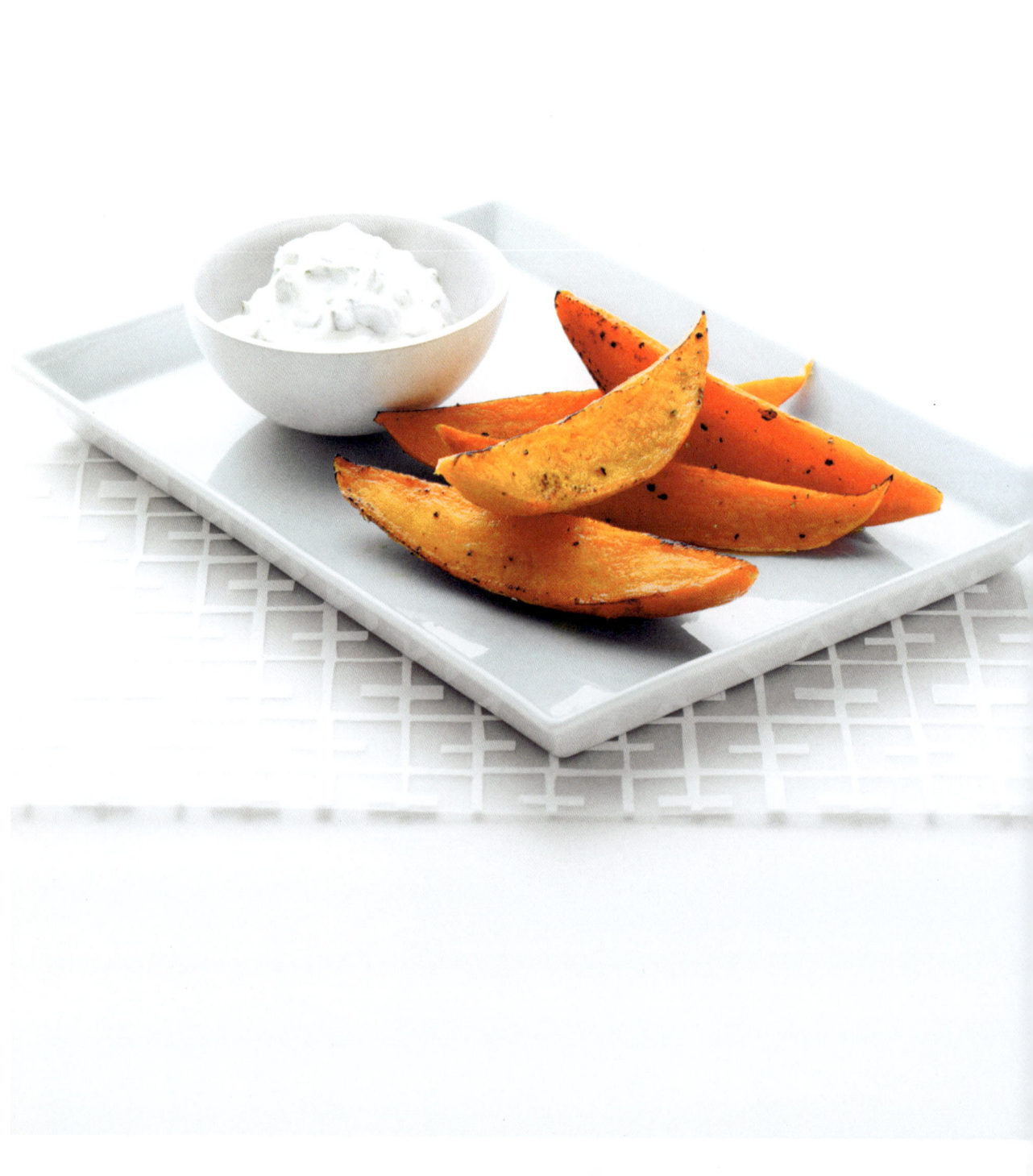

065 SWEET POTATO WEDGES

SERVES 4
PREPARATION
10 minutes
COOKING
40 minutes

STORAGE
You can refrigerate
for up to 2 days.

- 4 large sweet potatoes, peeled and chopped into wedges
- 4–6 tbsp olive oil
- ½ tsp sea salt, or to taste
- 1 tsp freshly ground black pepper
- 25g/1oz/⅓ cup chopped fresh coriander (cilantro)
- ½ tsp celery salt
- 225g/8oz/1 cup plain Greek yogurt

1. Preheat the oven to 220°C/425°F/gas mark 7. Place the sweet potato wedges in a large oven-proof dish. Cover with the olive oil and season to taste with salt and pepper. Bake in the oven for 30–40 minutes or until the potato is soft.

2. Mix the coriander (cilantro) and celery salt into the yogurt and serve in a small bowl as a dip for the sweet potato wedges.

066 VEGGIE DIPPERS

SERVES 2
PREPARATION
10 minutes

STORAGE
You can store the vegetables for 24 hours if you keep them in cold water and refrigerate.

- 100g/3½oz/½ cup sour cream
- 1 handful chives, finely chopped
- 3 carrots, peeled and cut into strips
- 100g/3½oz/½ cup sugar snap peas
- 55g/2oz radishes
- ½ cucumber, cut into strips
- ½ red (bell) pepper, deseeded and cut into strips
- ½ yellow (bell) pepper, deseeded and cut into strips
- 6 celery stalks, topped and tailed and cut into strips

1. In a small bowl, mix together the sour cream and chives.

2. Place the sour cream mixture in the centre of a large platter and arrange all the vegetable pieces around it, alternating the colours.

067 LEBANESE SPINACH

SERVES 2-4
PREPARATION
10 minutes
COOKING
20 minutes

STORAGE
Best eaten immediately.

1 onion, halved and sliced
olive oil, for frying
500g/1lb 2oz fresh spinach, roughly chopped
200ml/7fl oz/scant 1 cup plain yogurt
1 clove garlic, crushed
1 tbsp fresh mint leaves, chopped
2 large slices bread, chopped into cubes
2 tbsp pine kernels, toasted
sea salt and freshly ground black pepper to taste

1. Gently sweat the onion in a large heavy saucepan with a little oil until soft. Add the spinach, heat through, cover and very gently simmer until soft, about 10 minutes. Season to taste.

2. Make a dressing by whisking together the yogurt, garlic and mint. Season and set aside.

3. Fry the bread with a little oil in a frying pan (skillet) until golden to make croutons, then place half of them in a serving bowl, add the cooked spinach, followed by the yogurt dressing. Top with the remaining croutons and garnish with toasted pine kernels. Serve immediately.

068 CELERY SMACKERS

SERVES 2
PREPARATION
5 minutes

STORAGE
You can refrigerate for up to 24 hours.

4 celery stalks, topped and tailed and cut into chunks
115g/4oz/½ cup hummus
25g/1oz/⅓ cup chopped fresh coriander (cilantro)

1. Fill the groove in the celery chunks with the hummus, wiping away any excess.

2. Put the filled chunks on a plate and scatter the coriander (cilantro) on top.

069 CHEESY CELERY STALKS

SERVES 2
PREPARATION
2 minutes

STORAGE
Make on the day.

2–4 celery stalks
2–4 tbsp low-fat cream cheese (flavour of choice)

1) Cut the celery stalks into halves or thirds, depending on their length, then simply spread the cream cheese into the grooves running down the pieces of celery.

070 SUMMER CRUDITÉS

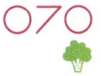

SERVES 2–4
PREPARATION
15 minutes
COOKING
10 minutes

1 red (bell) pepper, halved
100g/3½oz chanterelle mushrooms
oil, for frying
2 carrots
1 small raw beetroot (beet)
2 celery stalks
½ cucumber
4 artichoke hearts, sliced
10 red radishes, kept whole
1 pinch sea salt and black pepper
1 tbsp red wine vinegar
3 tbsp walnut oil
2 tsp fresh tarragon, chopped
1 tbsp pumpkin seeds, toasted

1) Grill (broil) the (bell) pepper until the skin becomes black and charred. Cover with a damp dish towel and leave to cool.

2) Meanwhile, stir-fry the chanterelle mushrooms in a little oil in a frying pan (skillet) over a medium heat.

3) Cut the carrots, beetroot (beet), celery and cucumber into thin 10-cm/4-in long sticks. Skin the cooled (bell) pepper and cut the flesh into long sticks, too. Arrange the crudités on two large plates.

3) To make the dressing, dissolve the salt and pepper in the vinegar, add the walnut oil and the tarragon and whisk. Drizzle the dressing over the crudités and garnish with toasted pumpkin seeds. Serve with toast.

071 SOY-COATED NUTS AND SEEDS

SERVES 4
PREPARATION 5 minutes
COOKING 10 minutes

STORAGE Make in advance and keep in an airtight container for up to 1 week.

200g/7oz/scant 2 cups mixed unsalted nuts and seeds: peanuts (skins rubbed off), almonds, cashews, walnuts, hazelnuts, brazils, sunflower, hemp, pumpkin or linseeds
1–2 tsp soy sauce

1. Preheat the oven to 170°C/325°F/gas mark 3. Place the nuts on a baking sheet and roast for about 6 minutes. Add the seeds and roast for another 2–4 minutes until they smell toasted and are golden; watch carefully as they burn easily.

2. Remove from the oven and transfer to a bowl. Leave to cool slightly then drizzle with the soy sauce, turning the nuts and seeds with a spoon until they are coated.

072 SOAKED ALMONDS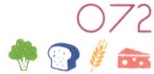

SERVES 4
PREPARATION 5 minutes + 12 hours soaking

STORAGE Store the almonds in water for 3 days, but replace the water frequently during that time.

175g/6oz/1 cup whole almonds
85g/3oz/½ cup dried almonds

1. Place the whole almonds in a large bowl and then fill the bowl with enough water to cover all the almonds.

2. Put the bowl in the fridge for 12 hours. After the first six hours, drain the water and replace with fresh water.

3. After 12 hours, drain the water, add the dried almonds and serve in a small snack bowl.

073 SAVOURY SPICY POPCORN

SERVES 4
PREPARATION
2 minutes
COOKING
3 minutes

STORAGE
Make in advance and keep in an airtight container for up to 3 days.

1 tbsp sunflower oil
70g/2½oz popping corn
1 tsp Cajun spice mix

① Heat the oil in a saucepan, then add the popping corn in a single layer. Cover the pan with a lid and cook over a medium heat, shaking the pan frequently, until the corn has popped. Do not lift the lid until it has finished popping.

② Transfer the popcorn to a large bowl and sprinkle the spice mix over the top. Turn the popcorn with a spoon until it is coated in the spices. Leave to cool.

074 ALMOND BUTTER BITES

SERVES 2
PREPARATION
5 minutes

STORAGE
Keep for up to a month in an airtight container.

175g/6oz/1 cup roasted whole almonds
2 tbsp olive oil
55g/2oz/⅔ cup roasted whole almonds, chopped
2 slices wholegrain bread

① Place the whole almonds into a food processor or blender and process until the nuts are finely ground. Add the olive oil and mix until smooth.

② Transfer to a small bowl and stir in the chopped almonds.

③ Spread liberally onto each slice of bread.

075 PESTO PIZZA

SERVES 4
PREPARATION
10 minutes
COOKING
20 minutes

STORAGE
Store leftovers in the fridge for up to 2 days.

2 pizza bases
4 tbsp pesto
20 cherry tomatoes, halved
20 sun-dried tomatoes, chopped
200g/7oz spinach, sautéed
200g/7oz feta cheese or marinated tofu, cubed
oregano, sea salt and black pepper to taste
200g/7oz mozzarella cheese, grated

1) Preheat the oven to 240°C/475°F/gas mark 9 and heat a large baking sheet.

2) Cover the prepared bases with the pesto. Top with the cherry tomatoes, sun-dried tomatoes, spinach and feta or tofu. Sprinkle with oregano, season and sprinkle with mozzarella cheese.

3) Bake in the hot oven for approximately 20 minutes. Serve hot with a side salad.

076 TOMATO AND GARLIC PIZZA

SERVES 4
PREPARATION
10 minutes
COOKING
15 minutes

STORAGE
Store leftovers in the fridge for up to 2 days.

8 fresh ripe tomatoes, chopped
2 pizza bases
8 cloves garlic, sliced and mixed with 2 tbsp olive oil
200g/7oz mozzarella cheese, cut into cubes
20 black olives
sea salt and black pepper to taste
4 tbsp fresh basil, chopped

1) Preheat the oven to 240°C/475°F/gas mark 9 and heat a large baking sheet.

2) Spread the tomatoes over the pizza bases and add a pinch of salt. Top with the garlic and oil mixture, cheese cubes and olives. Season and bake in a hot oven for approximately 15 minutes.

3) Garnish with the basil and more black pepper. Serve hot.

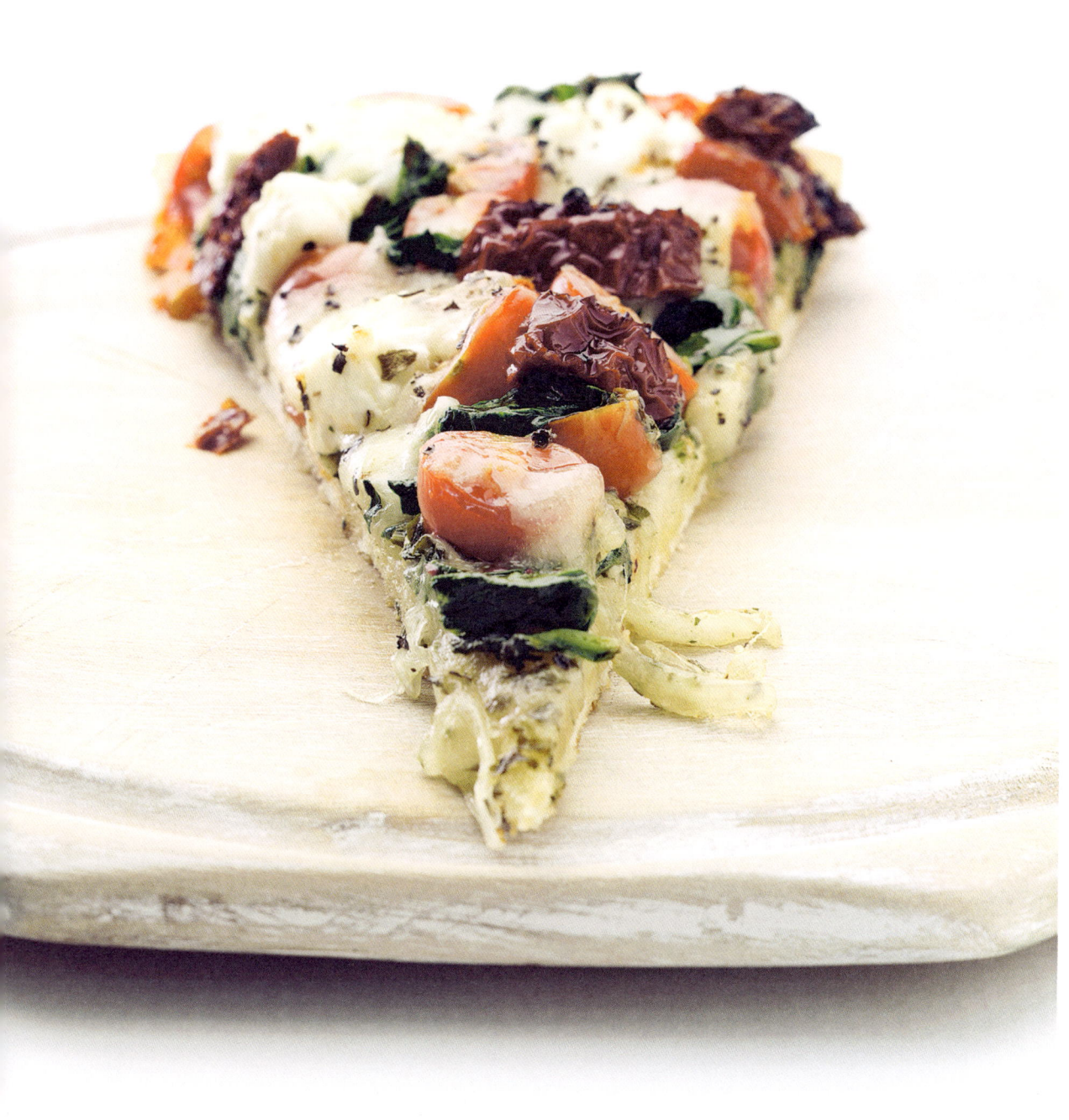

077 PIZZA MARGHERITA

SERVES 4
PREPARATION 5 minutes
COOKING 10–15 minutes

STORAGE Store leftovers in the fridge for up to 2 days.

- 4 tbsp passata (sieved tomatoes)
- 2 pizza bases
- 4 fresh ripe plum tomatoes, sliced
- oregano to taste
- 200g/7oz mozzarella cheese, grated

1. Preheat the oven to 240°C/475°F/gas mark 9 and heat a large baking sheet.

2. Spread the passata (sieved tomatoes) over the pizza bases. Add the plum tomatoes and plenty of oregano. Season to taste. Sprinkle the grated cheese over the pizzas.

3. Bake in the hot oven for 10–15 minutes. Serve hot.

078 PIZZA GRILL

SERVES 2
PREPARATION 10 minutes
COOKING 8 minutes

STORAGE Store leftovers in the fridge for up to 2 days.

- ½ French baguette (halved lengthways) or 2 bagels (split) or 2 pitta breads
- 2 tbsp passata (sieved tomatoes)
- 100g/3½oz mozzarella cheese, grated
- 1 tomato, sliced
- 1 small red onion, sliced
- ½ red (bell) pepper, sliced
- 1 small fresh hot chilli, sliced
- 2 cloves garlic, crushed
- 1 tbsp fresh basil, chopped

1. Preheat the grill (broiler) and toast the underside of the bread.

2. Spread the passata (sieved tomatoes) over the untoasted side of the bread. Cover with the grated cheese and the remaining topping ingredients (except the basil), and season. Grill for 4–5 minutes, or until the cheese has melted.

3. Garnish with the fresh basil and serve hot.

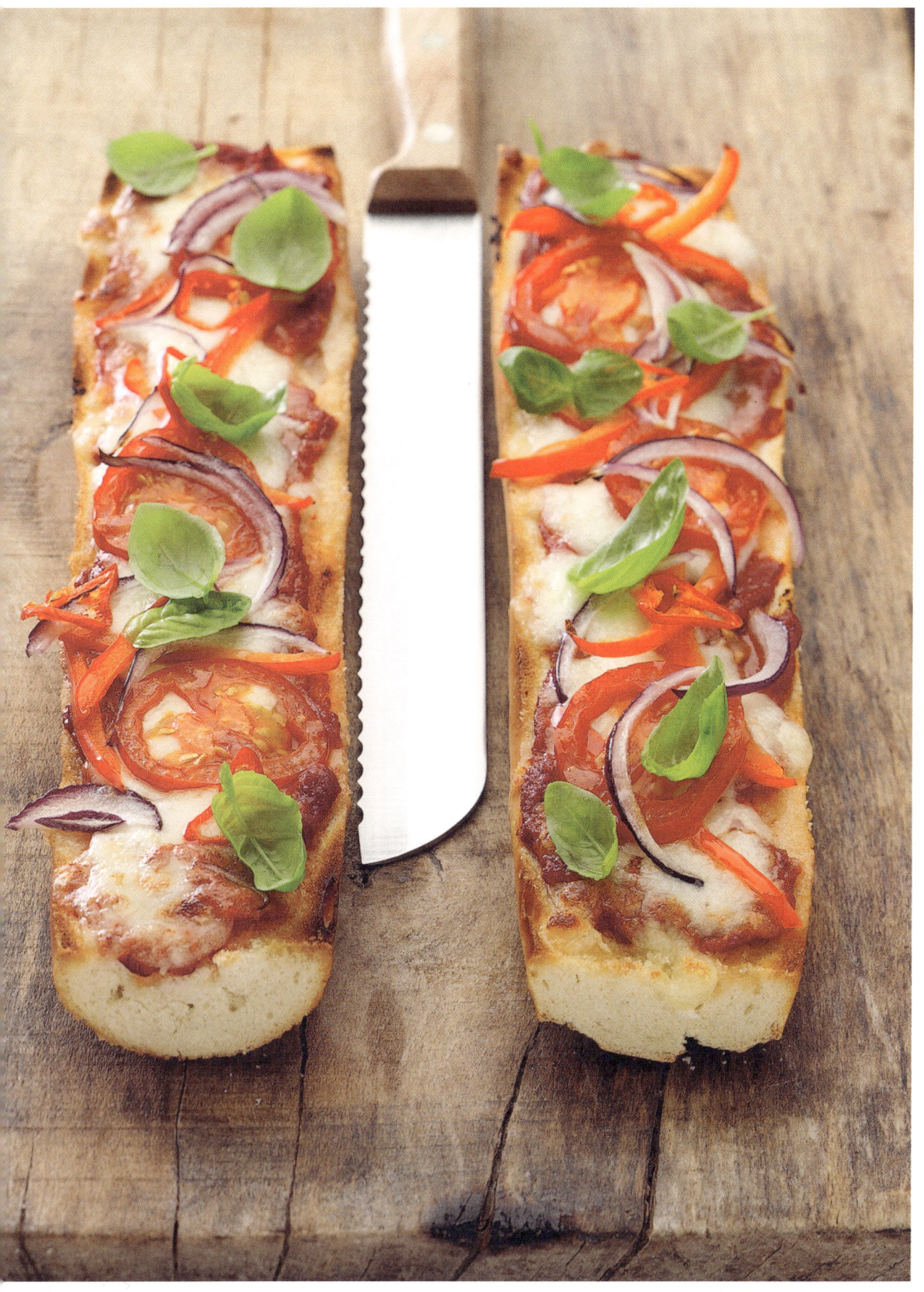

079 TORTILLA DIPPERS with TOMATO SALSA

SERVES 4
PREPARATION 10 minutes
COOKING 20 minutes

STORAGE Make the salsa in advance and keep in the fridge for up to 3 days or freeze for up to 1 month. Cook the tortilla wedges on the day.

4 wholemeal tortillas
4 tsp olive oil

TOMATO SALSA
2 tbsp olive oil
2 cloves garlic, crushed
350ml/12fl oz/1½ cups passata (sieved tomatoes)
1 tbsp sun-dried tomato paste
½ tsp sugar
2 tomatoes, deseeded and cut into small pieces (optional)

1. To make the tomato salsa, heat the oil in a saucepan. Fry the garlic for 1 minute, stirring to prevent it burning. Add the passata (sieved tomatoes), tomato paste and sugar, then bring to the boil. Reduce the heat to low, half-cover the pan with a lid and simmer for 15 minutes. Stir the sauce occasionally to prevent it sticking to the bottom of the pan. Leave to cool then stir in the fresh tomatoes, if using.

2. Cut the tortillas in half and then into three or four wedges. Heat the oil in a frying pan (skillet) and fry the wedges in batches for about 2 minutes on each side until golden and crisp. When cool, serve with the salsa.

080 QUICK TOMATO SOUP

SERVES 4
PREPARATION 5 minutes
COOKING 10 minutes

8 large tomatoes, stalks removed, quartered and blended
2 tsp tamari
2 pinches of ground coriander
2 tsp maple syrup
2 pinches of Chinese five-spice powder
2 tbsp fresh oregano, chopped
sea salt and black pepper to taste

1. Place all of the ingredients in a saucepan. Gently heat through, stirring often, and simmer for 5 minutes. Season and serve.

081 SOCCA NIÇOISE (GLUTEN-FREE FLATBREAD)

SERVES 4
PREPARATION
5 minutes
COOKING
20 minutes

STORAGE
Best eaten immediately. Leftovers will keep for up to 5 days in the fridge.

500g/18oz/4 cups chickpea (gram) flour
600ml/21fl oz/2½ cups cold water
600ml–1 litre hot water
sea salt and black pepper to taste
olive oil, for sprinkling and frying

1. Preheat the oven to 250°C/500°F/gas mark 10.

2. Place the chickpea (gram) flour in a heavy saucepan and slowly stir in the cold water until smooth. Place the saucepan over a moderate heat and gradually add the hot water and salt to taste, stirring continuously. Lower the heat and continue to stir until the mixture starts to form a ball of dough.

3. Spread out the dough evenly in an oiled, shallow baking tin (pan). Sprinkle with olive oil and black pepper. Bake in the hot oven for 10 minutes until slightly crisp. Cool and slice into pieces.

4. Gently fry the socca pieces in a little oil in a frying pan (skillet). Drain on paper towels and serve hot with a tomato salad.

082 HALF-MOON PASTRIES

SERVES 2-4
PREPARATION
10 minutes
COOKING
15 minutes

1 package ready-made shortcrust pastry, rolled out thinly
500g/1lb 2oz fresh spinach, curly kale or Swiss chard, chopped
2 tbsp lemon juice
2 tbsp olive oil, plus extra for greasing
½ tsp allspice
pinch of salt
1 tsp sumac (optional)

1. Preheat the oven to 200°C/400°F/gas mark 6.

2. Cut the pastry into approximately 10cm/4in rounds with a biscuit cutter.

3. Place the spinach, curly kale or Swiss chard in a bowl and mix in the remaining ingredients. Place a large spoonful of filling on each pastry round and fold each one into a half-moon shape. Firmly pinch together the edges of each pastry and place them on a greased baking sheet.

4. Bake in the middle of the hot oven until brown, about 15 minutes. Serve with a salad.

083 CAJUN SALMON AND CUCUMBER ROLL

SERVES 1
PREPARATION 5 minutes
STORAGE Make on the day. Keep chilled until ready to eat.

60g/2¼oz canned salmon, skin removed
¼–½ tsp mixed Cajun spices
squeeze of lemon juice
crusty brown bread roll
1 tsp mayonnaise
5 slices cucumber

1. Spoon the salmon into a bowl and mix with the spices. Squeeze some lemon juice over the top.

2. Cut the bread roll in half and spread one side with the mayonnaise. Spoon the salmon on top, followed by the cucumber slices. Place the other half of the roll on top.

084 NUT BUTTER AND BANANA BAGEL

SERVES 1
PREPARATION 15 minutes
COOKING 5 minutes
STORAGE The nut butter is enough for 8 servings. Make the nut butter in advance and keep in the fridge for up to 2 weeks. Assemble on the day.

1 sesame seed bagel
½ small banana, thinly sliced

NUT BUTTER
55g/2oz/½ cup unsalted cashew nuts
55g/2oz/½ cup unsalted peanuts
4–5 tbsp sunflower or rapeseed oil
½ tsp salt

1. Lightly toast the cashews and peanuts in a dry frying pan (skillet) over a medium-low heat for 4–5 minutes, turning regularly, until the nuts smell slightly toasted and are a light golden colour.

2. Leave the nuts to cool and rub off the brown papery skin covering the peanuts, if necessary. Put the nuts, oil and salt in a food processor and blend to a coarse paste. Place the nut butter in a lidded jar in the fridge.

3. Cut the bagel in half and spread the nut butter over one half. Arrange the slices of banana on top and cover with the other bagel half.

085 CREAM CHEESE AND DATE BAGEL

SERVES 1
PREPARATION 5 minutes

STORAGE
Make on the day.

2 ready-to-eat dried dates
1 tbsp low-fat cream cheese
1 cinnamon bagel

1. Snip the dates into small pieces using scissors. Mix the dates into the cream cheese.

2. Cut the bagel in half and spread the date and cream cheese filling in the middle.

086 CHEESE, APPLE AND CHUTNEY BAP

SERVES 1
PREPARATION 15 minutes
COOKING 30 minutes

STORAGE
Make the chutney in advance and keep in an airtight jar in the fridge for up to 2 weeks. Assemble on the day.

2–3 tbsp grated mature Cheddar cheese
½ small apple, cored and grated
1 seeded wholemeal bap

CHUTNEY
4 tomatoes, roughly chopped
1 large apple, peeled, cored and roughly chopped
1 onion, grated
5 tbsp white wine vinegar
55g/2oz/¼ cup sugar

1. Put all the chutney ingredients in a saucepan. Bring to the boil, then reduce the heat, cover and simmer for 5 minutes. Uncover the pan, then cook for a further 20 minutes. Leave to cool and spoon into a lidded jar.

2. Mix together the cheese, apple and 2 teaspoons of the chutney. Cut the bap in half and add the filling.

087 CINNAMON POPCORN

SERVES 2
PREPARATION
5 minutes
COOKING
10 minutes

STORAGE
Store for up to 3 days in an airtight container.

2 tbsp olive oil
55g/2oz/⅓ cup popping corn
55g/2oz butter
1 tsp ground cinnamon

1. Heat the olive oil in a medium saucepan. Pour in the corn, put a lid on the pan and shake it over the heat until the popping stops.

Remove from the heat, leaving the lid on for a few minutes.

2. Melt the butter in a small non-stick saucepan. Add the cinnamon and stir.

3. Pour the popcorn into a serving bowl and drizzle with the cinnamon butter.

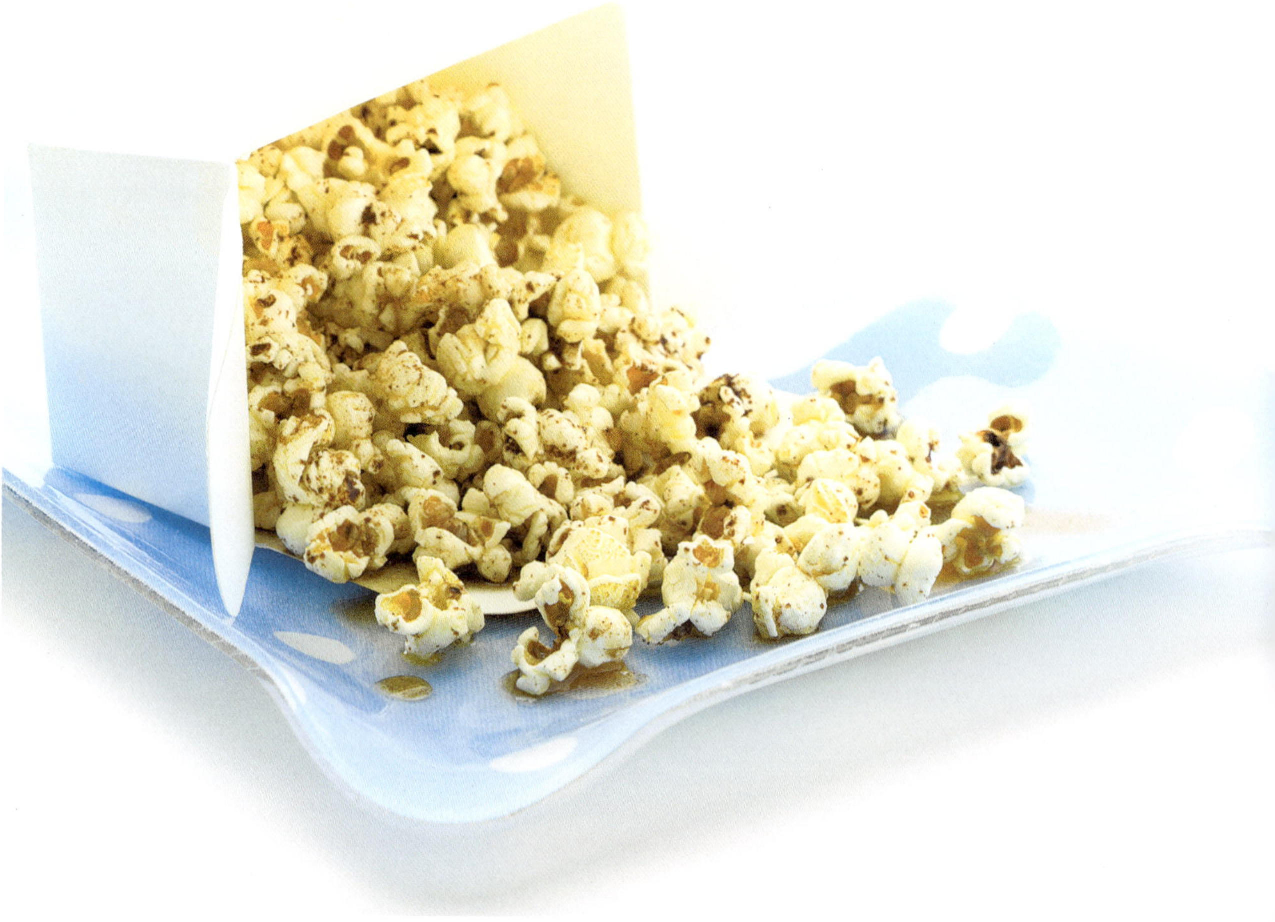

088 CHEWY DATE BARS

MAKES 16
PREPARATION 20 minutes
COOKING 45 minutes

STORAGE Make in advance and keep in an airtight container for up to 1 week.

125g/4½oz unsalted butter, plus extra for greasing
200g/7oz/1½ cups chopped ready-to-eat dried dates
125g/4½oz/1 cup wholemeal (whole wheat) flour
1 tsp baking powder
115g/4oz/½ cup light soft brown sugar
125g/4½oz/generous 1 cup whole porridge (rolled) oats
4 tbsp sunflower seeds

1. Grease the sides and line the base of a 28 x 18cm/11 x 7in baking tin (pan). Put the dates and 225ml/8fl oz/scant 1 cup water in a saucepan and bring to the boil. Reduce the heat and simmer, half-covered, for 20 minutes until the dates are very soft and the water has been absorbed. Purée the dates in a blender and leave to cool. Preheat the oven to 180°C/350°F/gas mark 4.

2. Meanwhile, mix together the flour, baking powder, sugar, oats and seeds in a mixing bowl. Rub in the butter until the mixture is soft and crumbly. Spoon three-quarters into the greased tin (pan) and press down to make an even layer.

3. Spoon the date mixture over the oats in an even layer, sprinkle with the remaining oat mixture and press down lightly. Bake for 25 minutes until golden, then leave in the tin (pan) to cool. Cut into 16 squares and remove from the tin (pan).

089 TOFFEE APPLE CRISPS

MAKES 10
PREPARATION
10 minutes
COOKING
15 minutes

STORAGE
Can be stored in an airtight container for up to 2 weeks.

55g/2oz butter
2 tbsp black molasses
2 tbsp golden syrup
115g/4oz/1 cup porridge (rolled) oats
2 apples, grated

1) Preheat the oven to 170°C/325°F/gas mark 3. Place the butter, molasses and syrup in a small saucepan and melt over a low heat. Put the oats and grated apple in a mixing bowl, add the melted mixture and stir.

2) Put teaspoon-size balls of the mixture onto a greased baking sheet and bake for 15 minutes, or until golden brown. Cool and serve.

090 APPLE FLAPJACKS

MAKES 10
PREPARATION
15 minutes
COOKING
35 minutes

STORAGE
Make in advance and keep in an airtight container for up to 1 week.

100g/3½oz unsalted butter, plus extra for greasing
100g/3½oz/scant ½ cup light soft brown sugar
4 tbsp golden syrup
250g/9oz/heaped 2 cups whole porridge (rolled) oats
1 tbsp sesame seeds
1 tbsp pumpkin seeds
2 tbsp sunflower seeds
1 apple, cored and grated

1) Preheat the oven to 180°C/350°F/Gas 4. Grease the sides and line the base of a 20cm/8in square tin (pan). Melt the butter in a saucepan with the sugar and syrup over a low heat, stirring occasionally; do not allow the mixture to boil.

2) Put the oats, seeds and apple in a mixing bowl and pour in the buttery syrup. Stir until everything is mixed together.

3) Spoon the oat mixture into the prepared tin (pan) and bake for 25–30 minutes until golden and lightly crisp. Cut into 10 bars while still warm and leave in the tin (pan) until cool.

091 TAHINI AND CHOCOLATE FUDGE

MAKES 30–36 PIECES
PREPARATION
15 minutes + 3 hours chilling

STORAGE
Store in the fridge for up to 1 week or in the freezer for up to 1 month.

25g/1oz/¼ cup sesame seeds
200g/7oz/2 cups almonds
6 dates, chopped
½ tsp ground cinnamon
2 tbsp desiccated (dried shredded) coconut
1 tbsp ground flaxseeds
6 tbsp tahini (sesame paste)
6 tbsp honey or agave nectar
150g/5½oz plain chocolate, melted
olive oil, for greasing

1 Put the sesame seeds and almonds in a food processor and process until finely ground. Add the dates, cinnamon, coconut and flaxseeds and process to form a coarse paste. Transfer the mixture to a bowl.

2 Mix the tahini (sesame paste), honey or agave nectar and chocolate until blended. Add to the almonds and stir well to form a sticky dough.

3 Lightly grease and line a 32 x 20cm/13 x 8in tin (pan) with oil and press the mixture into the tin (pan). Chill in the fridge for 2–3 hours until firm, then cut into 30–36 small bars and serve.

092 CHOCOLATE FRUIT TRUFFLES

MAKES 10–12
PREPARATION
15 minutes
COOKING
30 minutes

STORAGE
Keep in the fridge for up to 4 days.

100g/3½oz/¾ cup dried apricots, chopped
60g/2¼oz/½ cup dates, chopped
100g/3½oz plain chocolate (75% cocoa solids), melted
2 tbsp ground flaxseeds
2 tbsp sesame seeds
4 tbsp ground almonds
25g/1oz chopped mixed nuts or desiccated (dried shredded) coconut, for coating

1 Process the apricots, dates and chocolate in a food processor to form a thick paste. Add the flaxseeds, sesame seeds and almonds and stir until a stiff, sticky dough forms.

2 Roll the mixture into 10–12 small balls and roll them in the chopped nuts or coconut to coat. Chill for 30 minutes until firm, then serve.

093 HOT PEAR SOUP

SERVES 4
PREPARATION
5 minutes
COOKING
22 minutes

STORAGE
Store in the fridge for up to 5 days.

1kg/2lb 3oz ripe pears, peeled, cored and chopped
2 tsp fresh ginger, grated
4 tbsp grapeseed oil
2 tbsp lemon juice
600ml/21fl oz/2½ cups water
sea salt and black pepper to taste

1. Gently stir-fry the pears and the ginger in a saucepan with the oil for 1 minute. Add the lemon juice and stir for a further 30 seconds. Add the water, bring to the boil, cover and simmer for 20 minutes.

2. Allow to cool slightly before blending in a blender. Season and serve hot or cold.

094 BLUEBERRY YOGO-POPS

SERVES 4
PREPARATION
10 minutes + 2 hours freezing

STORAGE
Use the yogo-pops within a month of freezing.

500g/1lb 2oz/2½ cups plain yogurt
150g/5½oz frozen blueberries
juice of ½ lime

1. In a bowl mix together the yogurt, blueberries and lime juice. Pour into ice-lolly (popsicle) moulds and then add the sticks.

2. Place in the freezer for a minimum of 2 hours before serving.

SNACKS | 77

095 PINEAPPLE AND MINT FROZEN YOGURT

SERVES 4
PREPARATION
10 minutes + 4 hours freezing

STORAGE
Freeze for up to 3 months. Place in the fridge for 30 minutes before serving.

350g/12oz pineapple, cut into pieces
150g/5oz/scant 2/3 cup plain yogurt
1 tsp lime juice
2 tsp finely chopped mint

1. Freeze the pineapple pieces for 3–4 hours until solid.

2. Blend the frozen pineapple, yogurt, lime juice and mint in a blender until the mixture forms a thick, creamy 'ice cream'.

3. Serve immediately or pour into a shallow freezerproof container and freeze until required.

096 BLACKBERRY AND APPLE ICICLES

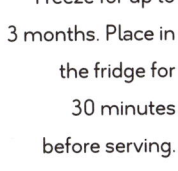

SERVES 4
PREPARATION
20 minutes + freezing

STORAGE
Freeze for up to a month.

250ml/9fl oz/1 cup water
115g/4oz/1/2 cup brown sugar
2 apples, peeled, cored and diced
115g/4oz/1/2 cup frozen blackberries
juice of 2 limes

1. Pour the water into a saucepan, add the sugar and stir until dissolved.

2. Add the apples, blackberries and lime juice to the water. Let simmer for 5–7 minutes until the mixture thickens slightly.

3. Remove from the heat and cool for an hour. Pour into ice-lolly (popsicle) moulds and freeze.

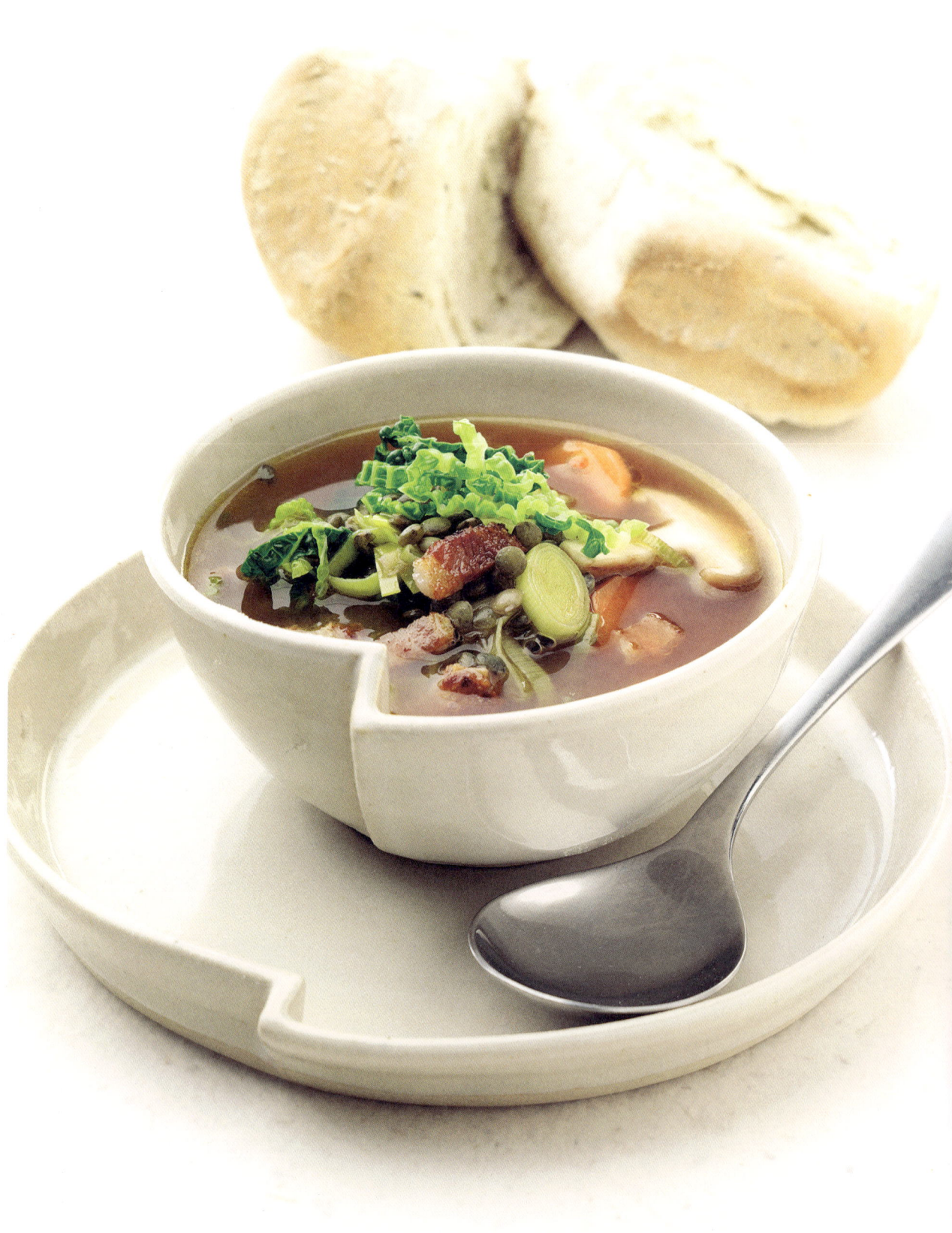

Soups, Salads & Sides

Nourishing soups keep well and are great for making in advance – ideal for busy family life: either chill, or freeze in portions and reheat on the day. Vegetable, bean, pasta or noodle soups, such as Chunky Italian Soup (see page 86), make complete meals, providing both protein and carbs. Purée soups for children who dislike "bits" or won't eat vegetables, as the smooth texture will disguise the ingredients.

The salads in this chapter range from substantial meals in their own right (Salmon Niçoise on page 112 or Chicken Caeser Salad on page 109) to perfect side dishes (Spicy Sweet Potatoes on page 127 or Mixed Bean Salad on page 121). Many would also make ideal additions to a lunchbox – be sure to keep them well chilled so they stay fresh and crisp.

097 WINTER VEGETABLE SOUP

SERVES 4
PREPARATION
15 minutes
COOKING
20–25 minutes

STORAGE
Make in advance and keep in the fridge for up to 3 days or freeze in single portions.

150g/5½oz/¾ cup Puy lentils
6 tbsp olive oil
2 small leeks, sliced
150g/5½oz smoked bacon, diced
2 carrots, sliced
2 slices celeriac (celery root), diced
24 shiitake mushrooms, sliced
200g/7oz cabbage, finely sliced
2l/70fl oz/8½ cups veg stock
2 bay leaves
2 tsp thyme
2 tbsp tomato purée (paste)

1. Boil the lentils in a saucepan with twice their volume of water for 20 minutes, or until almost tender.

2. Meanwhile, gently heat the oil in a saucepan, add the leek and the smoked bacon and stir-fry for 2 minutes. Add the carrot, celeriac (celery root), shiitake and cabbage and continue to stir-fry for a further 5 minutes. Stir in the stock, bay leaves, thyme and tomato paste and bring to the boil.

3. Drain the partially-cooked lentils and add them to the saucepan. Bring the soup to the boil again, and simmer for 10 minutes, or until the lentils are soft. Remove the bay leaves, season and serve with warm, crusty bread rolls.

098 SPINACH AND CHICKPEA SOUP

SERVES 4
PREPARATION
10 minutes
COOKING
25 minutes

STORAGE
Make in advance and keep in the fridge for up to 3 days or freeze in single portions.

4 tbsp olive oil, plus for frying
2 bay leaves
¼ tsp cayenne pepper
2 tsp ground cumin
2 tsp turmeric
500g/18oz chickpeas, canned
500g/18oz spinach, finely chopped
1.5l/52fl oz/6½ cups veg stock
1 head garlic
1 whole onion, peeled
2 slices of bread, crumbled
4 tbsp fresh parsley, chopped
4 cloves garlic, crushed
sea salt to taste

1. Heat the oil in a pan and fry the bay leaves and spices for 30 seconds. Add the chickpeas and fry for 5 minutes, then add the spinach and fry for a minute. Add the stock, whole garlic, onion and a little salt. Cover and simmer for 15 minutes.

2. Heat a little oil in a frying pan (skillet) and fry the crumbled bread and the parsley for 2 minutes.

3. Blend the crushed garlic with a little of the soup to make a paste. Add to the soup and remove the whole garlic, onion and bay leaves. Season and serve.

SOUPS, SALADS & SIDES

099 HAM AND BARLEY BROTH

SERVES 4
PREPARATION
10 minutes + soaking
COOKING
55 minutes

STORAGE
Make in advance and keep in the fridge for up to 3 days or freeze in single portions.

100g/3½oz pearl barley
1 tbsp olive oil
1 large leek, finely sliced
1 large carrot, finely diced
85g/3oz pancetta or lean smoky bacon, diced
1 bay leaf
1 tsp dried mixed herbs
1.2l/40fl oz/5 cups veg stock
salt and freshly ground black pepper

1 Soak the barley in cold water for about 2 hours – this will help to speed up the cooking time. Drain and rinse.

2 Heat the olive oil in a large saucepan and fry the leek for 5 minutes, then add the carrot, pancetta or bacon and barley and cook for another 2 minutes.

3 Add the bay leaf, mixed herbs and stock and bring to the boil. Reduce the heat and simmer, half-covered, for 40–45 minutes, stirring occasionally, until the barley is tender. Remove the bay leaf and season to taste.

100 CALDO VERDE

SERVES 6
PREPARATION
15 minutes
COOKING
20 minutes

STORAGE
Make in advance and keep in the fridge for up to 3 days or freeze in single portions.

1.7l/60fl oz/7½ cups water or vegetable stock
100g/3½oz curly kale leaves, chopped
4 potatoes, diced
2 shallots, chopped
8 cloves garlic, chopped
200g/7oz spicy sausages, sliced
2 tbsp olive oil, plus extra for frying
sea salt and black pepper to taste

1 Bring the water or stock to the boil in a saucepan with the curly kale, potatoes, shallot, garlic and a little salt. Heat through and simmer for 20 minutes.

2 Meanwhile, fry the sausage slices in a frying pan (skillet) with a little oil. Set aside.

3 Blend the soup in a food processor or blender, check the seasoning and add the oil. Garnish with black pepper and spicy sausage slices, and serve hot with corn bread.

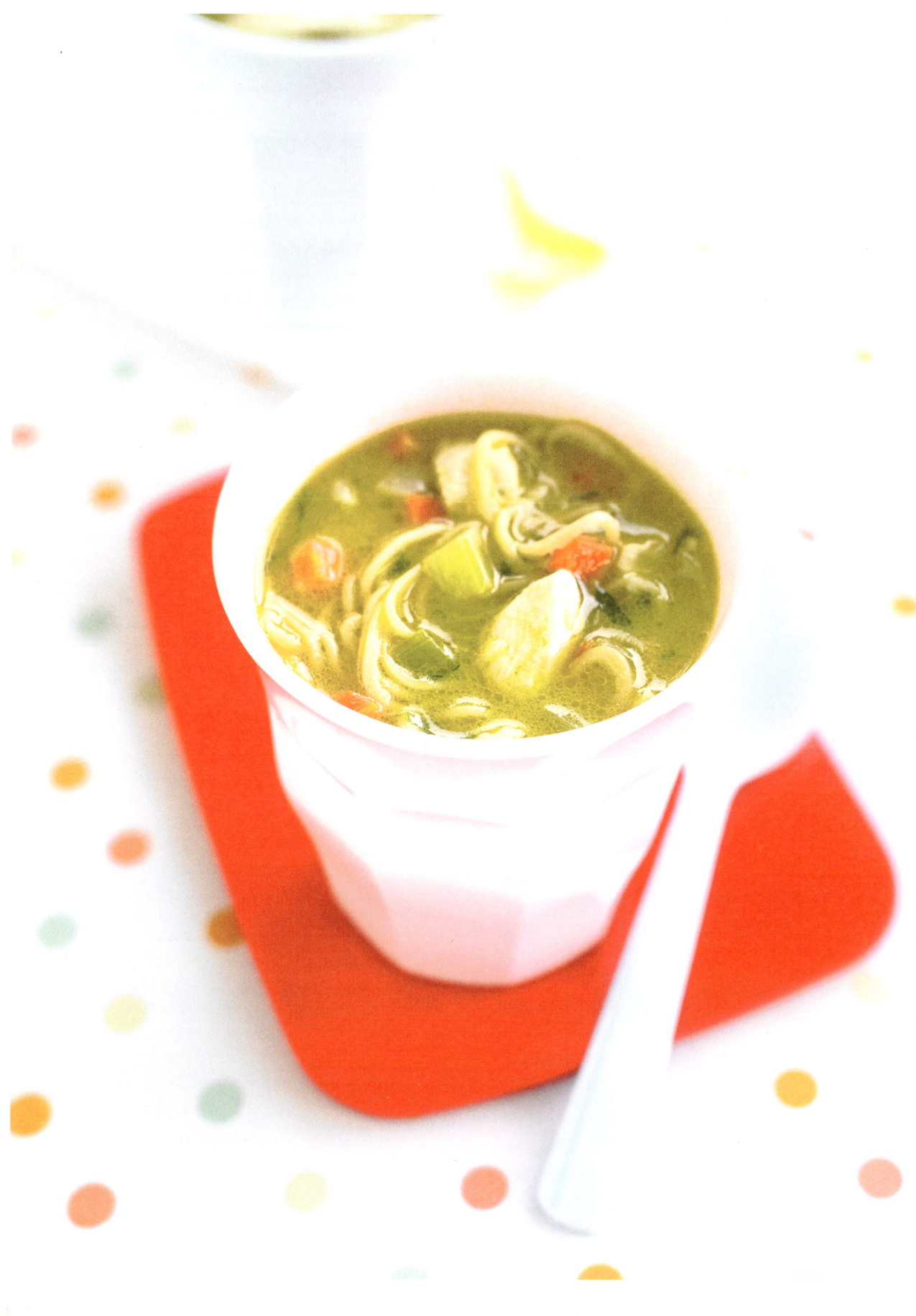

101 CHICKEN NOODLE SOUP

SERVES 4
PREPARATION
15 minutes
COOKING
35 minutes

STORAGE
Make in advance and keep in the fridge for up to 3 days or freeze in single portions (unless the chicken was frozen).

55g/2oz fine egg noodles
1 tbsp olive oil
1 onion, finely chopped
1 celery stalk, finely chopped
1 carrot, diced
1 bay leaf
200g/7oz skinless chicken breast, cut into bite-sized pieces
1.2l/40fl oz/5 cups chicken stock
2 tbsp reduced-fat crème fraîche
1 tbsp chopped flat-leaf parsley
salt and freshly ground black pepper

1. Cook the noodles following the package instructions until al dente; drain and rinse under cold water.

2. Put the oil in a large pan and add the onion. Half-cover the pan and sauté the onion for 7 minutes, stirring occasionally. Add the celery, carrot and bay leaf and sauté for another 3 minutes.

3. Add the chicken and sauté for 3–4 minutes, turning occasionally, until the chicken is golden all over.

4. Pour in the stock and bring to the boil, then reduce the heat and simmer for 20 minutes until the chicken is cooked. Stir in the crème fraîche and cooked noodles and warm through. Season and add the parsley, if using.

102 STEAMY SOUP

SERVES 4
PREPARATION
5 minutes
COOKING
20 minutes

STORAGE
You can refrigerate for up to 3 days or freeze for up to a month.

2 tbsp olive oil
600g/21oz chicken breast, roughly chopped
2 onions, peeled and diced
2 cloves garlic, peeled and crushed
2l/70fl oz/8½ cups water
8 tsp vegetable bouillon powder
750g/1lb 11oz canned sweetcorn

1. Heat the oil in a wok or large frying pan (skillet). Add the chicken and cook until lightly browned. Then add the onion and garlic and sauté for another 1–2 minutes.

2. Add the water, vegetable bouillon powder and sweetcorn, simmer for 10 minutes and then remove from heat and allow to cool for 5 minutes.

3. Pour the mixture into a blender and process until smooth. Return to the pan to reheat and serve.

103 TURKEY NOODLE SOUP

SERVES 4
PREPARATION
15 minutes
COOKING
15 minutes

STORAGE
Leftovers will keep in the fridge for up to 1 day.

150g/5½oz wholewheat noodles
750ml/26fl oz/3 cups turkey stock
1cm/½in fresh ginger, grated
1 clove garlic, crushed
1 tsp soft brown sugar
1 sachet instant miso soup powder
pinch of Chinese five-spice powder
2 tbsp tamari
100g/3½oz beansprouts
60g/2¼oz shiitake mushrooms, sliced
60g/2¼oz mangetout (snow peas), trimmed and sliced
150g/5½oz/1 cup sweetcorn
250g/9oz roast turkey, shredded
2 tbsp chopped coriander (cilantro)

1. Cook the noodles according to the package instructions. Set aside.

2. Pour the stock into a large pan. Add the ginger, garlic, sugar, miso soup, five-spice powder and tamari. Bring to the boil, then reduce the heat and simmer for 2 minutes.

3. Add the beansprouts, mushrooms, mangetout (snow peas), sweetcorn and turkey and simmer for 5 minutes.

4. Divide the noodles among four bowls. Ladle on the soup, sprinkle with the coriander (cilantro) leaves and serve.

104 PEA AND MINT SOUP WITH PANINIS

SERVES 4
PREPARATION
5 minutes
COOKING
20 minutes

STORAGE
You can refrigerate for up to 3 days or freeze for up to a month.

50g/2oz butter
12 spring onions (scallions), chopped
1.2l/40fl oz/5 cups water
560g/20oz/5 cups peas
50g/2oz/⅔ cup mint leaves
8 tsp vegetable bouillon powder
4 paninis
4 sprigs mint

1. Melt the butter in a medium saucepan over a low heat. Add the spring onions (scallions) and sauté for 30 seconds and then add the water, peas, mint and bouillon powder. Leave to simmer for 10 minutes.

2. Meanwhile, cut the paninis in half and toast lightly under a grill. Remove from the heat and leave to cool for 10 minutes.

3. Pour the soup into a blender and process until smooth. Pour into individual bowls, garnish each with a sprig of mint and serve with the toasted paninis on the side.

105 SMOKY BUTTER BEAN SOUP

SERVES 4
PREPARATION
10 minutes
COOKING
25 minutes

STORAGE
You can refrigerate for up to 3 days or freeze for up to a month.

2 leeks, sliced
4 tbsp olive oil
900g/2lb butter (lima) beans, cooked or canned
2l/70fl oz/8½ cups gluten-free veg stock
400g/14oz smoked haddock, skinned, boned and cubed
sea salt and black pepper to taste
2 tbsp fresh dill, finely chopped

(1) Gently stir-fry the leek in a saucepan with the oil until soft. Add the butter (lima) beans. Then mash the beans a little and stir-fry for a further 3–5 minutes. Pour in the stock and bring to the boil. Cover and simmer for 5 minutes. Add the smoked haddock and simmer for a further 10 minutes. Season, garnish with chopped fresh dill and serve with soft bread.

106 GREEN GIANT SOUP

SERVES 4
PREPARATION
10 minutes
COOKING
35 minutes

STORAGE
Make in advance and keep in the fridge for up to 3 days or freeze in single portions.

1 tbsp olive oil
1 large leek, finely chopped
1 celery stalk, thinly sliced
1 bay leaf
2 large sprigs mint (optional)
2 potatoes, peeled and cubed
1.2l/40fl oz/5 cups gluten-free veg stock
250g/9oz/heaped 2 cups frozen petits pois
120ml/4fl oz/½ cup milk (optional)

(1) Heat the oil in a large saucepan and fry the leek for 5 minutes until softened. Add the celery, bay leaf, mint, if using, and potatoes and cook, half-covered, for 3 minutes.

(2) Pour in the stock and bring to the boil. Reduce the heat, half-cover and simmer for 20 minutes. Add the peas and cook for another 5 minutes until the vegetables are tender.

(3) Purée in a blender or using a hand-held blender. Return to the pan and stir in the milk, if using, or more stock and heat through gently. Season to taste.

107 CHUNKY ITALIAN SOUP

SERVES 4–6
PREPARATION
15 minutes
COOKING
30 minutes

STORAGE
Make in advance and keep in the fridge for up to 3 days or freeze in single portions.

55g/2oz/½ cup small pasta shapes, such as conchigliette (small shells)
1 tbsp olive oil
1 onion, chopped
1 celery stalk, chopped
1 large carrot, diced
1 tsp dried oregano
2 bay leaves
1.2l/40fl oz/5 cups veg stock
100ml/3½fl oz/scant ½ cup passata (sieved tomatoes)
100g/3½oz/scant 1 cup canned chickpeas (garbanzo beans), drained and rinsed

1) Cook the pasta following the instructions on the package until al dente; drain and rinse under cold running water.

2) Meanwhile, put the oil in a large saucepan and add the onion. Half-cover the pan and sauté the onion for 7 minutes, stirring occasionally. Add the celery, carrot oregano and bay leaf and sauté for another 3 minutes.

3) Pour in the stock and passata (sieved tomatoes) and add the chickpeas. Bring to the boil, then reduce the heat and simmer, half-covered, for 15 minutes. Add the pasta, stir and cook for another 5 minutes.

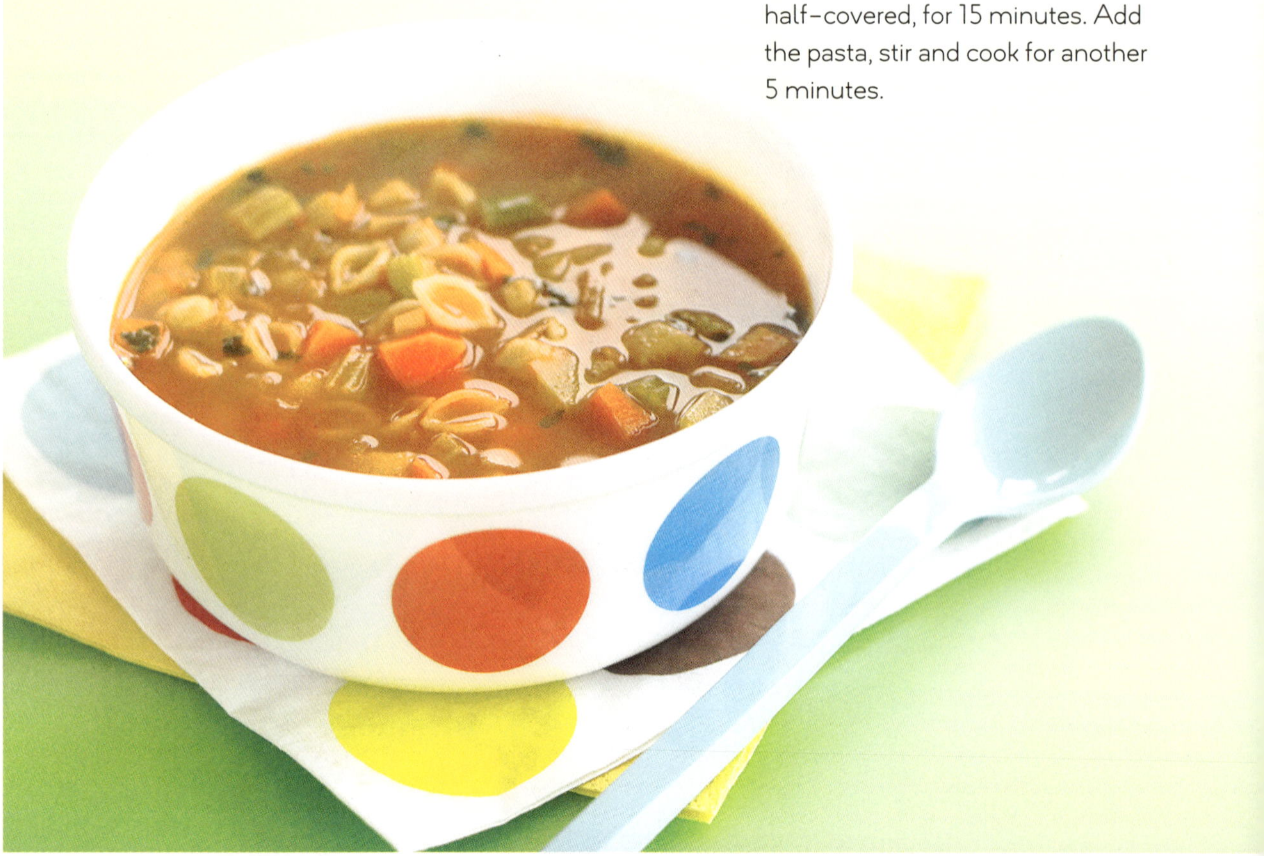

108 SPICY CARROT and LENTIL SOUP

SERVES 4
PREPARATION
15 minutes
COOKING
50 minutes

STORAGE
Make in advance and keep in the fridge for up to 3 days or freeze in single portions.

1 tbsp sunflower oil
1 large onion, chopped
1 celery stalk, finely chopped
4 carrots, thinly sliced
140g/5oz/⅔ cup split red lentils
1 tsp ground cumin
1 tbsp mild curry powder
1.2l/40fl oz/5 cups gluten-free vegetable stock
salt and freshly ground black pepper

1. Heat the oil in a large saucepan and fry the onion over a medium-low heat for 7 minutes, half-covered, until softened. Add the celery and carrots and cook for another 3 minutes. Rinse the lentils.

2. Stir in the spices and lentils and cook, stirring, for 1 minute, then pour in the stock. Bring to the boil then reduce the heat and simmer, half-covered, for 35 minutes until the lentils are very soft and mushy. Occasionally skim off any foam created by the lentils during cooking.

3. Purée in a blender or using a hand-held blender. Season to taste.

109 HALLOWE'EN SOUP

SERVES 4
PREPARATION
15 minutes
COOKING
30 minutes

STORAGE
Make in advance and keep in the fridge for up to 3 days or freeze in single portions.

1 tbsp olive oil
1 onion, chopped
1 carrot, chopped
1 celery stalk, chopped
350g/12oz peeled pumpkin or butternut squash, cut into chunks
1 bay leaf (optional)
1 tsp dried mixed herbs (optional)
2 sprigs rosemary
1 tbsp curry powder (optional)
1.2l/40fl oz/5 cups gluten-free vegetable stock
salt and freshly ground black pepper

1. Heat the oil in a large pan and fry the onion for 7 minutes, then add the carrot, celery and pumpkin or squash. Half-cover the pan and cook for another 3 minutes.

2. Add the herbs (and curry powder for a spicy soup) and stock. Bring to the boil, then reduce the heat and simmer, half-covered, for 20 minutes until the vegetables are tender.

3. Remove the bay leaf and rosemary. Purée in a blender. Season to taste.

110 MISO AND TOFU BROTH

SERVES 4
PREPARATION
10 minutes
COOKING
5 minutes

STORAGE
Make on the day.

200g/7oz fine egg noodles
4 sachets instant miso soup powder
2 carrots, cut into very thin strips
4 spring onions (scallions), cut into thin strips
4 tsp soy sauce
4 tsp toasted sesame seeds
3-cm/1-in piece fresh ginger, peeled and cut into thin strips
16 x 1-cm/$\frac{1}{2}$-in cubes soft tofu
sprinkling of nori flakes (optional)
pinch of dried chilli flakes (optional)

1. Cook the noodles following the package instructions; drain.

2. Rehydrate the instant miso soup powder sachets in a saucepan, following the package instructions.

3. Add the cooked noodles, carrots, spring onions (scallions), soy sauce, sesame seeds, ginger, tofu, nori flakes and chilli, if using, and heat through for 1 minute.

111 BEETROOT CREAM SOUP

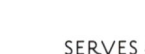

SERVES 4
PREPARATION
15 minutes
COOKING
55 minutes

STORAGE
Leftovers will keep in the fridge for up to 1 day or in the freezer for up to 1 month.

500g/1lb 2oz raw beetroot (beets), scrubbed
1 tbsp olive oil
1 onion, chopped
2 cloves garlic, chopped
2 celery stalks, chopped
3 carrots, chopped
750ml/26fl oz/3 cups veg stock
200g/7oz creamed coconut, chopped
2 tsp cider vinegar
freshly ground black pepper
4 tsp pumpkin seeds, to serve

1. Put the beetroot (beets) in a large saucepan. Cover with boiling water and bring back to the boil. Reduce the heat and simmer, covered, for 30–40 minutes until tender. Drain, then rub off the peel, holding the beetroot (beets) under cold water to avoid burning your fingers. Chop when cool.

2. Heat the oil in the rinsed-out pan. Add the onion, garlic, celery and carrots and cook for 1–2 minutes. Stir in the stock and coconut. Bring to the boil, reduce the heat and simmer for 10 minutes until the vegetables are tender. Add the beetroot (beets).

3. Purée the soup in a blender, then return it to the pan. Add the cider vinegar. Reheat gently for 2–3 minutes and add pepper to taste. Serve sprinkled with the pumpkin seeds.

112 TOMATO AND CHICKPEA SOUP

SERVES 4
PREPARATION
10 minutes
COOKING
20 minutes

STORAGE
Leftovers will keep in the fridge for up to 2 days or in the freezer for up to 3 months.

1 tbsp olive oil
1 red onion, chopped
1 clove garlic, crushed
pinch of cayenne pepper
pinch of ground allspice
¼ tsp ground cumin
400g/14oz canned chickpeas (garbanzo beans), drained and rinsed
350ml/12fl oz/scant 1½ cups passata (sieved tomatoes)
250ml/9fl oz/1 cup veg stock
4 sun-dried tomatoes in oil, drained and finely chopped
freshly ground black pepper
1 tbsp chopped parsley

1 Heat the oil in a saucepan. Add the onion and garlic, and cook for 2–3 minutes. Stir in the cayenne, allspice and cumin and cook gently for a further 3 minutes until the onion is softened.

2 Stir in the chickpeas (garbanzo beans), passata (sieved tomatoes), stock and sun-dried tomatoes. Bring to the boil, then reduce the heat and simmer for 10 minutes, or until the soup has thickened slightly.

3 Season the soup to taste with black pepper, stir in the parsley and serve.

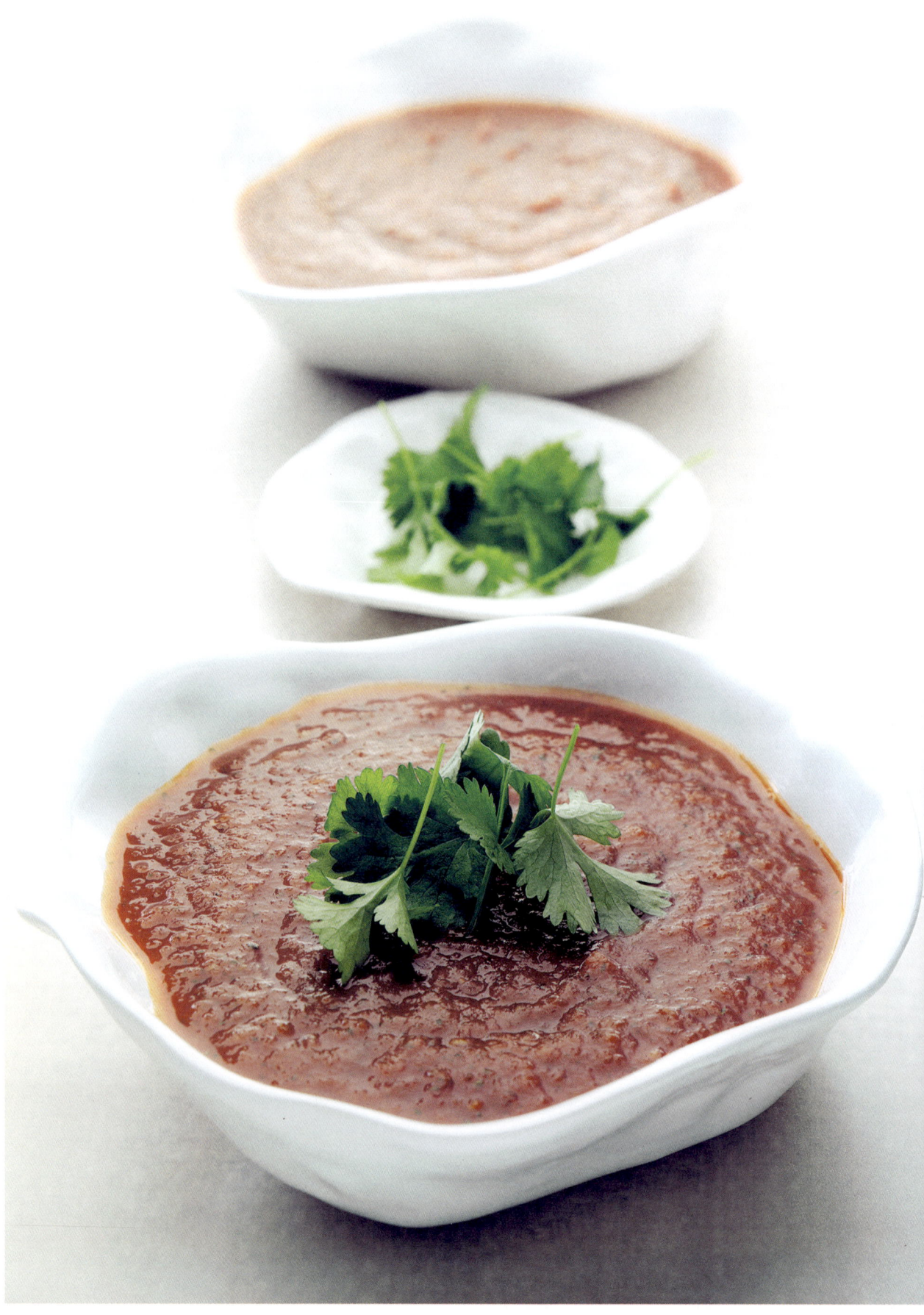

SOUPS, SALADS & SIDES | 91

113 TOMATO SOUP with FRESH CORIANDER

SERVES 4
PREPARATION
10 minutes
COOKING
20 minutes

STORAGE
Make in advance and keep in the fridge for up to 3 days or freeze in single portions.

1kg/2lb 3oz ripe tomatoes, quartered and stalks removed
2 red onions, chopped
2 cloves garlic, chopped
4 tbsp olive oil
500ml/17fl oz/2 cups veg stock
2 tsp raw cane sugar
large handful fresh coriander (cilantro) leaves, chopped
sea salt and black pepper to taste
4 tbsp tamari
2 tsp fresh ginger, finely chopped

1) Gently sauté the tomatoes, onion and garlic in a saucepan with the oil for approximately 10 minutes. Add the stock, sugar and half of the coriander (cilantro) leaves and season with a little salt and pepper. Bring to the boil, cover and gently simmer for 10 minutes.

2) Remove from the heat and blend in a blender, then add the tamari (wheat-free soy sauce) and ginger and heat through.

3) Check the seasoning and serve hot or cold, garnished with the remaining half of the coriander (cilantro) leaves.

114 SUMMER TOMATO SOUP

SERVES 4
PREPARATION
10 minutes
COOKING
5 minutes

STORAGE
Make in advance and keep in the fridge for up to 3 days or freeze in single portions.

1kg/2lb 3oz fresh ripe tomatoes, quartered
2 spring onions (scallions), finely chopped
1 large bunch fresh basil, finely chopped
sea salt and black pepper to taste

1) Blend the tomatoes in a food processor or blender, then gently heat them in a saucepan.

2) Add the spring onions (scallions) and the basil, and season. Serve hot or cold.

115 CREAMY TOMATO AND LENTIL SOUP

SERVES 4–6
PREPARATION
15 minutes
COOKING
35 minutes

STORAGE
Make in advance and keep in the fridge for up to 3 days or freeze in single portions.

85g/3oz/$\frac{1}{3}$ cup split red lentils
1 tbsp olive oil
1 large onion, chopped
1 carrot, chopped
400ml/14fl oz/1$\frac{2}{3}$ cups passata (sieved tomatoes)
900ml/1$\frac{1}{2}$ pints/3$\frac{3}{4}$ cups gluten-free veg stock
1 bay leaf
4 tbsp reduced-fat crème fraîche
salt and freshly ground black pepper

1 Rinse the lentils, put in a saucepan, cover with water and bring to the boil. Reduce the heat and simmer, half-covered, for 15 minutes until tender. Drain and set aside.

2 Meanwhile, heat the oil in a large saucepan. Add the onion and fry, half-covered, for 7 minutes, then add the carrot. Fry the vegetables, half-covered, for another 3 minutes, stirring occasionally.

3 Add the passata (sieved tomatoes), stock, cooked lentils and bay leaf. Bring to the boil, then reduce the heat and simmer, part-covered, for 20 minutes until the vegetables are tender.

4 Purée in a blender or using a hand-held blender. Stir in the crème fraîche, season to taste and heat through gently.

SOUPS, SALADS & SIDES | 93

116 SPRING GREENS BROTH

SERVES 2–4
PREPARATION
10 minutes
COOKING
20 minutes

STORAGE
You can refrigerate for up to 2 days or freeze for a month.

1 tbsp olive oil
8 spring onions (scallions), chopped
1 onion, peeled and sliced
2 cloves garlic, peeled and crushed
175g/6oz/$2/3$ cup cabbage greens, shredded
175g/6oz/$1 1/2$ cups spinach, chopped
55g/2oz/$1/3$ cup sunflower seeds
4 tsp green pesto
750ml/26fl oz/3 cups water
4 tsp vegetable bouillon powder
25g/1oz/$1/3$ cup chopped parsley

1. Heat the oil in a saucepan. Add the spring onions (scallions), onion and garlic and sauté for 2 minutes. Add the remaining ingredients (except the parsley), cover with a lid and simmer for 15 minutes.

2. Remove from the heat, place in a blender and process until smooth. Pour into individual bowls, garnish each with a sprinkle of parsley, and serve.

117 CARROT AND PARSNIP SOUP

SERVES 4
PREPARATION
10 minutes
COOKING
15 minutes

STORAGE
You can refrigerate for up to 3 days or freeze for a month.

1 tbsp olive oil
1 onion, peeled and diced
1 tsp coriander seeds
4 carrots, peeled and sliced
4 parsnips, peeled and sliced
1 tsp ground cinnamon
500ml/17fl oz/2 cups water
3 tsp vegetable bouillon powder
25g/1oz/$1/3$ cup chopped parsley

1. Heat the oil in a saucepan, add the onion and sauté until lightly browned.

2. Add the coriander seeds, carrots, parsnips, cinnamon, water, and bouillon powder. Simmer for 15 minutes or until the vegetables are soft.

3. Pour the soup into a blender and process until smooth. Divide into individual bowls and garnish each with a sprinkle of parsley.

118 CURRIED CARROT SOUP

SERVES 4
PREPARATION 10 minutes
COOKING 15 minutes

STORAGE You can refrigerate for up to 3 days or freeze for a month.

4 tbsp olive oil
4 cloves garlic, crushed
2 tsp curry powder
1 small green chilli, deseeded and chopped
2 potatoes, chopped
900g/2lb carrots, chopped
2 tsp finely chopped fresh root ginger
1.2l/42fl oz/5 cups veg stock
2 oranges, halved and squeezed
2 lemons, halved and squeezed
sea salt and black pepper to taste
sugar or maple syrup to taste (optional)

1. Gently heat the oil in a large casserole dish, add the garlic, curry powder and chilli and fry over a medium heat for 1 minute. Then add the chopped potato and the chopped carrots and stir-fry until they are well coated in the spices. Add the fresh ginger and stir-fry for a further minute before adding the stock. Bring to the boil, cover and simmer until the carrots are soft.

2. Remove from the heat, add the juice from the orange and the lemon, and season. Blend in a food processor or blender and check the seasoning (you may need to add a little sugar or maple syrup, depending on taste). Serve hot.

119 PUMPKIN SOUP

SERVES 2-4
PREPARATION 15 minutes + cooling
COOKING 20 minutes

STORAGE You can refrigerate for up to 3 days or freeze for up to a month.

2 tbsp olive oil
2 onions, peeled and diced
800g/1lb 12oz pumpkin
1.2l/40fl oz/5 cups water
8 tsp vegetable bouillon powder
2 tsp grated nutmeg
1 tsp ground cinnamon
1 tsp freshly ground black pepper

1. Heat the oil in a large saucepan, add the onion and pumpkin and sauté for 4 minutes, stirring occasionally. Add the water, bouillon powder, nutmeg and cinnamon.

2. Cover the pan and simmer for 10–15 minutes, until the pumpkin is soft. Remove from the heat and let cool for 10 minutes.

3. Pour into a blender and process until smooth. Serve in individual bowls and garnish with ground black pepper.

120 SWEET CHESTNUT SOUP

SERVES 2-4
PREPARATION
15 minutes
COOKING
25 minutes

STORAGE
You can refrigerate for up to 3 days or freeze for a month.

600g/21oz sweet chestnuts, peeled
2l/70fl oz/8½ cups water or stock
2 shallots, finely chopped
2 slices of celeriac (celery root), diced
4 tbsp olive oil
4 tbsp vegetable margarine or butter, diced
sea salt and black pepper to taste

1. Boil the sweet chestnuts in a saucepan with the water or stock for 5–10 minutes until they begin to disintegrate.

2. Meanwhile, gently sauté the shallot and the celeriac (celery root) with the oil in a frying pan (skillet) over a medium heat until they begin to brown. Add the shallots and the celeriac (celery root) to the pan with the chestnuts and cook for a further 10 minutes. Blend and season (adding a little more water or stock if necessary). Stir in the margarine or butter, check the seasoning and serve hot.

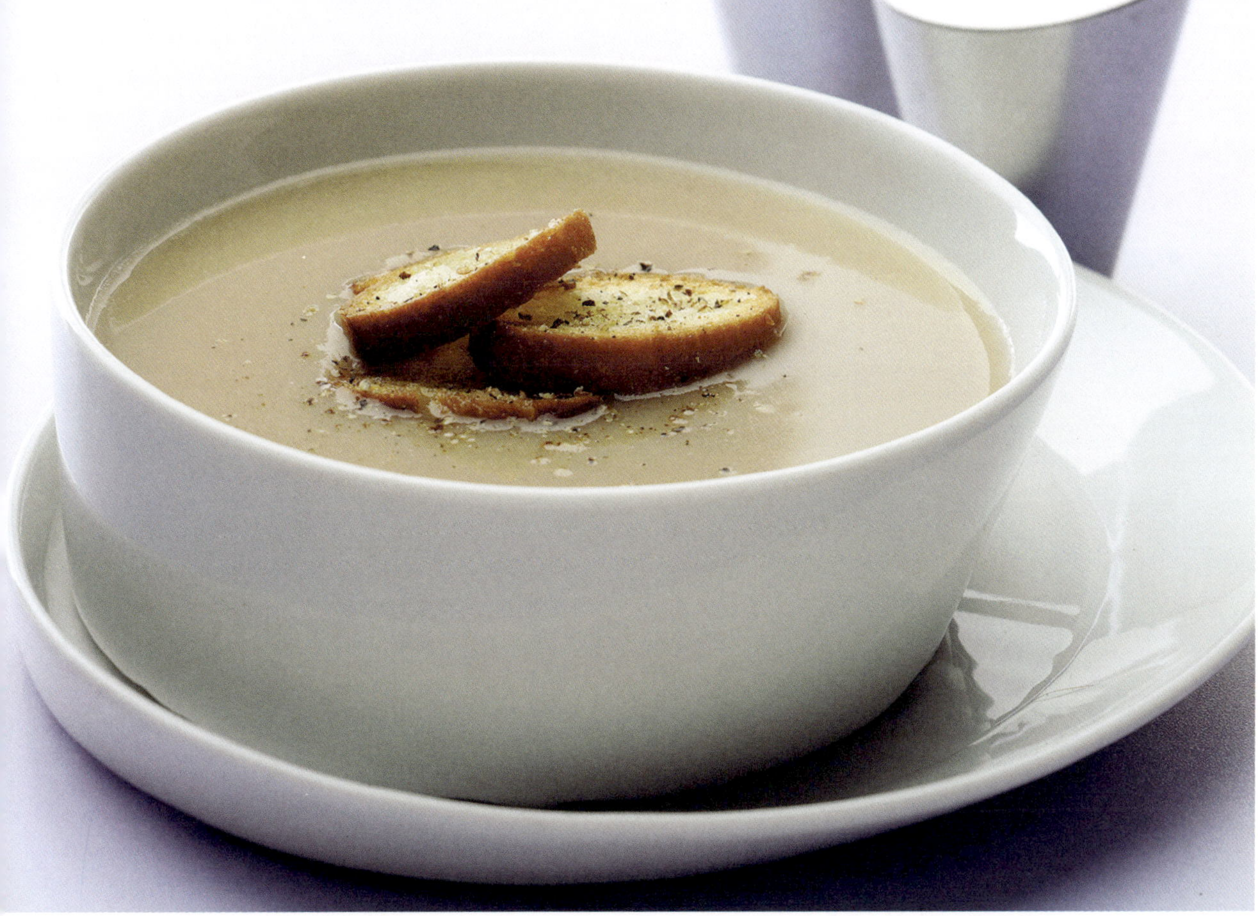

121 SPICY BEETROOT SOUP

SERVES 4
PREPARATION 15 minutes
COOKING 18 minutes
STORAGE You can refrigerate for up to 3 days or freeze for up to a month.

2 tbsp grapeseed oil
2 tsp ground cumin
1 cinnamon stick
1 tsp ground cloves
2 tsp freshly ground black pepper
500g/18oz raw beetroot (beets), diced
500g/18oz tomatoes, diced
1l/35fl oz/4¼ cups veg stock or water
sea salt to taste
100ml/3½fl oz/scant ½ cup crème fraîche or coconut cream

1. Heat the oil in a saucepan, add the spices and stir for 10 seconds. Add the beetroot (beets), stir for a further 30 seconds, then add the tomatoes. Stir-fry for 1 minute before adding the stock or water. Bring to the boil and simmer for 15 minutes, then season.

2. Take off the heat, remove the cinnamon stick, blend in a blender and add the crème fraîche or coconut cream. Serve with croutons or toast.

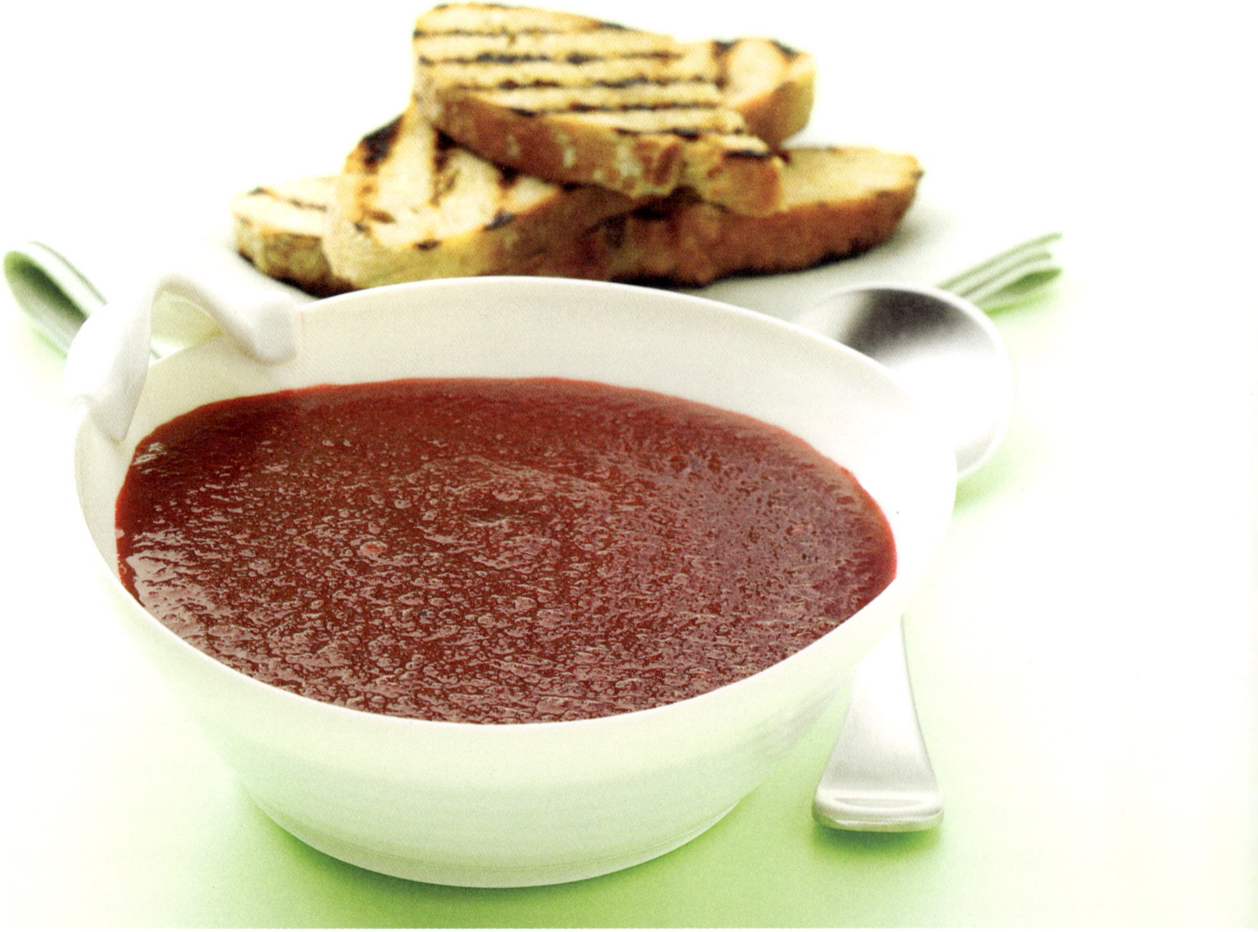

SOUPS, SALADS & SIDES | 97

122 BROCCOLI AND ALMOND SOUP

SERVES 4
PREPARATION
5 minutes
COOKING
20 minutes

STORAGE
You can refrigerate for up to 3 days or freeze and use within a month.

1 tbsp olive oil
1 onion, peeled and diced
1l/35fl oz/4¼ cups water
4 tsp vegetable bouillon powder
115g/4oz/¾ cup whole almonds
250g/9oz broccoli, cut into small florets

1) Heat the oil in a medium saucepan, add the onion and gently fry until golden. Add the water, bouillon powder, almonds and broccoli florets.

2) Simmer for 10 minutes and then remove from the heat and leave to cool for 5 minutes. Pour the mixture into a blender, give it a whiz and then serve in individual bowls.

123 SWEETCORN CHOWDER

SERVES 2
PREPARATION
10 minutes
COOKING
35 minutes

STORAGE
Make in advance and keep in the fridge for up to 3 days or freeze in single portions.

1 tbsp sunflower oil
1 large onion, chopped
1 carrot, chopped
2 potatoes, peeled and cubed
3-4 sweetcorn cobs, corn sliced off or 400-g/14-oz can sweetcorn, drained
1 bay leaf
900ml/32fl oz/3¾ cups gluten-free veg stock
300ml/10fl oz/1¼ cups milk
salt and freshly ground black pepper

1) Heat the oil in a large saucepan and fry the onion for 7 minutes, half-covered, until softened. Add the carrot, potatoes, fresh corn (if using) and bay leaf and cook, half-covered, for another 3 minutes.

2) Pour in the stock, bring to the boil, reduce the heat and simmer for 10 minutes. Add the canned sweetcorn (if using) and simmer for a further 15 minutes, stirring occasionally.

3) Pour in the milk, gently heat through, then season to taste. Serve chunky, semi-chunky or smooth, as preferred.

124 SWEET POTATO AND PUMPKIN SOUP

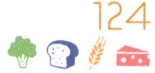

SERVES 2-4
PREPARATION
15 minutes
COOKING
20 minutes

STORAGE
Make in advance and keep in the fridge for up to 3 days or freeze in single portions.

4 tbsp olive oil
1 red onion, chopped
600g/21oz pumpkin, peeled, deseeded and chopped
2 small sweet potatoes, peeled and chopped
1.7l/60fl oz/7½ cups veg stock
400ml/14fl oz/1⅔ cups coconut milk
sea salt and black pepper to taste
2 tbsp fresh coriander (cilantro) leaves, chopped

1. Heat the oil in a saucepan and gently stir-fry the onion, pumpkin and sweet potato for 3 minutes. Add the stock and the coconut milk, and season. Bring to the boil, cover and simmer for 15 minutes.

2. Check the seasoning and garnish with fresh coriander (cilantro). Serve with corn bread.

125 MINESTRONE

SERVES 2-4
PREPARATION
15 minutes
COOKING
20 minutes

STORAGE
Make in advance and keep in the fridge for up to 3 days or freeze in single portions.

4 tbsp olive oil
2 small onions, chopped
2 carrots, chopped
½ fennel bulb or 2 celery stalks, chopped
2 courgettes (zucchini), chopped
2 handfuls white cabbage, finely shredded
500g/18oz ripe tomatoes, blended
1l/35fl oz/4¼ cups veg stock
sea salt and black pepper to taste
4 tbsp small pasta shapes
100g/3½oz white beans, cooked or canned
1 large bunch parsley and basil, finely chopped
2 cloves garlic, crushed
a little Parmesan (optional)

1. Heat the oil in a large heavy saucepan and gently stir-fry the onion, carrot, fennel, courgette (zucchini) and cabbage (don't let them brown). Add the tomatoes and stock, and season. Bring to the boil, add the pasta, cover and simmer for 10 minutes.

2. Add the beans, parsley, basil and garlic. Heat through, check the seasoning, sprinkle with Parmesan (if using) and serve.

126 PASTA AND SUN-DRIED TOMATO SOUP

SERVES 2
PREPARATION
10 minutes
COOKING
15 minutes

STORAGE
Make in advance and keep in the fridge for up to 3 days or freeze in single portions.

2l/70fl oz/8½ cups veg stock
2 handfuls pasta shapes
2 handfuls sun-dried tomatoes, finely chopped
2 spring onions (scallions), finely chopped
2 small courgettes (zucchini), finely chopped
8–10 mushrooms, sliced
2 tbsp parsley, finely chopped
2 tbsp fresh basil, finely chopped
sea salt and black pepper to taste
1 lemon, sliced

1. Bring the stock to the boil in a saucepan with the pasta and the rest of the ingredients (except for the lemon). Simmer for 10–15 minutes, until the pasta is cooked.

2. Garnish with slices of lemon and serve with thick slices of bread.

127 MEXICAN AVOCADO SOUP

SERVES 4
PREPARATION
10 minutes
COOKING
15 minutes

STORAGE
Make in advance and keep in the fridge for up to 3 days or freeze in single portions.

2 onions, finely chopped
4 tbsp corn oil
2 tbsp wheat flour
2l/70fl oz/8½ cups veg stock
2 large avocados, peeled, pitted and mashed
¼ tsp cayenne pepper
200ml/7fl oz/scant 1 cup almond milk or single (light) cream
sea salt to taste
1 yellow (bell) pepper, finely chopped
1 red (bell) pepper, finely chopped
2 tsp paprika

1. Gently fry the onion in a heavy saucepan with the oil. Sprinkle with the flour and stir-fry until the onion is well coated. Continue to stir, and slowly add the stock. Bring to the boil, add the avocado and the cayenne pepper and gently simmer for 5 minutes.

2. Stir in the almond milk or cream, season with salt and serve garnished with red and yellow (bell) pepper and paprika.

128 SOUPE AU PISTOU

SERVES 2
PREPARATION
15 minutes
COOKING
25 minutes

STORAGE
Make in advance and keep in the fridge for up to 3 days or freeze in single portions.

SOUP
olive oil for frying
2 small leeks, sliced
2 onions, halved and sliced
2 cloves garlic, chopped
6 tomatoes, peeled and chopped
2l/70fl oz/8½ cups veg stock
1 large handful green beans, chopped
2 small celery stalks, sliced
2 potatoes, diced
200g/7oz white beans, cooked or canned
4 tbsp small macaroni pasta
sea salt and black pepper to taste

PISTOU
2 handfuls fresh basil leaves, chopped
5 cloves garlic
a little olive oil
Parmesan to taste
a little sea salt

1) Heat a little oil in a heavy saucepan and gently fry the leek, onion and garlic until soft. Add the tomatoes and cook for 5 minutes. Pour in the stock and bring to the boil. Add the remaining soup ingredients (except for the macaroni) and simmer until the vegetables are cooked.

2) Add the macaroni, bring to the boil and cook until the macaroni is soft, then season.

3) Meanwhile, prepare the pistou by placing the basil and the garlic in a mortar with the oil, Parmesan and salt. Mash to a thick paste and add to the soup just before serving.

129 GAZPACHO DEL CAMPO

SERVES 4
PREPARATION 10 minutes
COOKING 10 minutes
STORAGE Make in advance and keep in the fridge for up to 3 days or freeze in single portions.

1 cucumber
500g/18oz tomatoes
2 small red onions
1 green (bell) pepper
2 cloves garlic
6 tbsp olive oil
2 tbsp lemon juice
4 tbsp red wine vinegar
sea salt and black pepper to taste
1 large handful fresh dill, finely chopped

① Finely chop a quarter of each of the vegetables and set aside.

② In a food processor or blender, blend the remaining vegetables with the garlic, oil, lemon juice and vinegar to a thick, smooth consistency. Season and chill well.

③ Garnish with the finely chopped vegetables and fresh dill. Serve with a few ice cubes in each bowl, and croutons.

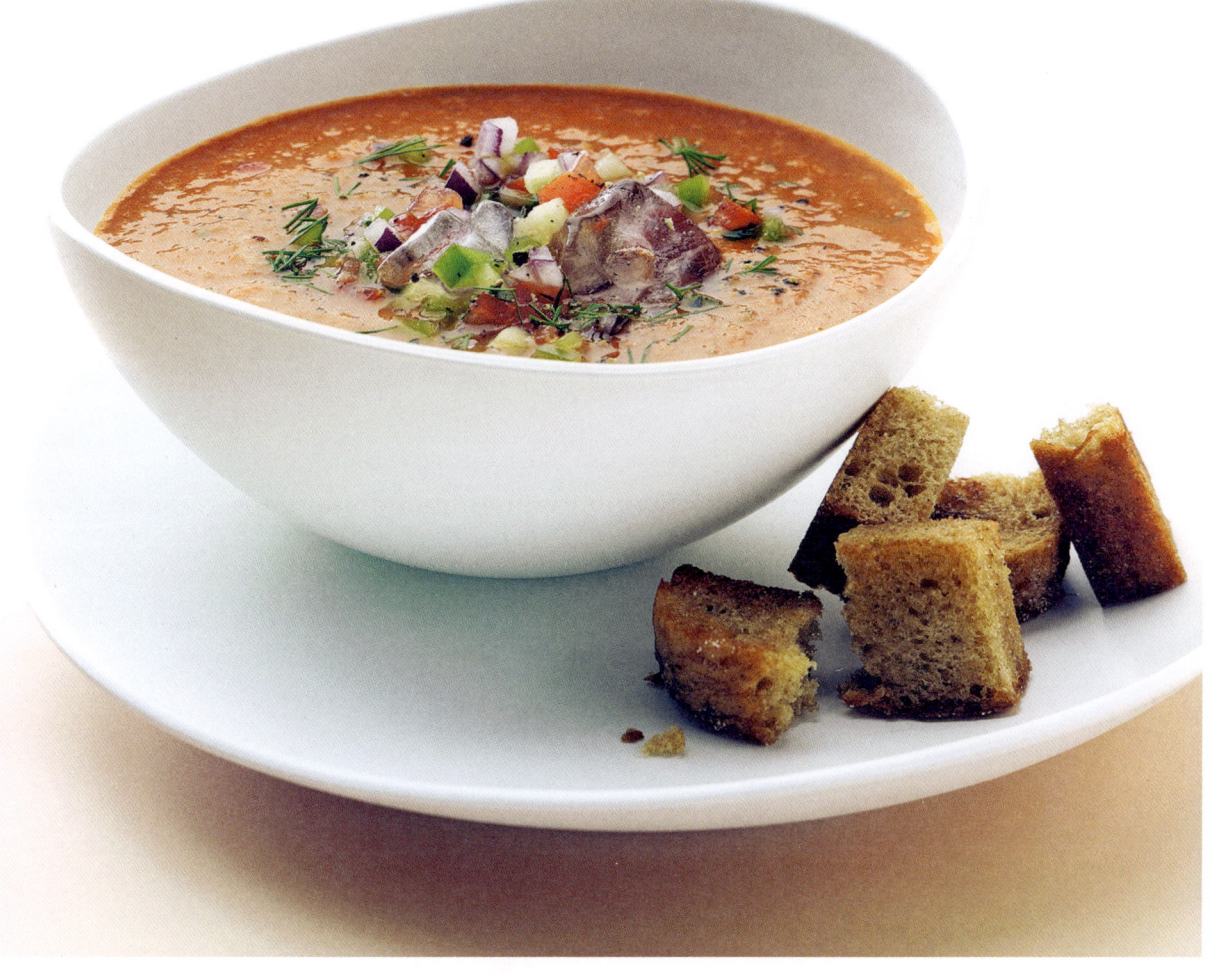

130 JAPANESE SPINACH SOUP

SERVES 4
PREPARATION
10 minutes
COOKING
15–20 minutes

STORAGE
Make in advance and keep in the fridge for up to 3 days or freeze in single portions.

2 tbsp grapeseed oil
2 shallots, sliced
2 small carrots, finely chopped
250g/9oz tofu, diced
8 medium mushrooms, sliced
200g/7oz spinach, chopped into strips
4 tsp tamari
10-cm/4-in strip kombu seaweed
½ tsp raw cane sugar
2 tsp mirin (Japanese rice wine) or dry sherry (optional)
2l/70fl oz/8½ cups water
sea salt and black pepper to taste
1 tsp sesame oil
2 tsp lemon juice
lemon peel, cut into strips to garnish

1. Heat the grapeseed oil in a saucepan, add the shallots, carrots and tofu cubes and stir-fry for 1 minute. Add the mushrooms and stir for a further minute, then add the spinach and continue to stir over a medium heat until the spinach is wilted.

2. Add the remaining ingredients (except for the sesame oil, lemon juice and lemon peel). Bring to the boil and simmer for 10 minutes. Finally, add the sesame oil and lemon juice. Check the seasoning and serve garnished with strips of lemon peel.

131 LEEK AND POTATO SOUP

SERVES 4
PREPARATION
10 minutes
COOKING
20 minutes

STORAGE
Make in advance and keep in the fridge for up to 3 days or freeze in single portions.

4 tbsp olive oil
4 leeks, sliced
4 potatoes, diced
2l/70fl oz/8½ cups veg stock
sea salt and black pepper to taste

1. Gently heat the oil in a saucepan, add the leeks and the potatoes and sauté for 3 minutes, then add the stock. Heat through and simmer for 15 minutes.

2. Season and serve with croutons.

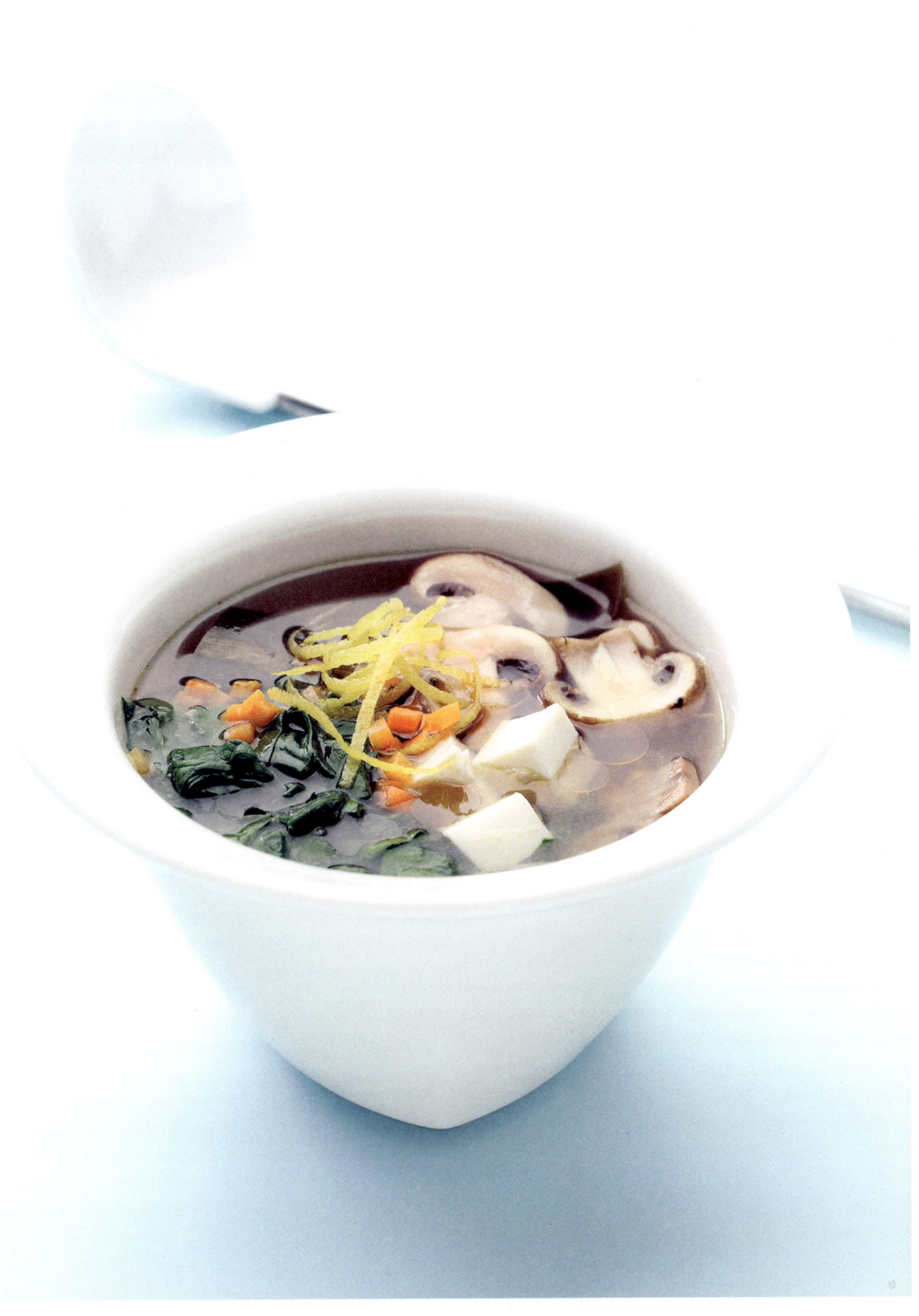

132 CHINESE SOUP with SHIITAKE & NOODLES

SERVES 4
PREPARATION
5 minutes
COOKING
6–10 minutes

STORAGE
Make in advance and keep in the fridge for up to 3 days or freeze in single portions.

4 tbsp olive oil
2 spring onions (scallions), chopped
250g/9oz tofu
200g/7oz shiitake mushrooms, sliced
10 pieces bamboo shoots, cut into squares
2 small carrots, sliced into sticks
2l/70fl oz/8½ cups veg stock
4 tbsp tamari
4 tbsp dry sherry
¼ tsp Chinese five-spice powder
1 large bunch watercress, chopped
2 tsp sesame oil
1 large handful noodles

1. Gently heat the oil in a heavy saucepan and stir-fry the spring onions (scallions) for 30 seconds. Add the tofu, shiitake, bamboo shoots and carrot and stir-fry for 2 minutes before adding the stock, tamari, sherry, five-spice powder and watercress. Bring to the boil. Add the oil and noodles. Cover, remove from the heat and leave for 2 minutes until the noodles are cooked, and serve.

133 CHINESE CORN SOUP

SERVES 4
PREPARATION
10 minutes
COOKING
15 minutes

STORAGE
Make in advance and keep in the fridge for up to 3 days or freeze in single portions.

2 tsp fresh ginger, finely chopped
4 tsp tamari
4 tsp dry sherry
1.5l/52fl oz/6½ cups veg stock
300g/10½oz sweetcorn
1 cinnamon stick
2 tsp cornflour (cornstarch) dissolved in a little cold water
2 tsp almond butter
2 eggs, beaten (optional)
sea salt and black pepper to taste
1 large bunch chives, finely chopped

1. Marinate the ginger in the tamari and sherry in a bowl.

2. Bring the stock to the boil in a heavy saucepan, add the sweetcorn, cinnamon, marinated ginger and a little salt. Simmer for 10 minutes. Slowly add the dissolved cornflour (constarch) and the almond butter while stirring continuously. Then add the egg (if using), season, heat through and serve garnished with chives.

134 AUTUMN VEGETABLE SOUP

SERVES 4
PREPARATION
15 minutes
COOKING
10–15 minutes

STORAGE
Make in advance and keep in the fridge for up to 3 days or freeze in single portions.

2l/70fl oz/8½ cups gluten-free veg stock
2 leeks, sliced
2 slices celeriac (celery root), diced
2 carrots, sliced
2 potatoes, diced
2 slices pumpkin, diced
6 tomatoes, blended
200g/7oz green beans, chopped
2 cloves garlic, crushed
4 tbsp olive oil
sea salt and black pepper to taste
4 tbsp fresh parsley, chopped

1. Bring the stock to the boil in a large heavy saucepan with the leek, celeriac (celery root), carrot, potato and pumpkin and simmer for 5 minutes. Then add the tomatoes, together with the green beans, garlic and oil, and season. Cook for a further 5–10 minutes.

2. Add the chopped parsley, check the seasoning and serve with wholemeal (whole wheat) bread.

135 CREAMY PARSNIP SOUP

SERVES 4
PREPARATION
15 minutes
COOKING
15 minutes

STORAGE
Make in advance and keep in the fridge for up to 3 days or freeze in single portions.

4 tbsp olive oil
4 tsp mustard powder
1kg/2lb 3oz parsnips, chopped
2 cooking apples, peeled, cored and chopped
2l/70fl oz/8½ cups veg stock
2 tbsp tamari
2 tsp thyme
sea salt and black pepper to taste
200ml/7fl oz/scant 1 cup plain or soya yogurt

1. Gently heat the oil in a large saucepan. Stir in the mustard powder and let it dissolve. Add the parsnips and the apple and stir-fry for a few minutes, then add the stock and bring to the boil. Cover and simmer for 10 minutes. Add the tamari and the thyme, and season.

2. In a food processor or blender, blend the soup to a rich, creamy texture, check the seasoning and serve with a spoonful of plain or soya yogurt in each bowl.

136 PEACH AND PROSCIUTTO SALAD

SERVES 2-4

PREPARATION
10 minutes

COOKING
6 minutes

STORAGE
You can store the salad for up to 24 hours in the fridge.

- 12 slices prosciutto (Parma ham)
- 4 peaches with skins, cut into three, stone removed
- 225g/8oz/1 cup mangetout (snow peas), chopped
- 225g/8oz/2 cups baby spinach, chopped
- 1 red onion, peeled and sliced
- 115g/4oz/1 cup cherry or baby plum tomatoes, cut in half
- ½ cucumber, grated
- 3 tbsp olive oil
- 1 tbsp balsamic vinegar
- 4 sprigs mint

1. Preheat the grill (broiler) to medium. Wrap a slice of prosciutto (Parma ham) around each peach piece. Bake under the grill (broiler) for 3–6 minutes until lightly browned.

2. Meanwhile, place the mangetout (snow peas) and spinach in a salad bowl. Add the red onion, tomatoes and cucumber, and stir together well, adding the olive oil and balsamic vinegar.

3. Divide the salad equally between four plates. Place three of the peach and prosciutto (Parma ham) wraps on top of each salad and garnish with a sprig of mint.

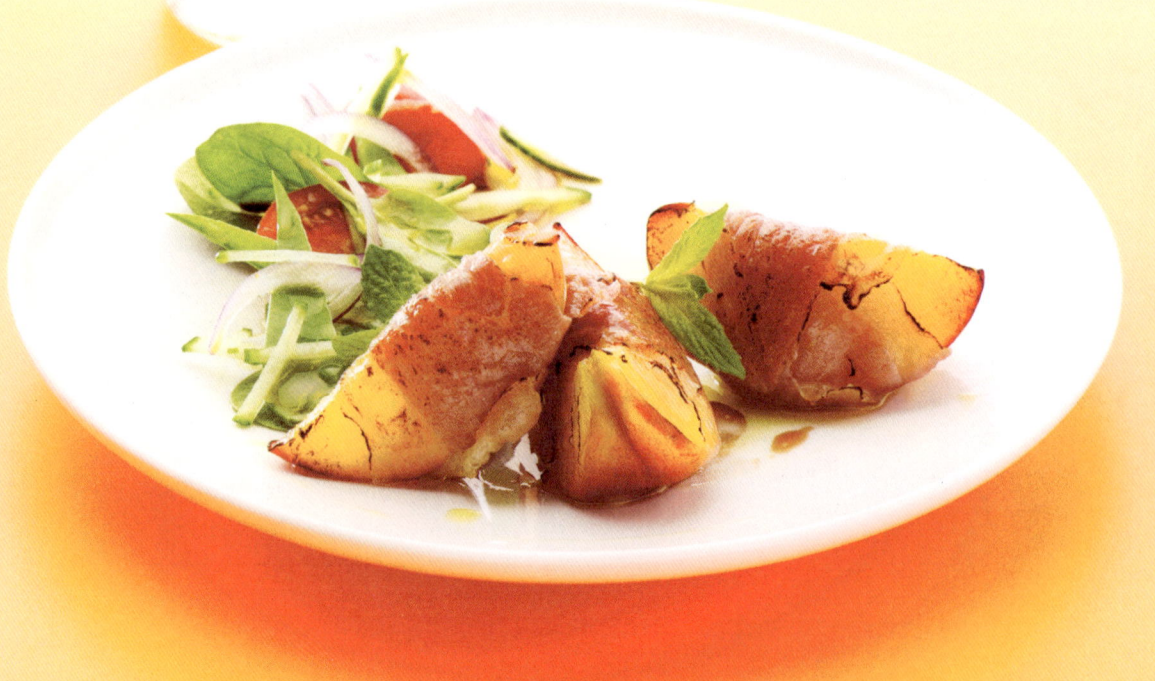

137 HAM, BEAN AND PINEAPPLE SALAD

SERVES 2–4
PREPARATION
10 minutes

STORAGE
Make in advance and keep in the fridge for up to 3 days. Keep chilled until ready to eat.

350g/12oz canned pineapple, cut into chunks
300g/10½oz thickly cut good-quality ham, cubed
200g/7oz canned cannellini beans, drained and rinsed

DRESSING
2 tbsp natural juice from the canned pineapple
3 tbsp extra-virgin olive oil
4 tsp white wine vinegar
1 tsp Dijon mustard

1) Mix together the ingredients for the dressing.

2) Put the pineapple, ham and beans in a bowl, then pour the dressing over the top. Toss the salad well to coat it thoroughly in the dressing.

138 SCANDINAVIAN POTATO AND SAUSAGE SALAD

SERVES 4
PREPARATION
10 minutes
COOKING
10 minutes

STORAGE
Make in advance and keep in the fridge for up to 3 days. Keep chilled until ready to eat.

olive oil, for stir-frying
2 red onions, halved and sliced
400g/14oz spicy sausages, sliced
2 small courgettes (zucchini), finely sliced
2 tsp fresh thyme
2 tsp Dijon mustard
4 tsp plain (all-purpose) flour
6 tbsp red wine vinegar
2 tsp maple syrup
sea salt and black pepper to taste
1 large handful lettuce leaves
500g/18oz new potatoes, halved and boiled
16 grape tomatoes, halved
20 gherkins

1) Gently heat 3 tablespoons of oil in a frying pan (skillet). Add the onion and the sausages and stir-fry for 3 minutes, then add the courgette (zucchini) and stir-fry for a further 2 minutes. Mix in the thyme, mustard and flour and cook over a low heat for 1 minute. Add the vinegar, maple syrup and a little more oil, and continue to stir while the mixture thickens. Season and turn off the heat.

2) Arrange the lettuce leaves on serving plates and top with the halved potatoes and the sausage mixture. Garnish with grape tomatoes and gherkins, and serve immediately.

139 SAUSAGE AND BARLEY SALAD

SERVES 4
PREPARATION
15 minutes + 6 hours soaking
COOKING
20 minutes

STORAGE
Make in advance and keep in the fridge for up to 3 days or freeze for up to 1 month. Keep chilled until ready to eat.

100g/3½oz/heaped ½ cup pearl barley
6 good-quality sausages, or vegetarian alternative
2 tbsp olive oil
2 cloves garlic, finely chopped
1 tsp dried oregano
4 tbsp canned tomatoes
salt and freshly ground black pepper

1. Soak the barley for 6 hours or overnight; drain and rinse.

2. Preheat the grill (broiler) to medium and line the grill pan with foil. Grill (broil) the sausages, turning them occasionally, for 20 minutes until cooked through and browned. Leave to cool.

3. Meanwhile, heat the oil in a frying pan (skillet) and fry the garlic for 1 minute, stirring. Add the oregano, tomatoes and barley and cook for 10 minutes, stirring occasionally. Remove from the heat and leave to cool.

4. Slice the sausages and stir into the barley mixture.

140 QUICK AND EASY BEAN AND HAM SALAD

SERVES 4
PREPARATION
10 minutes
COOKING
3 minutes

STORAGE
Leftovers will keep in the fridge for up to 4 days.

3 tbsp olive oil
2 spring onions (scallions), chopped
2 cloves garlic, crushed
½ red chilli, deseeded and chopped
2 tomatoes, deseeded and chopped
400g/14oz canned cannellini beans, drained and rinsed
400g/14oz canned butter (lima) beans, drained and rinsed
2 tbsp flaxseed oil
2 tbsp lemon juice
3 tbsp chopped parsley leaves
75g/2½oz lean ham, cut into slivers

1. Heat 1 tbsp of the olive oil in a frying pan (skillet) and sauté the spring onions (scallions), garlic and chilli for 1 minute until soft. Toss in the tomatoes and beans and warm through for 2 minutes, then transfer to a bowl.

2. Whisk together the remaining olive oil, flaxseed oil, lemon juice and parsley. Toss through the salad, scatter the ham on top and serve.

141 CHICKEN CAESER SALAD

SERVES 4
PREPARATION
15 minutes
COOKING
12 minutes

STORAGE
Make the day before and keep in the fridge overnight. Assemble on the day. Keep chilled until ready to eat. The dressing will keep in the fridge for up to 1 week.

500g/18oz new potatoes
4 tsp olive oil
300g/10½oz chicken breast, cut into large bite-sized pieces
4 Cos lettuce leaves, shredded
4 tomatoes, seeded and diced

DRESSING
3 tbsp mayonnaise
3 tbsp extra-virgin olive oil
4 tsp lemon juice
2 small cloves garlic, crushed
1 tsp Dijon mustard
½ tsp gluten-free Worcestershire sauce
4 tbsp finely grated Parmesan

1. Cook the potatoes in boiling water for about 12 minutes, until tender; drain and set aside to cool.

2. Meanwhile, heat the olive oil in a frying pan (skillet) and fry the chicken for 5–6 minutes, turning occasionally, until golden and cooked through. Leave to cool.

3. Put the dressing ingredients in a blender and process until smooth and creamy.

4. Put the Cos lettuce in a bowl and add the potatoes, tomatoes and chicken. Spoon over enough of the dressing to coat the salad.

142 THAI CHICKEN SALAD

SERVES 4
PREPARATION
15 minutes

STORAGE
Leftovers will keep in the fridge for up to 1 day.

2 cooked chicken breasts, shredded
1 carrot, cut into julienne
1 red (bell) pepper, sliced
¼ small white cabbage, shredded
3 spring onions (scallions), finely chopped
4 shiitake mushrooms, sliced
50g/1¾oz beansprouts
2 tbsp chopped mint
2 tbsp fresh coriander (cilantro)

DRESSING
2 tsp fish sauce
2 tbsp lime juice

2 tbsp honey or agave nectar
2 tsp tamari
1 tbsp omega oil or flaxseed oil

1. Layer the chicken, carrot, (bell) pepper, cabbage, spring onions (scallions), mushrooms and beansprouts in a large bowl. Sprinkle with the mint and coriander (cilantro).

2. Whisk the dressing ingredients in a small bowl, then pour over the salad. Toss lightly and serve.

143 SALMON, MANGO AND ASPARAGUS SALAD

SERVES 4
PREPARATION
10 minutes
COOKING
10 minutes

STORAGE
Best eaten immediately. Leftovers will keep in the fridge for up to 1 day.

600g/21oz salmon fillet, flaked
2 tbsp olive oil
400g/14oz asparagus spears, trimmed and chopped
4 handfuls lamb's lettuce
1 fennel bulb, sliced
2 mangoes, peeled and cubed
2 spring onions (scallions), finely chopped
200ml/7fl oz plain or soya yogurt
2 tsp Dijon mustard
sea salt and black pepper to taste

1. Stir-fry the salmon in a frying pan (skillet) with the oil for 2–3 minutes, until it begins to brown.

2. Blanch the asparagus in a pan of boiling water with a little salt for 2–3 minutes, drain and set aside.

3. Divide the lamb's lettuce between serving plates. Add the fried salmon, asparagus, fennel, mango and spring onion (scallion).

4. To make the dressing, place the yogurt in a small bowl, add the mustard and salt and pepper. Mix well and pour over the salads.

144 PRAWN PASTA SALAD

SERVES 4
PREPARATION
10 minutes
COOKING
12 minutes

STORAGE
Make in advance and keep in the fridge for up to 2 days. Assemble on the day. Keep chilled until ready to eat.

200g/7oz/2 cups pasta shells
230g/8oz cooked peeled small prawns (shrimp), defrosted if frozen
12 cherry tomatoes, quartered
crisp lettuce leaves, such as Cos, shredded

DRESSING
2 tbsp mayonnaise
2 tsp lemon juice
2 tbsp tomato ketchup
4 drops Tabasco (optional)
salt and freshly ground black pepper

1. Bring a large saucepan of salted water to the boil. Add the pasta, stir and cook following the package instructions until al dente. Drain well and refresh under cold water.

2. Put the prawns (shrimp) and tomatoes in a bowl with the pasta and season with pepper.

3. Mix the dressing ingredients together and spoon over the salad. Turn the salad with a spoon to coat it well.

4. Serve the salad on a bed of shredded lettuce.

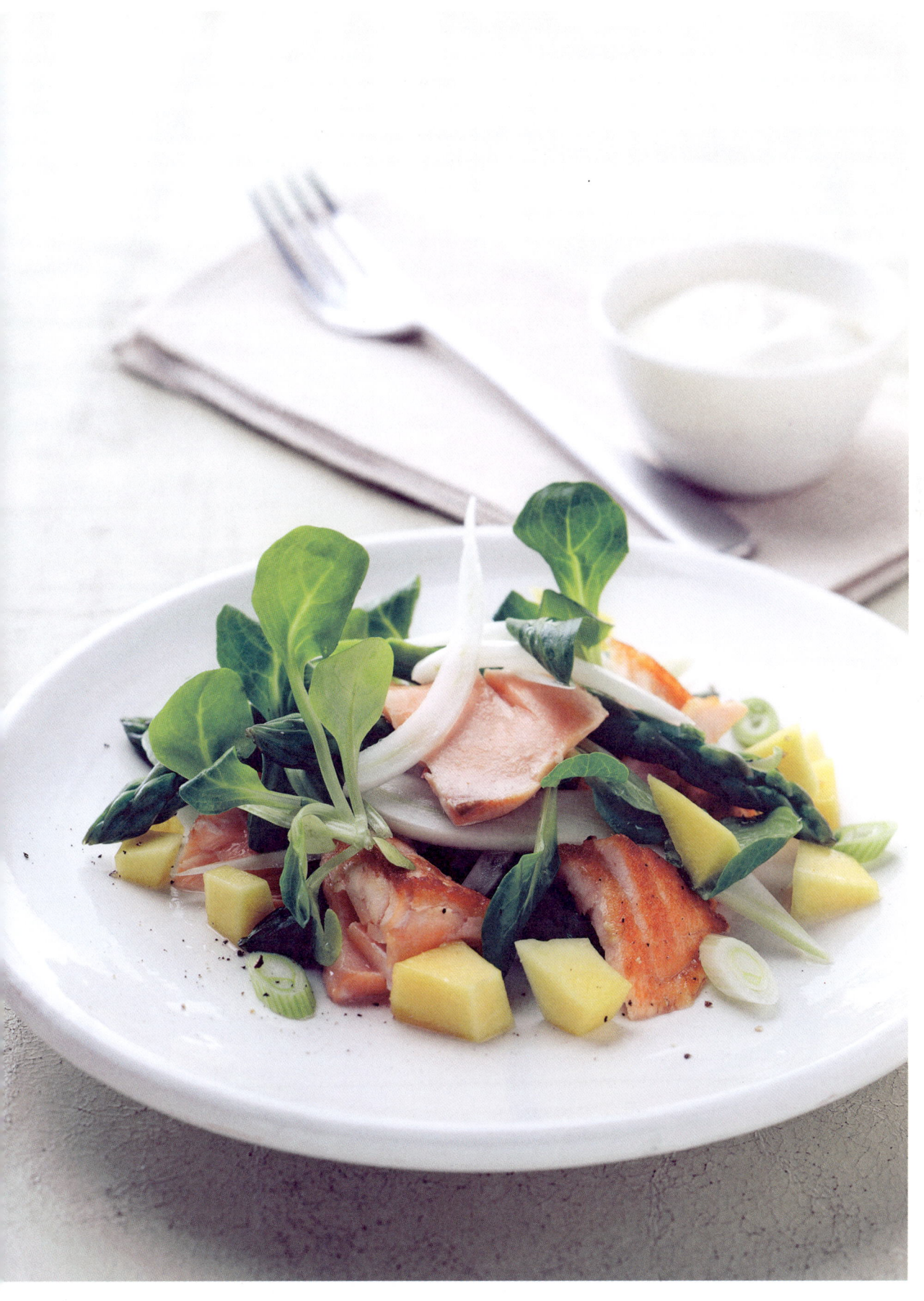

145 SALMON NIÇOISE SALAD

SERVES 4
PREPARATION 15 minutes
COOKING 25 minutes

STORAGE
Leftovers will keep in the fridge for up to 1 day.

6 new potatoes
75g/2½oz green beans
2 Little Gem lettuces, leaves separated
150g/5½oz cherry tomatoes, halved
16 pitted black olives, halved
6 anchovy fillets, chopped
3 tsp olive oil
4 salmon fillets, about 100g/3½oz each
1 avocado
2 tsp lime juice
4 hard-boiled eggs, quartered

DRESSING
1 tsp Dijon mustard
2 tbsp red wine vinegar
pinch of sugar
6 tbsp omega oil or flaxseed oil

1. Boil the new potatoes for 15 minutes until tender. Drain and halve. Meanwhile, cook the green beans in boiling water for 3–4 minutes until beginning to soften, then drain. Put the potatoes, green beans, lettuce leaves, tomatoes, olives and anchovies in a salad bowl and set aside.

2. Pour the oil over the salmon. Heat a griddle (grill) pan over a medium heat. Cook the salmon for 4–5 minutes. Turn and cook for 1 minute until cooked through, then drain on paper towels.

3. Slice the avocado and add it to the salad with the lime juice and eggs. Whisk the dressing ingredients together, pour it over the salad and serve topped with the salmon.

146 MACKEREL, APPLE AND POTATO SALAD

SERVES 4
PREPARATION 15 minutes
COOKING 12 minutes

500g/18oz new potatoes, scrubbed and halved if large
170g/6oz smoked mackerel fillets (or salmon or trout)
2 small red apples, cored and diced
4 celery stalks, finely chopped

DRESSING
3 tbsp mayonnaise
2 tbsp extra-virgin olive oil
4 tsp creamed horseradish
2 tsp lemon juice, plus a little extra for the apple

1. Cook the potatoes in a pan of boiling water for about 12 minutes, until tender; drain and set aside to cool.

2. Meanwhile, mix together the

ingredients for the dressing with 1 tbsp water until smooth and creamy.

③ Peel the skin off the mackerel and break into large chunks. Toss the apple in a little lemon juice to prevent it turning brown. Put the apple in a bowl with the mackerel, potatoes and celery.

③ Spoon the dressing over the top. Turn the salad until it is coated in the dressing.

STORAGE
Make the day before and keep in the fridge overnight. Assemble on the day. Keep chilled until ready to eat.

147 COOL BULGUR TABOULEH

SERVES 4
PREPARATION
10 minutes
COOKING
10 minutes

200g/7oz/1¼ cups bulgur wheat
200g/7oz smoked salmon, diced or chickpeas, cooked or sprouted
4 spring onions (scallions), chopped
1 large lemon, peeled and diced
2 tbsp each of fresh parsley, mint and dill, chopped
4 tomatoes, diced
200g/7oz/1½ cups green peas, fresh or defrosted
2 Little Gem lettuces
4 tsp red wine vinegar
large pinch of raw cane sugar
large pinch each of sea salt and black pepper
2 tsp Dijon mustard
4 tbsp wheatgerm oil

① Put the bulgur wheat in a small saucepan with twice its volume of water and a little salt. Bring to the boil and simmer for 8–10 minutes, or until soft. Drain in a sieve.

② In a large bowl, combine the bulgur, smoked salmon or chickpeas (garbanzo beans), spring onions (scallions), lemon, herbs, tomatoes and peas. Mix well.

③ Divide the lettuce leaves between serving plates and cover with the bulgur mixture.

④ To make the dressing, mix the vinegar, sugar, salt, pepper and mustard in a bowl, and slowly whisk in the oil. Sprinkle the dressing over the salads and serve.

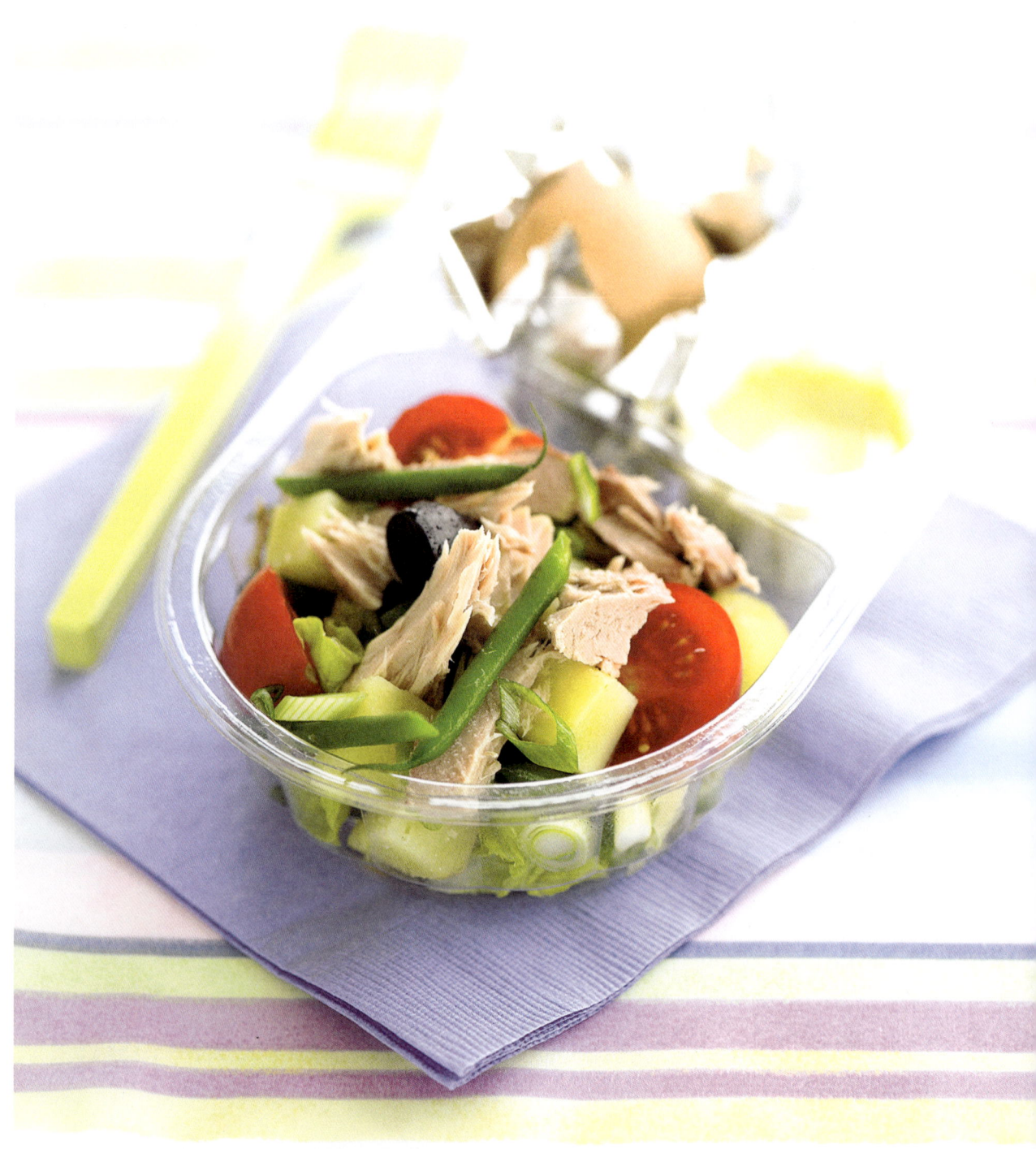

148 TUNA NIÇOISE

SERVES 4
PREPARATION 15 minutes

STORAGE Prepare the ingredients the day before and keep in the fridge overnight. Assemble on the day. Keep chilled until ready to eat.

- 4 large Cos lettuce leaves, roughly sliced
- 230g/8oz cooked fine green beans, halved
- 12 small new potatoes, cooked and cut into cubes
- 12 cherry tomatoes, halved
- 4 spring onions (scallions), sliced
- 24 pitted black olives, halved
- 600g/21oz canned tuna, drained
- 4 hard-boiled free-range eggs

DRESSING:
- 2 tbsp extra-virgin olive oil
- 1 tsp white wine vinegar
- ½ clove garlic, crushed
- 3 tbsp mayonnaise

1. Arrange the Cos lettuce in the serving bowl. Place the green beans on top, then add the potatoes, tomatoes, spring onions (scallions) and olives. Flake the tuna and sprinkle it on top.

2. Whisk together the ingredients for the dressing. Drizzle it over the salad.

3. When ready to eat, peel the eggs and serve with the salad.

149 PRAWN SALAD LUNCHBOWL

SERVES 4
PREPARATION 10 minutes

STORAGE Make the day before and keep in the fridge overnight. Assemble on the day. Keep chilled until ready to eat.

- 170g/6oz crisp lettuce leaves such as Cos, thickly sliced
- 230g/8oz canned beans of choice, drained and rinsed
- 4 carrots, finely grated
- 24 slices of cucumber
- 100g/3½oz/¾ cup canned sweetcorn, drained
- 460g/1lb cooked peeled prawns (shrimp)

DRESSING
- 1 tbsp extra-virgin olive oil
- 2 tsp mayonnaise
- ½ clove garlic, crushed
- 1 tsp lemon juice
- salt and freshly ground black pepper

1. Mix together the ingredients for the dressing and set aside until ready to use.

2. Arrange the salad ingredients in layers: salad leaves, beans, carrot, cucumber, sweetcorn and prawns (shrimp). Spoon the dressing over the salad when ready to eat.

150 AVOCADO AND SEAFOOD SALAD

SERVES 4
PREPARATION
15 minutes

STORAGE
Make the dressing the day before and keep in the fridge overnight. Assemble on the day. Keep chilled until ready to eat.

2 avocados, halved, pitted, peeled and sliced
4 beef tomatoes, sliced
½ cucumber, sliced
4 tbsp mixed seaweed, soaked for 10 minutes and boiled until tender
200g/7oz prawns (shrimp), cooked and peeled
juice of 1 lemon
200g/7oz/scant 1 cup plain yogurt
1 large bunch chives, finely chopped
2 tsp tomato ketchup
a few drops Tabasco sauce
sea salt and black pepper to taste

1. Arrange the avocado slices on serving plates. Pile the tomato and cucumber slices on top. Sprinkle with the boiled seaweed and garnish with the prawns (shrimp).

2. Make a dressing by mixing the lemon juice, yogurt, chives, tomato ketchup and Tabasco sauce in a bowl. Season and spoon over the salad. Serve with French baguette.

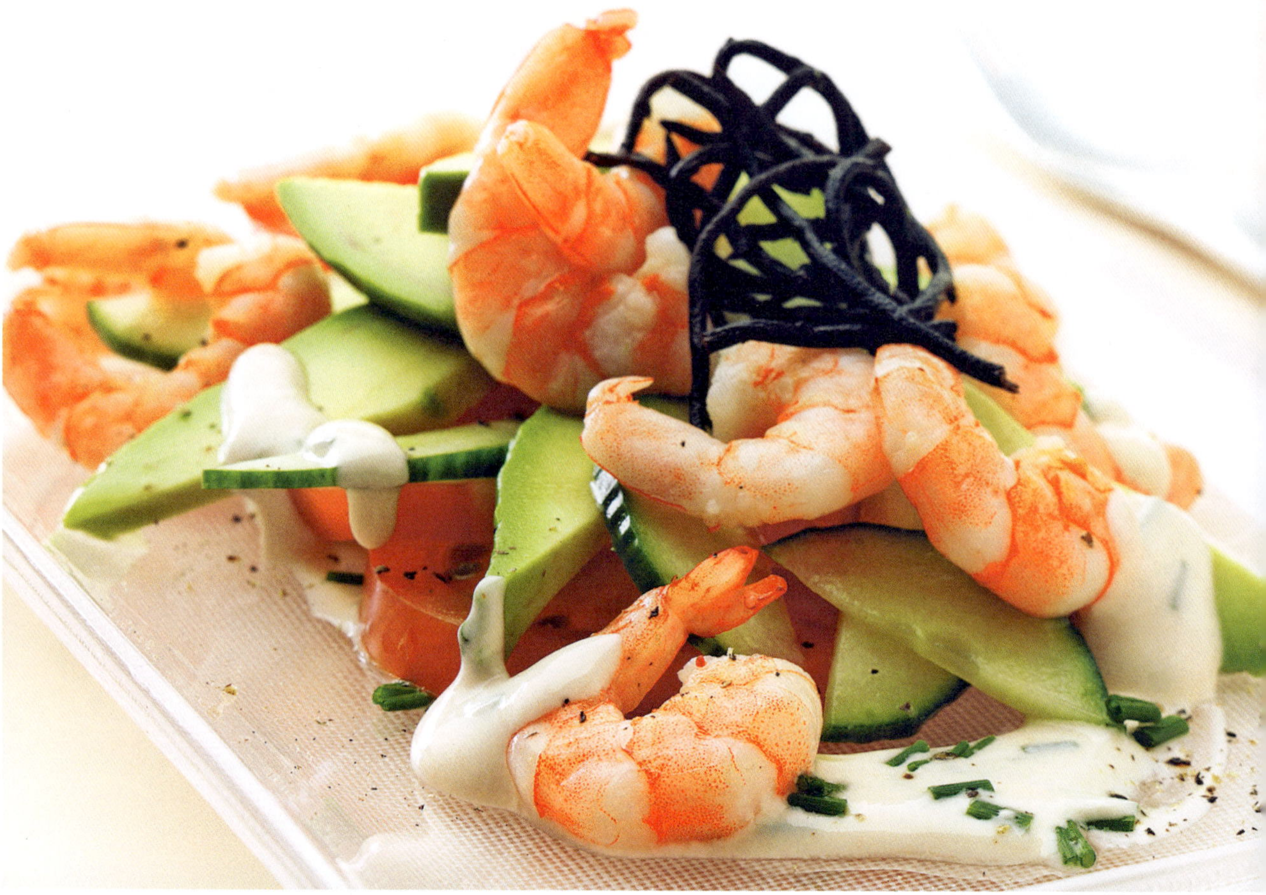

151 SEAFOOD TABOULEH

SERVES 4
PREPARATION 20 minutes

STORAGE Store in the fridge for up to 2 days.

400g/14oz/2¼ cups couscous
1 tsp Tabasco sauce mixed with 2 tbsp olive oil
200g/7oz/1½ cups green peas, fresh or defrosted
2 courgettes (zucchini), finely sliced
4 tbsp mixed seaweed, soaked for 10 minutes and boiled until tender
200g/7oz cooked prawns (shrimp)
2 small spring onions (scallions), finely chopped
2 cloves garlic, crushed
4 tbsp fresh mint, finely chopped
1 lemon, peeled and diced
sea salt and black pepper to taste

1 Put the couscous in a small saucepan with twice its volume of boiling water and a little salt. Cover and leave to stand for 10 minutes.

2 Mix in the Tabasco sauce, followed by the peas, courgette (zucchini), seaweed, prawns (shrimp), spring onions (scallions), garlic, mint and lemon. Season and serve.

152 GERMAN SALAD

SERVES 4
PREPARATION 10 minutes

STORAGE Store in the fridge for up to 2 days.

400g/14oz new potatoes, boiled and coarsely chopped
2 red apples, cored and chopped
2 tbsp mayonnaise
2 large gherkins, sliced diagonally
4 small herring fillets
4 tbsp fresh parsley, chopped
2 beetroot (beets), cooked and sliced
1 small red onion, finely sliced
4 tsp white wine vinegar
1 tsp mustard
2 tbsp walnut oil
sea salt and black pepper to taste

1 Place the boiled potatoes and the apple in a salad bowl and mix in the mayonnaise. Top with the gherkins and herring. Garnish with fresh parsley, cooked beetroot (beets) and red onion.

2 Make a dressing by whisking together the vinegar, mustard, oil, salt and pepper, and sprinkle over the salad just before serving.

153 ROCKET AND TROUT SALAD

SERVES 4
PREPARATION
10 minutes

STORAGE
Store in the fridge for up to 2 days.

1 large bunch rocket (arugula) or curly kale, chopped
1 handful radicchio leaves
2 pears, cored and sliced
1 handful chopped walnuts
300g/10½oz smoked trout
6 tbsp plain yogurt
2 tbsp lemon juice
2 tsp grated horseradish
4 tsp tamari
sea salt and black pepper to taste

1. Place the salad leaves in a large bowl. Add the pears and the walnuts.

2. Cut the trout into chunks and add to the salad.

3. Make a dressing by mixing the yogurt, lemon juice, horseradish and tamari in a bowl. Pour over the salad and gently toss. Season and serve with fresh bread.

154 ITALIAN FLAG SALAD

SERVES 4
PREPARATION
10 minutes

STORAGE
Prepare the tomato and mozzarella the day before and keep in the fridge overnight. Assemble on the day.

2 avocados, pitted, peeled and sliced
lemon juice, for brushing
4 tomatoes, seeded and diced
160g/5½oz mozzarella cheese, cut into chunks
basil leaves (optional)

DRESSING:
4 tbsp extra-virgin olive oil
4 tsp balsamic vinegar
freshly ground black pepper

1. Place the avocado in a serving bowl (or, if not serving immediately, in a plastic container that has a lid, making sure it is quite a tight fit), then brush a little lemon juice over the top to prevent it turning brown.

2. Arrange the tomato and mozzarella on top of the avocado, then sprinkle with a few basil leaves, if using.

3. Whisk together the dressing ingredients, and pour over the salad just before serving.

155 ROYAL COUSCOUS

SERVES 4
PREPARATION 10 minutes
COOKING 5 minutes

STORAGE
Store in the fridge for up to 2 days.

300g/10½oz/scant 2 cups couscous
100g/3½oz coconut, freshly grated or desiccated (dried shredded)
1 tsp sea salt
400ml/14fl oz/1⅔ cups boiling water
2 tbsp olive oil
150g/5½oz pine nuts
2 tbsp tamari
2 Little Gem lettuce, shredded
20 dried apricots, chopped
20 sun-dried tomatoes, chopped

DRESSING
2 tbsp lemon juice
2 cloves garlic, crushed
4 tsp Dijon mustard
6 tbsp olive oil
sea salt and black pepper to taste

1. Place the couscous in a medium bowl. Mix in the coconut and salt. Pour the boiling water over the couscous and leave to stand for a few minutes. When the water is absorbed, add the oil and mix well.

2. Dry-roast the pine nuts in a frying pan (skillet). When they start to brown, add the tamari, remove from the heat and stir until the kernels are well coated.

3. Mix together the dressing ingredients and season to taste.

4. Divide the lettuce between serving plates. Add the couscous, then the apricots, sun-dried tomatoes and roasted pine nuts. Top with the dressing and serve.

156 BLACKBERRY AND APPLE ICICLES

SERVES 4
PREPARATION
10 minutes

STORAGE
Make the day before and keep in the fridge overnight, with the dressing separate. Assemble on the day.

170g/5½oz mixed sprouted beans and seeds, such as alfalfa, chickpeas, mung beans, aduki beans and lentils
8 radishes, thinly sliced
2 carrots, grated
1 small red onion, diced

DRESSING
2 tbsp extra-virgin olive oil
4 tsp sesame oil
2 tsp grated fresh ginger
2 tsp tamari
4 tsp rice vinegar or lemon juice

1. Mix together the ingredients for the dressing; set aside.

2. Put the sprouted beans and seeds, radishes, carrot and red onion in a bowl. Pour the dressing over the salad and turn to coat the ingredients in the dressing.

157 MIXED BEAN SALAD

SERVES 4

PREPARATION
10 minutes

STORAGE
Make in advance and keep in the fridge for up to 2 days.

- 400-g/14-oz can mixed beans, drained and rinsed
- 1 red (bell) pepper, seeded and diced
- 1 celery stalk, sliced
- 2 spring onions (scallions), sliced
- 2 tbsp chopped mint (optional)
- 1 apple, cored and diced
- squeeze of lemon juice

DRESSING
- 2 tbsp extra-virgin olive oil
- 2 tsp white wine vinegar
- ½ tsp mustard powder
- ¼ tsp sugar
- salt and freshly ground black pepper

1. Mix together the dressing ingredients in a small bowl.

2. Put the beans in a serving bowl with the red (bell) pepper, celery, spring onions (scallions) and mint, if using.

3. Put the diced apple in another bowl, add the lemon juice, toss to prevent the apple browning, then add to the salad.

4. Pour the dressing over the salad, then toss until everything is mixed together.

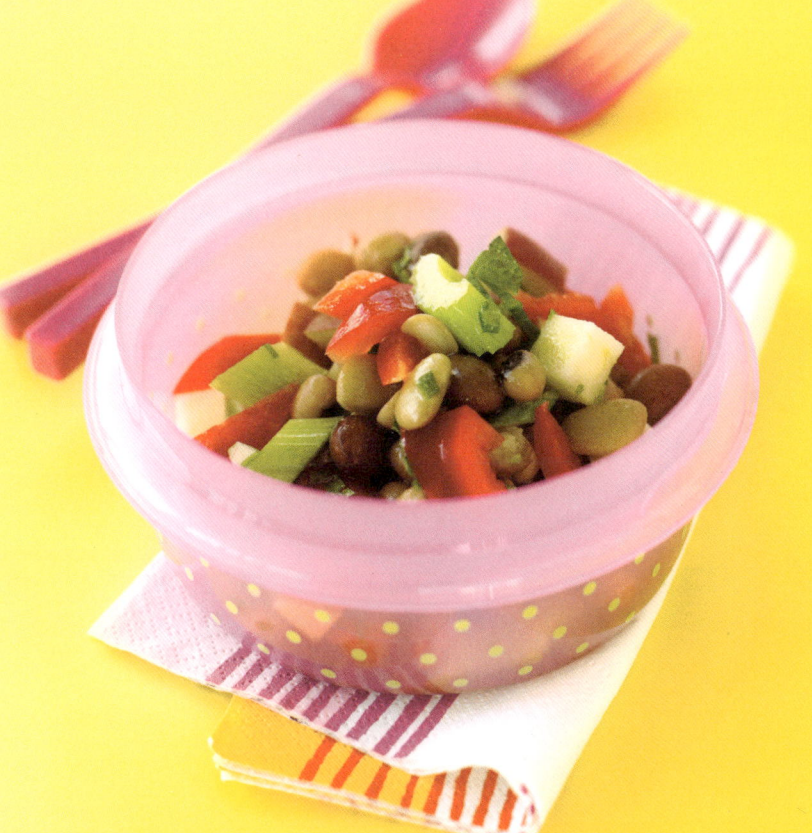

158 APPLE COLESLAW

SERVES 4
PREPARATION
10 minutes

STORAGE
Make in advance
and keep in the
fridge for up to
3 days.

55g/2oz red or white cabbage, grated
1 large carrot, grated
2 spring onions (scallions), finely sliced
1 apple, cored and grated

DRESSING
1 tbsp extra-virgin olive oil
1 tsp lemon juice
1 tbsp mayonnaise

1. Mix the cabbage, carrot, spring onions (scallions) and apple together in a bowl.

2. Whisk the oil and lemon juice together, then stir in the mayonnaise. Spoon the dressing over the salad and stir until combined.

159 CARROT, RAISIN AND PINENUT SALAD

SERVES 4
PREPARATION
10 minutes
COOKING
3 minutes

STORAGE
Make in advance
and keep in the
fridge for up to 3
days.

2 heaped tbsp pine nuts
2 large carrots, grated
2 heaped tbsp raisins

DRESSING
3 tbsp extra-virgin olive oil
2 tsp fresh lemon juice
1/2 tsp ground cumin

1. Put the pine nuts in a dry frying pan (skillet) and toast them over a medium heat for about 3 minutes, turning them occasionally, until slightly golden – take care as they can easily burn. Leave the nuts to cool, then place in a bowl with the carrots and raisins.

2. Mix together the dressing ingredients and pour over the salad before serving, turning until coated in the dressing.

SOUPS, SALADS & SIDES | 123

160 MELON AND HALLOUMI SALAD

SERVES 4
PREPARATION
5 minutes
COOKING
6 minutes

STORAGE
Make the day before and keep in the fridge overnight.

olive oil, for brushing
12 slices halloumi cheese, rinsed and patted dry
4 large wedges melon
mint leaves, chopped (optional)

DRESSING
4 tbsp extra-virgin olive oil, plus extra for brushing
4 tsp fresh lemon juice

1. Lightly brush a frying pan (skillet) with oil and heat. When the pan is hot, put the halloumi in the pan and cook for about 2–3 minutes on each side until light golden. Cut each slice into quarters.

2. Remove the skin from the melon and cut into chunks. Combine with the halloumi.

3. Combine the dressing ingredients and pour over the salad with some mint, if using, turning to coat the leaves.

161 GREEK SALAD

SERVES 4
PREPARATION
10 minutes

STORAGE
Make in advance and keep in the fridge for up to 2 days.

170g/5½oz feta cheese, rinsed, patted dry and cut into cubes
4 tomatoes, deseeded and cut into chunks
20-cm/8-in piece cucumber, cut into chunks
½ small red onion, thinly sliced
16 black olives (optional)
2 tbsp chopped mint or oregano leaves (optional)

DRESSING:
4 tbsp extra-virgin olive oil
4 tsp fresh lemon juice

1. Put the feta in a bowl with the tomatoes, cucumber, red onion and olives, if using.

2. Whisk together the oil and lemon juice and pour the dressing over the salad. Turn to coat the salad in the dressing and sprinkle with the mint or oregano, if using.

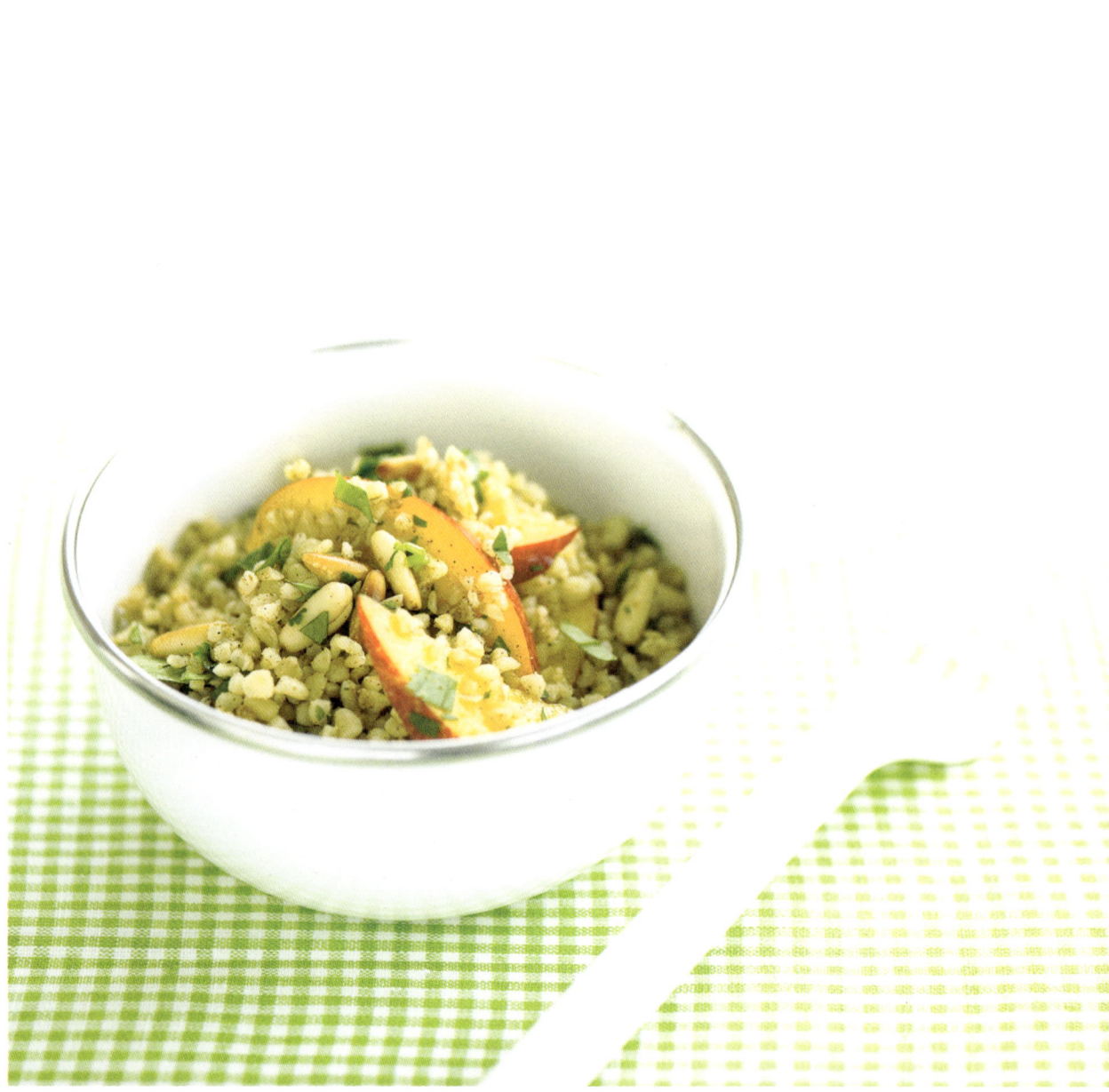

162 SPICY BULGUR SALAD with NECTARINES

SERVES 4
PREPARATION
10 minutes
COOKING
18 minutes

STORAGE
Make in advance and keep in the fridge for up to 3 days. Keep chilled until ready to eat.

100g/3½oz/½ cup bulgur wheat
475ml/16fl oz/2 cups veg stock
1 tbsp olive oil
2 cloves garlic, chopped
1 tsp ground cumin
1 tsp ground coriander
½ tsp ground cinnamon
1 ripe nectarine, pitted and sliced
3 tbsp toasted pine nuts (optional)
2 tbsp chopped fresh coriander (cilantro) (optional)
freshly ground black pepper

1. Put the bulgur wheat in a saucepan with the stock. Bring to the boil then reduce the heat, cover and simmer for 10–15 minutes until the stock is absorbed. Remove from the heat and leave the pan to stand for 5 minutes with the lid on.

2. Meanwhile, heat the oil in a frying pan (skillet) and fry the garlic for 1 minute, then add the spices and cook for another minute. Remove from the heat, add the wheat and stir to coat it in the spices. Transfer to a bowl and leave to cool.

3. Stir in the nectarine, pine nuts and coriander (cilantro), if using, and season with pepper.

163 TABOULEH

SERVES 4
PREPARATION
10 minutes
COOKING
15 minutes

STORAGE
Make in advance and keep in the fridge for up to 3 days. Keep chilled until ready to eat.

110g/4oz/⅔ cup bulgur wheat
6 small tomatoes, seeded and chopped
4 spring onions (scallions), finely chopped
10-cm/4-in piece cucumber, diced
6 tbsp chopped mint
6 tbsp chopped parsley
salt and freshly ground black pepper

DRESSING
2 tbsp extra-virgin olive oil
4 tbsp lemon juice

1. Put the bulgur wheat in a saucepan and cover it with cold water. Bring to the boil then reduce the heat, cover and simmer for 10–15 minutes until tender. Drain, if necessary, and leave to cool.

2. Put the bulgur wheat in a bowl with the tomatoes, spring onions (scallions), cucumber and herbs.

3. Mix together the olive oil and lemon juice and pour the dressing over the salad. Season and turn the salad to coat it in the dressing.

164 ORIENTAL RICE SALAD

SERVES 4
PREPARATION
10 minutes
COOKING
10 minutes

STORAGE
Make in advance and keep in the fridge for up to 2 days. Keep chilled until ready to eat.

200g/7oz/1 cup brown basmati rice
1 red (bell) pepper, diced
4 spring onions (scallions), sliced
6 baby sweetcorn, quartered
4 tbsp toasted sunflower and sesame seeds

DRESSING
4 tbsp sunflower oil
2 tbsp fresh apple juice
4 tsp tamari
4 tsp rice wine vinegar or white wine vinegar
1 tsp Chinese five-spice powder
2 tsp clear honey
1–2 tsp grated fresh ginger

1. Put the rice in a pan with plenty of salted water, bring to the boil, then simmer for 10 minutes, or until cooked. Drain, then rinse under cold running water until cold.

2. Put the cooked rice, red (bell) pepper, spring onions (scallions), baby sweetcorn and toasted seeds in a bowl.

3. Mix together the ingredients for the dressing, then pour over the salad, turning it gently until it is well coated.

165 CHINESE NOODLE SALAD

SERVES 4
PREPARATION
15 minutes
COOKING
5 minutes

STORAGE
Make in advance and keep in the fridge for up to 3 days.

140g/5oz medium egg noodles
2 carrots, cut into thin strips
10cm/4in cucumber, cut into batons
4 tomatoes, seeded and diced
4 spring onions (scallions), sliced
6 tbsp chopped coriander (cilantro)
2 tbsp toasted sesame seeds

DRESSING
2 tbsp olive oil
2 tsp toasted sesame oil
2 tsp soy sauce
2 tsp grated fresh ginger
2 small cloves garlic, crushed
2 tsp lemon juice

1. Cook the noodles following the package instructions; drain and refresh under cold running water. Meanwhile, mix together the ingredients for the dressing. Pour it over the noodles and leave to cool.

2. Put the noodles, carrots, cucumber, tomatoes, spring onions (scallions) and coriander (cilantro), if using, in a bowl, then toss with your hands to mix. Sprinkle with the sesame seeds.

SOUPS, SALADS & SIDES | 127

166 SPICY SWEET POTATOES

SERVES 4
PREPARATION
10 minutes
COOKING
10 minutes

STORAGE
Make in advance and keep in the fridge for up to 3 days.

560g/20oz orange-fleshed sweet potato, peeled and cut into bite-sized chunks
2 celery stalks, thinly sliced

DRESSING
2 tbsp low-fat plain yogurt
1½ tsp tandoori spice mix or curry powder
2 tsp smooth mango chutney
squeeze of lemon juice

1. Cook the sweet potato in plenty of boiling water for about 8–10 minutes until tender. Drain and refresh the potato under cold running water to stop it cooking any further.

2. Meanwhile, mix the dressing ingredients in a bowl.

3. Put the potato and celery in a bowl, spoon the dressing over the top and turn the salad with a spoon to coat it well.

167 PESTO PASTA SALAD

SERVES 4
PREPARATION
10 minutes
COOKING
12 minutes

STORAGE
Make the day before and keep in the fridge overnight.

200g/7oz/2 cups farfalle pasta
12 small broccoli florets
110g/4oz/scant 1 cup frozen petits pois
110g/4oz mature Cheddar cheese, cut into small chunks

DRESSING
2 tbsp mayonnaise
2–3 tbsp pesto
squeeze of lemon juice
freshly ground black pepper

1. Bring a large saucepan of salted water to the boil. Add the pasta, stir and cook following the package instructions until al dente. Drain well and refresh under cold running water.

2. Meanwhile, steam the broccoli for 4 minutes until only just tender – it should still be slightly crunchy. Add the peas about 1½ minutes before the end of the cooking time. Refresh the vegetables under cold running water.

3. Mix the dressing ingredients together, adding the pesto to taste, and season with pepper. Put the pasta, vegetables and Cheddar in a bowl and spoon the dressing over the top. Turn the salad with a spoon to coat it in the dressing.

168 TROPICAL SALAD

SERVES 4
PREPARATION
15 minutes

STORAGE
Best eaten immediately.

1 large butterhead lettuce, shredded
4 spring onions (scallions), thinly sliced
1 large bunch watercress, chopped
2 papayas, halved, deseeded, peeled and diced
2 mangoes, peeled and diced
2 avocados, halved, pitted, peeled and sliced
20 Brazil nuts, chopped
juice of 1 lime
5 tbsp walnut oil
sea salt and black pepper to taste

1. Arrange the salad ingredients on four large plates, in the order that is listed.

2. Sprinkle with the lime juice and walnut oil, season and serve with corn bread or tortillas.

169 KOREAN SALAD

SERVES 4
PREPARATION
15 minutes

STORAGE
Make in advance and keep in the fridge for up to 3 days.

4 medium carrots, cut into thin diagonal sticks
400g/14oz white radish (daikon), cut into thin diagonal sticks
1 cucumber, cut into diagonal sticks
1 tsp sea salt
2 tbsp rice vinegar
2 dashes tamari
large pinch of raw cane sugar
2 dashes Tabasco sauce
2 tbsp toasted sesame oil
4 tbsp almonds, chopped and toasted

1. Place the carrot, radish and cucumber sticks in a salad bowl. Sprinkle with the salt and mix well.

2. To make the dressing, whisk together the vinegar, tamari, sugar and Tabasco sauce. Then add the oil and whisk again.

3. Pour the dressing over the salad, garnish with the toasted almonds and serve with bread.

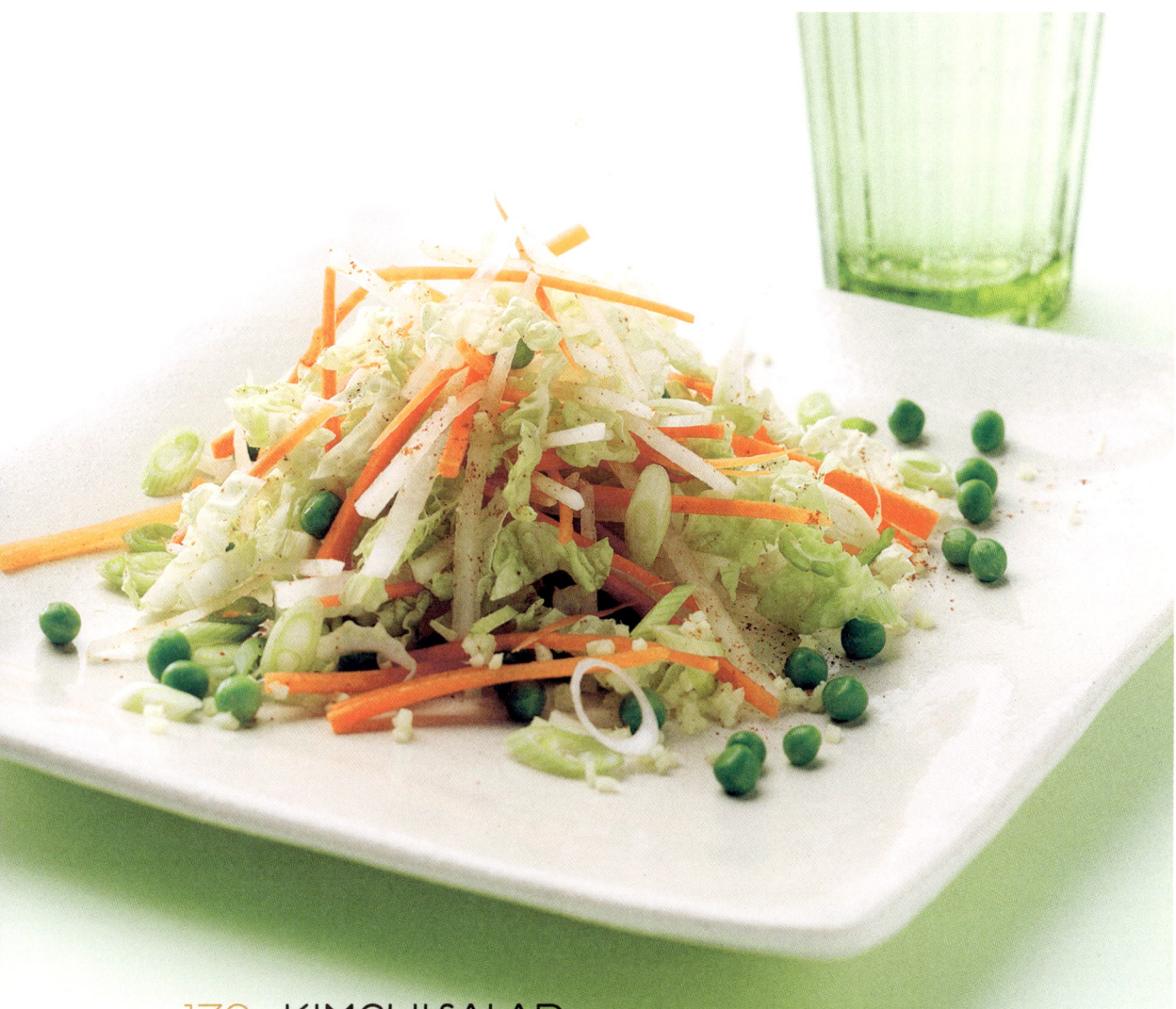

170 KIMCHI SALAD

SERVES 4
PREPARATION
10 minutes

STORAGE
Make in advance and keep in the fridge for up to 3 days.

- 2 small Chinese cabbages, finely chopped
- 2 small white radishes (daikon), finely chopped
- 2 tsp sea salt
- 1 tsp cayenne pepper
- 2 cloves garlic, finely chopped
- 2 tsp fresh ginger, finely chopped
- 4 spring onions (scallions), finely chopped
- 2 carrots, grated
- 200g/7oz/1 cup green peas, fresh or frozen, blanched

1. Place the Chinese cabbage and the white radish (daikon) in a salad bowl, sprinkle with the salt and cayenne pepper. Mix well, then add the garlic, ginger, spring onions (scallions), carrots and peas. Mix again and serve with toasted bread and pâté.

171 CRUNCHY COUNTRY SALAD

SERVES 4
PREPARATION 10 minutes
COOKING 5 minutes

STORAGE
Store in the fridge for 1 day only.

- 230g/8oz/1 cup broad (fava) beans
- 230g/8oz/2½ cups rocket (arugula)
- 1 red onion, peeled and sliced
- 2 cooked beetroot (beets), grated
- 4 celery stalks, grated
- 8 plum tomatoes, sliced
- 50g/2oz/⅔ cup sunflower seeds
- 8 tbsp olive oil
- 2 tsp horseradish sauce (ensure it's wheat- and gluten-free)
- 2 tsp honey
- 2 tsp dried oregano

1. Half fill a small saucepan with water, bring to the boil and add the broad (fava) beans. Cover and leave to simmer for 5 minutes until cooked. Remove from the heat, drain and leave to cool.

2. Place the rocket (arugula) in a large salad bowl, add the onion, beetroot (beets), celery, tomatoes and the cooled broad (fava) beans. Scatter the sunflower seeds on top.

3. In a bowl mix together the olive oil, horseradish, honey and oregano. Drizzle over the salad and serve.

172 BRIGHT BEAN SALAD

SERVES 4
PREPARATION 10 minutes
COOKING 5 minutes

STORAGE
Eat the salad fresh, immediately after it is made.

- 3 tbsp olive oil
- 2 courgettes (zucchini), sliced thinly
- leaves of 2 Little Gem lettuces
- 115g/4oz/½ cup alfalfa sprouts
- 2 small beetroot (beets), grated
- 400-g/14-oz can mixed beans, drained and rinsed
- 1 avocado, peeled and sliced
- 100g/3½oz cherry tomatoes, cut in half
- 1 tsp dried oregano
- 2 tbsp balsamic vinegar
- 25g/1oz/⅓ cup chopped parsley

1. Heat a large wok with 1 tablespoon of the olive oil. Sauté the courgettes (zucchini) until golden brown. Remove from the heat.

2. Arrange the lettuce leaves in a serving bowl and add the sprouts, beetroot (beets), mixed beans and avocado and then scatter the sliced tomatoes and courgettes (zucchini) on top.

3. Sprinkle the oregano, balsamic vinegar and remaining olive oil over the salad, garnish with the parsley and serve.

SOUPS, SALADS & SIDES | 131

173 SPANISH POTATO SALAD

SERVES 4
PREPARATION
10 minutes
COOKING
15 minutes

STORAGE
Best eaten immediately.

4 tbsp olive oil
2 tsp paprika
600g/21oz potatoes, sliced
1 Spanish onion, finely chopped
4 cloves garlic, chopped
sea salt and black pepper to taste
150ml/5fl oz/$^2/_3$ cup water
4 chicory (Belgian endive), sliced lengthways
2 tbsp walnut oil
2 tbsp red wine vinegar
1 large handful fresh parsley, chopped
300g/10$^1/_2$oz goat's cheese, sliced

1. Heat the oil in a frying pan (skillet), add the paprika and stir in the potatoes, onion and garlic. Season and stir-fry for 5 minutes. Add the water and bring to the boil. Cover and gently simmer for 10 minutes until the potatoes are tender.

2. Arrange the chicory (Belgian endive) on four plates, top with the potato slices and drizzle with the walnut oil and the vinegar. Check the seasoning, sprinkle with parsley and cheese, and serve.

174 SUMMER SALAD

SERVES 4
PREPARATION
15 minutes

STORAGE
Make in advance and keep in the fridge for up to 3 days.

2 tbsp walnut oil
2 tsp balsamic vinegar
2 tsp Dijon mustard
sea salt and white pepper to taste
2 Little Gem lettuce, shredded
1 small cauliflower, cut into small florets
2 green (bell) peppers, sliced
1 fennel bulb, finely chopped
2 carrots, cut into peelings
10 red radishes, sliced
200g/7oz/scant 1 cup broad (fava) beans, chopped
$^1/_2$ cucumber, finely sliced
1 large bunch watercress, chopped

1. To make the dressing, whisk the oil, vinegar, mustard, salt and pepper in a salad bowl.

2. Add the salad ingredients and gently toss in the dressing. Serve with bread.

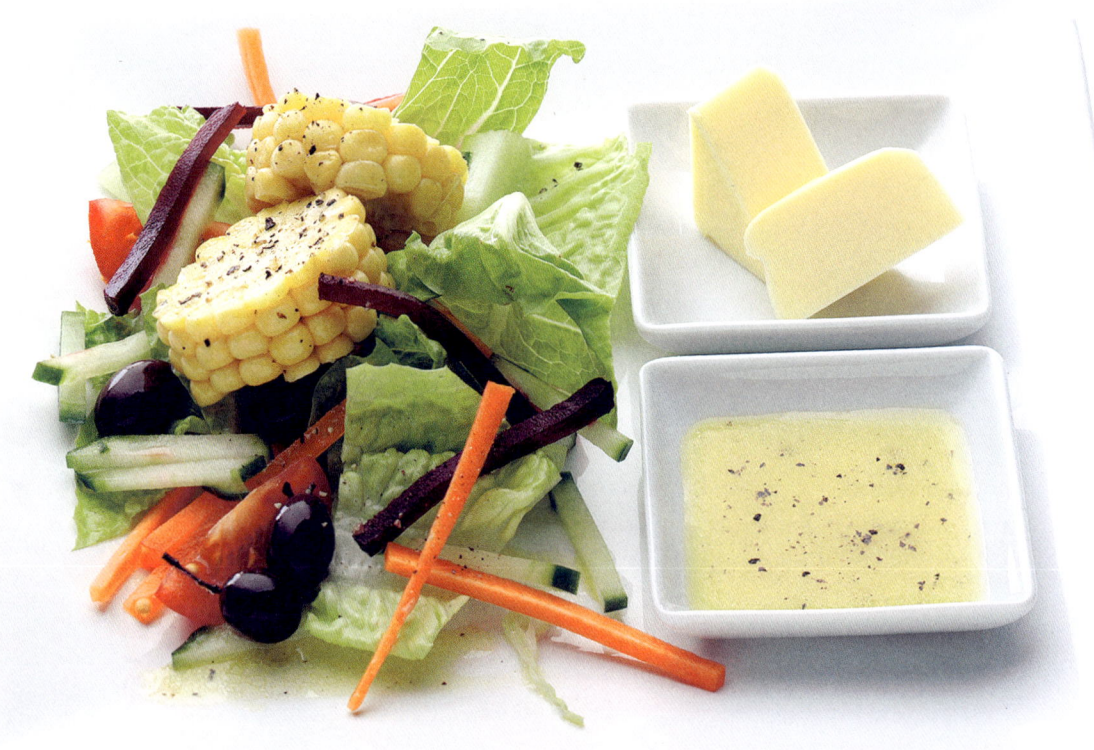

175 CORN-ON-THE-COB SALAD

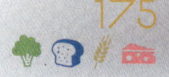

SERVES 4
PREPARATION
10 minutes
COOKING
5 minutes

STORAGE
Make in advance and keep in the fridge for up to 3 days.

4 corn-on-the-cob, peeled and sliced into chunks
1 large handful lettuce
1/2 cucumber, cut into sticks
4 tomatoes, cut into boats
2 small beetroot (beets), cut into sticks
4 carrots, cut into sticks
24 black olives, pitted
sea salt and black pepper to taste

DRESSING
2 tbsp lemon juice
2 cloves garlic, crushed
4 tsp Dijon mustard
6 tbsp olive oil
sea salt and black pepper to taste

1. Plunge the corn chunks into a saucepan of boiling water and cook for 3–5 minutes.

2. Mix the dressing ingredients and set aside.

3. Meanwhile, arrange the salad ingredients on four plates, in the order given. Top with the cooked corn, season and serve with the dressing drizzled over.

176 STUFFED TOMATO SALAD

SERVES 4
PREPARATION 10 minutes
COOKING 8 minutes
STORAGE Make in advance and keep in the fridge for up to 3 days.

400g/14oz fresh tuna, diced
2 tbsp lemon juice
8 tbsp olive oil
12 medium tomatoes, hollowed out (retain the flesh)
2 tbsp fresh basil, finely chopped
1 cucumber, finely diced
1 red (bell) pepper, finely diced
100g/3½oz red onion, chopped
24 black olives, halved and pitted
sea salt and black pepper to taste

1. Preheat the oven to 220°C/425°F/gas mark 7. Cook the tuna with 1 tablespoon of the lemon juice and 2 tablespoons of the olive oil in a small baking dish for 5–8 minutes.

2. To make a dressing, blend the scooped-out tomato flesh with the remaining lemon juice and olive oil, the basil and salt and pepper to a thick consistency and set aside.

3. Place the cooked tuna in a bowl with the cucumber, red (bell) pepper, red onion and olives. Mix in the dressing. Spoon the salad mixture into the hollowed-out tomatoes. Serve on a bed of green lettuce.

177 WARM PASTA SALAD

SERVES 4
PREPARATION 10 minutes
COOKING 10 minutes
STORAGE Make in advance and keep in the fridge for up to 3 days.

300g/10½oz tricolor pasta
2 thick slices celeriac (celery root), chopped into matchsticks
2 leeks, chopped into matchsticks
2 carrots, chopped into matchsticks
4 tbsp olive oil
juice of 1 lemon
sea salt and black pepper to taste
¼ tsp ground coriander
300g/10½oz smoked salmon, cut into strips
8 mushrooms, sliced and sprinkled with lemon juice
4 tsp fresh parsley, finely chopped

1. Cook the pasta in boiling water for 10–12 minutes, then set aside.

2. Blanch the celeriac (celery root), leek and carrot in a pan of boiling water for 1 minute. Drain and set aside.

3. Make a dressing by whisking the oil, lemon juice, salt, pepper and coriander in a bowl.

4. Mix the pasta, blanched vegetables, smoked salmon and mushrooms in a salad bowl. Add the dressing and gently toss. Garnish with parsley and serve.

178 AVOCADO AND MELON SALAD WITH CREAMY DRESSING

SERVES 4
PREPARATION
15 minutes

STORAGE
Best eaten immediately.

4 handfuls lettuce leaves
2 avocados, halved, pitted, peeled and sliced
1 small yellow melon, deseeded, peeled and sliced
16 sun-dried tomatoes, thinly sliced
200g/7oz cooked prawns (shrimp)
200ml/7fl oz/scant 1 cup plain or soya yogurt
2 tbsp olive oil
2 tbsp balsamic vinegar
2 tbsp tomato ketchup
1 tsp sea salt
plenty of black pepper
1 large bunch fresh dill

1 Arrange the lettuce leaves on serving plates. Add the avocado, followed by the melon, sun-dried tomatoes and prawns (shrimp).

2 To make a dressing, place the yogurt in a bowl, add the oil, vinegar, ketchup, salt and pepper and mix well. Spoon the dressing onto the salads.

3 Garnish with finely chopped dill and serve with crusty bread.

179 COLLIOURE SALAD

SERVES 4
PREPARATION
10 minutes
COOKING
30 minutes

STORAGE
Best eaten immediately.

6 red (bell) peppers
16 halved pieces of salsify
16 black olives
olive oil, for brushing and drizzling
2 tbsp red wine vinegar
2 cloves garlic, chopped
2 tbsp fresh parsley, finely chopped
black pepper to taste
4 hard-boiled eggs, quartered

1 Preheat the oven to 250°C/500°/gas mark 10.

2 Brush the (bell) peppers with oil, place them on a baking sheet and roast for 30 minutes, turning from time to time, until the skins are black and charred. Then peel off the skins (while they are still warm), deseed and cut into thick slices.

3 Arrange the salsify and olives like sunrays around the edge of a large plate and place the (bell) pepper slices in the middle of the plate. Drizzle with oil and vinegar, sprinkle with the garlic, parsley and black pepper and top with the eggs to serve.

180 WILD RICE SALAD

SERVES 4
PREPARATION 10 minutes
COOKING 10 minutes

STORAGE
Make in advance and keep in the fridge for up to 3 days.

400g/14oz/3¼ cups wild rice, cooked (200g/7oz/generous 1 cup uncooked)
200g/7oz baby spinach, chopped
1 red onion, finely chopped
200g/7oz fennel bulb, sliced
2 thick slices pineapple, chopped
2 tbsp lemon juice
2 tsp Dijon mustard
2 tsp maple syrup
sea salt and black pepper to taste
6 tbsp hazelnut oil
1 large handful beansprouts
50g/2oz/⅓ cup hazelnuts, chopped

1. Place the cooked rice in a salad bowl with the spinach, onion, fennel and pineapple and mix well.

2. To make the dressing, whisk the lemon juice, mustard, maple syrup, salt and pepper in a small bowl, slowly adding the oil. Pour the dressing over the rice salad, garnish with the beansprouts and hazelnuts, and serve.

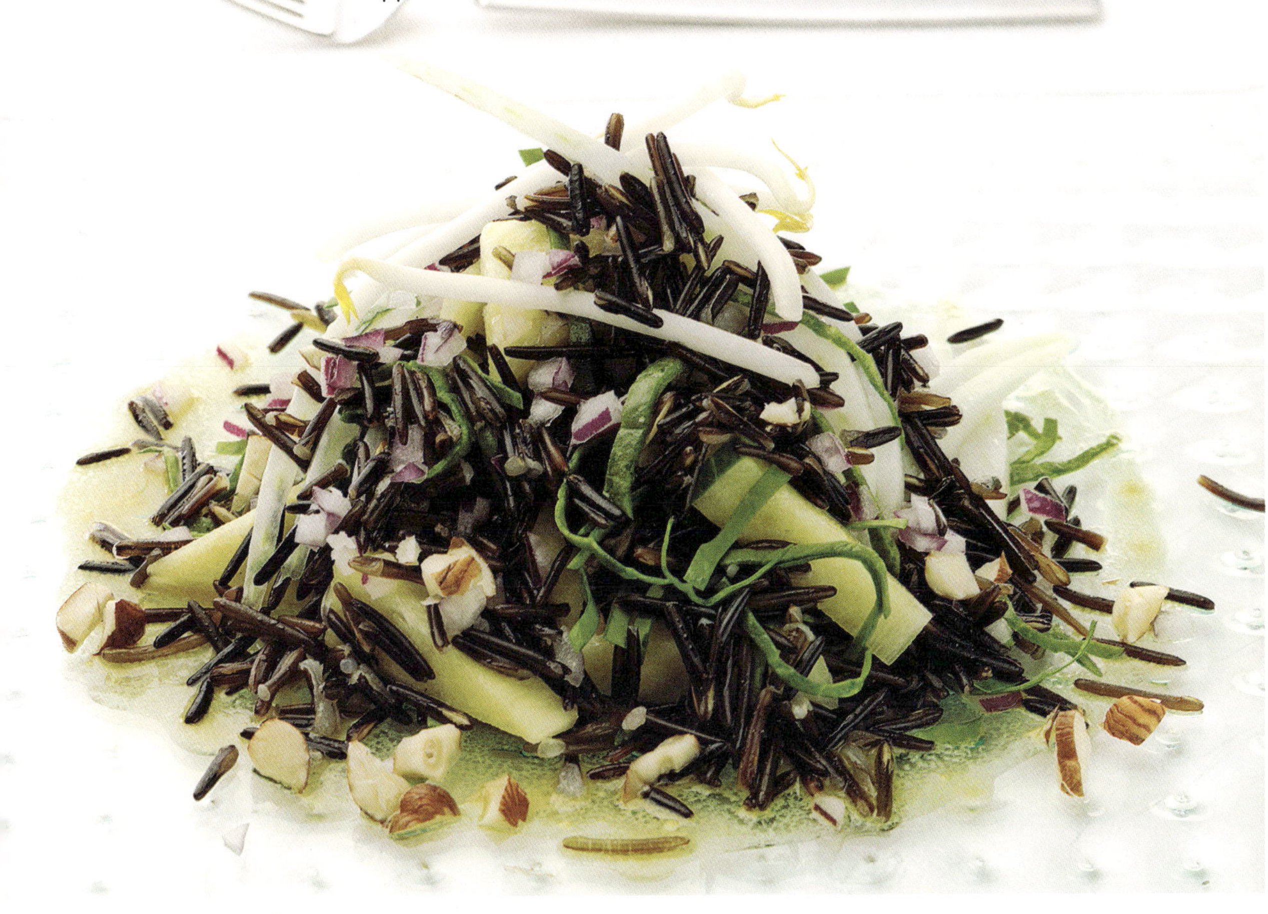

181 CARROT, DATE AND PECAN SALAD WITH GINGER DRESSING

SERVES 4
PREPARATION 15 minutes
STORAGE Make in advance and keep in the fridge for up to 3 days.

500g/1lb 2oz carrots, grated
150g/5½oz dates, pitted and chopped
150g/5½oz pecans, chopped
6 tbsp lemon juice
4 tsp fresh ginger, finely chopped
2 tsp liquid honey

1. Mix the carrots, dates and pecans in a salad bowl.

2. To make the dressing, pour the lemon juice into a small bowl and mix in the ginger and honey.

3. Mix the dressing with the salad and serve with pitta bread.

182 CARROT SALAD WITH ALMOND DRESSING

SERVES 4
PREPARATION 10 minutes
STORAGE Make in advance and keep in the fridge for up to 3 days.

500g/1lb 2oz carrots, grated
4 tbsp light almond butter
2 tsp red wine vinegar
2 tsp lemon juice
2 tsp Dijon mustard
sea salt and white pepper to taste
4 tbsp almonds, chopped
4 tbsp fresh parsley, finely chopped
1 large lettuce, shredded
300g/10½oz ham, sliced

1. Place the grated carrots in a salad bowl.

2. To make the dressing, whisk the almond butter, vinegar, lemon juice, mustard, salt and pepper in a small bowl. Slowly add water until you have a smooth, even consistency.

3. Add the dressing to the carrots, gently mix and top with the almonds and parsley. Divide the shredded lettuce between serving plates, add the slices of ham, top with the dressed salad and serve.

SOUPS, SALADS & SIDES | 137

183 CARROT SALAD WITH SUNFLOWER SEEDS AND PARSLEY

SERVES 4
PREPARATION
10 minutes

STORAGE
Make in advance and keep in the fridge for up to 3 days.

500g/1lb 2oz carrots, grated
4 tbsp sunflower seeds
4 tbsp lemon juice
4 tbsp sunflower oil
sea salt and black pepper to taste
4 tbsp fresh parsley, finely chopped

1. Mix the grated carrots and sunflower seeds in a bowl with the lemon juice and oil. Season and garnish with fresh parsley. Serve with toast and pâté.

184 SESAME ASIAN GREENS

SERVES 4
PREPARATION
5 minutes
COOKING
5 minutes

STORAGE
Refrigerate and use cold in a salad the following day.

3 tbsp sesame oil
350g/12oz pak choi (bok choy) leaves
1 tsp chopped fresh ginger
8 spring onions (scallions), chopped
225g/8oz/1 cup beansprouts
2 tbsp sesame seeds
2 tbsp tamari

1. Heat the oil in a wok, add the pak choi (bok choy) leaves and stir-fry for 2 minutes.

2. Add the ginger, spring onions (scallions) and beansprouts and stir continuously over a high heat for 2–3 minutes until the vegetables are tender.

3. Add the sesame seeds and tamari. Remove from the heat and serve in individual bowls.

185 LEBANESE MACARONI SALAD

SERVES 4
PREPARATION 10 minutes
COOKING 15 minutes
STORAGE Make in advance and keep in the fridge for up to 3 days.

- 450g/1lb macaroni pasta
- 200ml/7fl oz/scant 1 cup plain or soya yogurt
- 4 cloves garlic, crushed
- 2 tbsp fresh mint leaves, chopped
- sea salt and black pepper to taste
- 150g/5½oz pine nuts
- 2 tbsp olive oil
- 4 tsp tamari

1. Boil the macaroni in plenty of water with a little salt and oil until just tender. Meanwhile, mix the yogurt, garlic and mint in a bowl, and season.

2. Toast the pine nuts in a frying pan (skillet) with the oil until they begin to brown. Remove from the heat, quickly add the tamari and stir well..Set aside.

3. Drain the cooked macaroni, run it under cold water for a few seconds, and drain again. Place in a serving bowl and gently mix in the yogurt mixture. Garnish with the toasted pine nuts and serve.

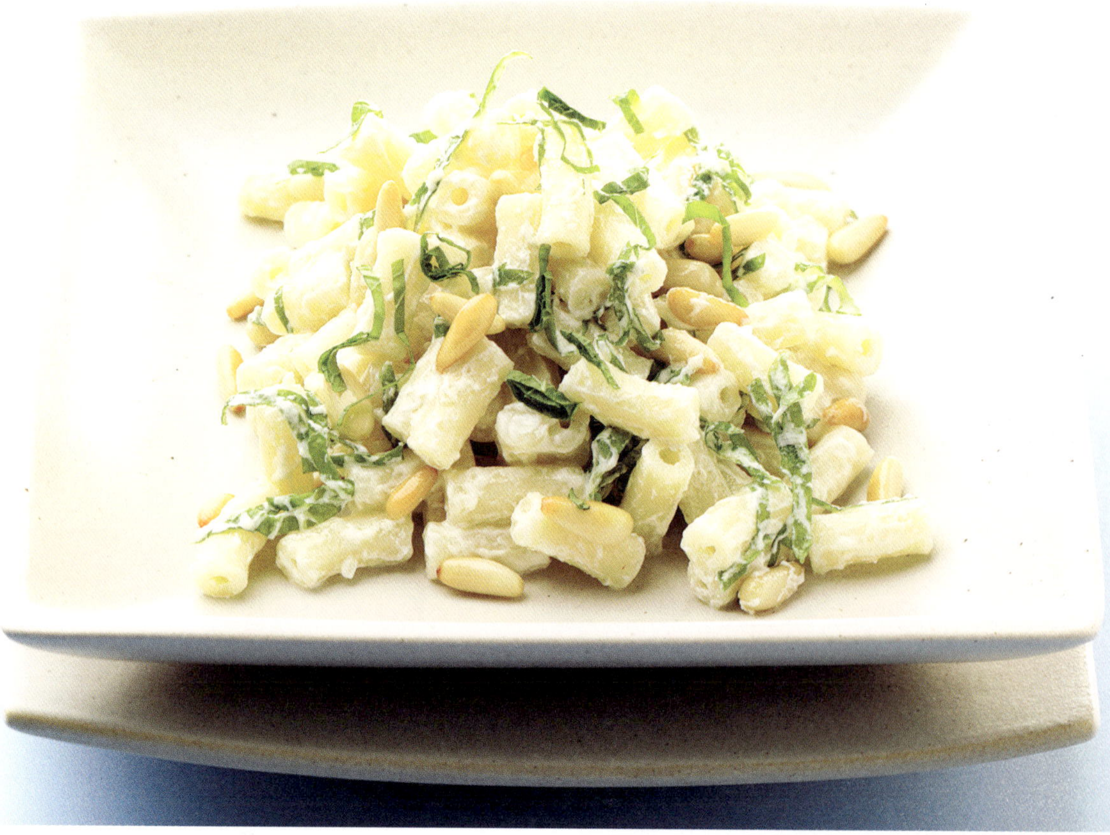

SOUPS, SALADS & SIDES | 139

186 AFRICAN-STYLE BROAD BEANS

SERVES 4
PREPARATION
5 minutes
COOKING
12 minutes

STORAGE
Make in advance and keep in the fridge for up to 3 days.

4 tbsp olive oil
4 tsp ground cumin
4 cloves garlic, chopped
500g/1lb 2oz fresh broad (fava) beans, shelled
6 tbsp lemon juice
4 tbsp fresh parsley, chopped
sea salt and cayenne pepper to taste
2 tsp paprika

1 Gently heat the oil in a heavy saucepan, add the cumin and the garlic and stir-fry for 15 seconds. Add the fresh broad (fava) beans and stir for a further 15 seconds, then add enough water to cover the beans, bring to the boil and simmer for approximately 10 minutes until the beans are soft. Add the lemon juice and the fresh parsley.

2 Mash some of the cooked beans with a spoon. Season and serve garnished with paprika on a bed of millet or couscous.

187 ASIAN ASPARAGUS

SERVES 4
PREPARATION
10 minutes
COOKING
12 minutes

STORAGE
Best eaten immediately.

1 large bunch green asparagus,
3 tbsp olive oil
1 tsp ground cumin
2 lemongrass stalks, finely sliced
4 tsp fresh ginger, finely chopped
4 medium carrots, cut into sticks
4 spring onions (scallions), sliced
2 tbsp tamarind paste dissolved in 200ml/7fl oz/1 cup hot water
1 large handful bean sprouts
2 tbsp tamari
2 tsp maple syrup
2 tbsp lemon juice
sea salt and black pepper to taste

1 Cut the asparagus into 5cm/2in pieces. Heat the oil in a wok. Add the spices, then the asparagus, carrots and spring onions (scallions) and stir-fry for 5 minutes. Add the dissolved tamarind paste. Simmer until the asparagus is tender, then add the beansprouts, tamari, maple syrup and lemon juice. Heat through, season to taste, and serve with rice or noodles.

188 BRAISED BRUSSELS SPROUTS

SERVES 4
PREPARATION
5 minutes
COOKING
22 minutes

STORAGE
Best eaten immediately.

500g/1lb 2oz Brussels sprouts, halved
2 tbsp olive oil
juice and zest of 1 orange
100g/3½oz smoked bacon, diced
2 medium carrots, diced
2 tsp wholegrain mustard
sea salt and black pepper to taste

1. Place the Brussels sprouts in a heavy saucepan with the rest of the ingredients. Bring to the boil, cover and very gently simmer until the Brussels sprouts are tender (about 20 minutes). Stir from time to time (adding a little water if necessary). Season and serve with rice.

189 BAKED CHICORY AND BEETROOT

SERVES 4
PREPARATION
10 minutes
COOKING
20 minutes

STORAGE
Leftovers will keep in the fridge for up to 2 days.

4 large chicory (Belgian endive), quartered lengthways
2 medium beetroot (beets), sliced
12 sun-dried tomatoes, sliced
100g/3½oz/1 cup chopped walnuts
4 tbsp olive oil
2 tbsp lemon juice
sea salt and black pepper to taste
1 large handful Gouda cheese, grated
4 tbsp breadcrumbs

1. Preheat the oven to 200°C/400°F/gas mark 6.
2. Place the quartered chicory (Belgian endive) and the beetroot (beet) slices in a shallow ovenproof dish. Scatter the sun-dried tomato slices and the walnuts on top, drizzle with the oil and lemon juice, and season. Top with the grated cheese and the breadcrumbs. Bake for 20 minutes (adding a little water if necessary) and serve.

190 MINTED POTATOES WITH HAZELNUTS

SERVES 4
PREPARATION
5 minutes
COOKING
20 minutes

600g/1lb 5oz new potatoes
100g/3½oz whole hazelnuts
2 sprigs mint, plus 2 tbsp chopped mint
25g/1oz butter

1. Bring a half-filled saucepan of water to the boil and add the potatoes, hazelnuts and 1 mint sprig. Simmer for 15–20 minutes, until the potatoes are soft. Drain

STORAGE
You can refrigerate for up to 3 days.

and add the butter and chopped mint, stirring until the butter is melted.

2) Pour into a serving dish and garnish with the remaining sprig of mint.

191 PROVENÇAL LEMON POTATOES

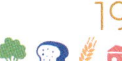

SERVES 4
PREPARATION
5 minutes
COOKING
12 minutes

1kg/2lb 3oz small new potatoes, kept whole and unpeeled
4 tbsp olive oil
1 lemon (unpeeled), chopped
2 tsp herbes de Provence
sea salt and plenty of black pepper

1) Boil the potatoes in lightly salted water until tender (approximately 10 minutes). Drain and set aside.

2) Heat the oil in a large pan, add the boiled potatoes, lemon and herbs. Stir continuously until the potatoes are well coated with herbs. Season and serve on a bed of fresh rocket (arugula).

192 COCONUT AND CLOVE RICE

SERVES 4
PREPARATION
5 minutes
COOKING
20 minutes

STORAGE
Refrigerate this dish overnight, but use within 24 hours.

300g/12oz/2 cups brown basmati rice
50g/2oz/$^2/_3$ cup desiccated (dried shredded) coconut
4 cloves
2 cardamom pods
1 tsp ground cinnamon
25g/1oz/$^1/_3$ cup chopped parsley

1) Half fill a saucepan with water, bring to the boil and add the rice and coconut. Cover and let simmer for 10 minutes. Drain the rice, wash with hot water, then return to the pan.

2) Add the remaining ingredients and a tablespoon of water, cover with the lid again and simmer over a low heat for 10 minutes, stirring occasionally, until the mixture is of rice-pudding consistency. Remove from the heat and serve, garnished with chopped parsley.

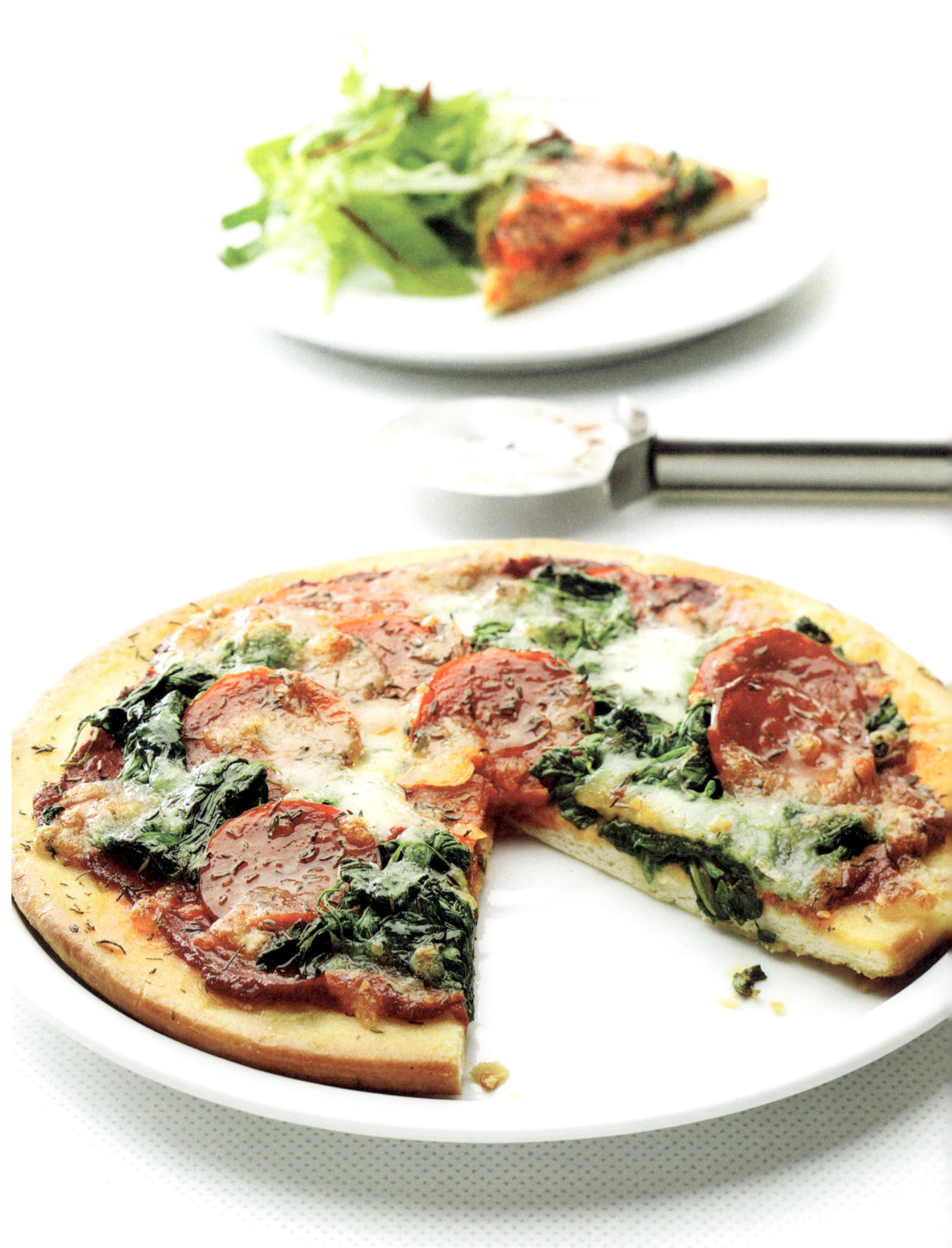

Lunches

Wholesome and packed with protein, vegetables or healthy whole grains, this range of delicious lunch recipes will keep the entire family happy, with enough variety to find something to suit everyone.

From light meals to eat at home to lunchbox fillers, here you will find ideas for any occasion. Perfect homemade pizzas (Feisty Fiesta Pizza on page 198) and nutritious hot treats such as Tuna and Onion Tortilla (see page 167) or Spicy Bean Burgers (see page 188) will sort out any midday slumps. And for those on the go, tasty sandwiches and wraps, such as Steak Ciabatta (see page 147) or Moroccan Turkey Wraps (see page 158), and clever meal-in-one ideas, such as Ham and Egg "Pies" (see page 150), make ideal solutions to avoid turning to unhealthy pre-packaged sandwiches or fat-laden fast-food fixes.

193 PEPPERONI PIZZA

SERVES 4
PREPARATION 10 minutes
COOKING 15 minutes
STORAGE Store leftovers in the fridge for up to 2 days.

175ml/6fl oz/¾ cup passata (sieved tomatoes)
4 pizza bases
400g/14oz fresh spinach, sautéed
4 cloves garlic, crushed
400g/14oz spicy sausage, sliced and fried
4 tsp each of thyme and oregano
sea salt and black pepper to taste
400g/14oz mozzarella cheese, grated

1. Preheat the oven to 240°C/475°F/gas mark 9 and heat a large baking sheet.

2. Spread 2-3 tablespoons of the passata over each prepared pizza base and top with the sautéed spinach, garlic and spicy sausage. Sprinkle with the herbs, season and top with the grated cheese.

3. Bake in the hot oven for approximately 15 minutes. Serve hot with a side salad.

194 SMOKED HAM AND PEPPER PIZZA

SERVES 4
PREPARATION 10 minutes
COOKING 15 minutes
STORAGE Store leftovers in the fridge for up to 2 days.

175ml/6fl oz/¾ cup passata (sieved tomatoes)
4 pizza bases
4 tsp thyme
4 tsp marjoram
4 bay leaves, crushed
4 cloves garlic, crushed
1 green (bell) pepper, finely sliced
1 red (bell) pepper, finely sliced
1 yellow (bell) pepper, finely sliced
200g/7oz smoked ham, thinly sliced
sea salt and black pepper to taste
400g/14oz mozzarella cheese, grated

1. Preheat the oven to 240°C/475°F/gas mark 9 and heat a large baking sheet.

2. Spread 2-3 tablespoons of the passata over each prepared pizza base. Sprinkle with the thyme, marjoram, bay leaf and garlic. Arrange the (bell) pepper slices and the smoked ham on top. Season, sprinkle with the grated cheese and bake in a hot oven for approximately 15 minutes. Serve hot with a side salad.

195 CALZONE

MAKES 8
PREPARATION 30 minutes
COOKING 40 minutes

STORAGE Make the day before and keep in the fridge overnight.

1 tbsp olive oil
1 onion, chopped
2 cloves garlic, chopped
1 large carrot, diced
1 small red (bell) pepper, seeded and diced
250g/9oz vegetarian mince
375ml/13fl oz/1½ cups passata (sieved tomatoes)
1 tsp dried oregano
2 tbsp tomato ketchup
freshly ground black pepper
115g/4oz mozzarella cheese, cut into small pieces

DOUGH
350g/12oz/3 cups white self-raising (self-rising) flour, plus extra for dusting
200g/7oz/1⅔ cups wholemeal self-raising (self-rising) flour
1 tsp salt
300ml/10fl oz/1¼ cups semi-skimmed (half-fat) milk
8 tbsp olive oil

1. Preheat the oven to 200°C/400°F/Gas 6. Heat the oil in a saucepan and fry the onion for 8 minutes, then add the garlic, carrot and red (bell) pepper and cook for another 3 minutes. Stir in the remaining ingredients (except the cheese) and bring to the boil. Simmer for 15 minutes, until reduced. Season well and leave to cool.

2. To make the dough, sift the flours and salt into a mixing bowl, adding any bran left in the sieve. Make a well in the middle and pour in the milk and oil. Mix with a fork until the ingredients start to come together into a dough (adding a little more milk if dry). Tip the dough out onto a floured work surface and knead briefly until it forms a smooth ball.

3. Divide the dough into eight pieces. Roll into thin discs about 12cm/4½in in diameter and divide the sauce and cheese between them.

4. Fold the discs in half, press the edges together and crimp to seal. Prick the top with a fork. Place on floured baking sheets and bake for 10–12 minutes until golden.

196 SMILEY FACE PIZZA

SERVES 4
PREPARATION
10 minutes
COOKING
15 minutes

STORAGE
You can refrigerate for up to 3 days.

4 cheese and tomato pizza bases
1 small red onion, peeled
200g/7oz/1⅓ cup goat's cheese
200g/7oz ham, sliced
1 red (bell) pepper, deseeded and cut into thin slices
1 yellow (bell) pepper, deseeded and cut into thin slices
4 olives, stuffed with pimento
2 tsp oregano
large handful of rocket (arugula)
20 cherry tomatoes, halved
balsamic vinegar

1. Preheat the oven to 220°C/425°F/gas mark 7. Place the pizza bases on a non-stick baking sheet.

2. Slice the red onion into rings. Remove the inner rings and place on the pizza base as eyes. Cut four slices from the goat's cheese and place beneath the onions as a nose.

3. Place a ham slice on the pizza in a curved line and top with a pepper strip to create a smile.

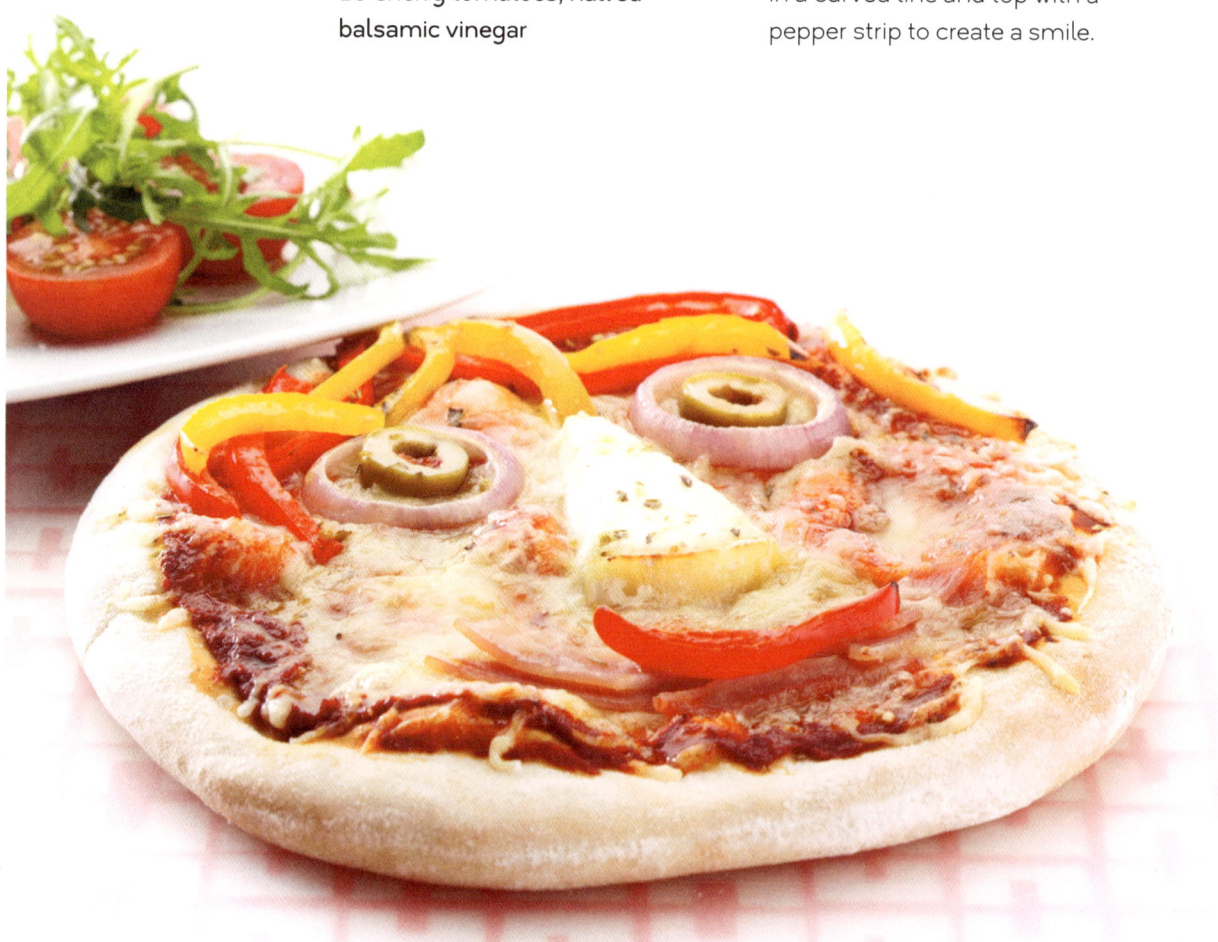

Alternate the coloured (bell) pepper strips for hair. Halve the stuffed olives and put these in the middle of the onion rings as pupils.

4. Sprinkle the pizzas with oregano, then bake in the oven for 15 minutes.

5. Put the rocket (arugula) and tomatoes in a salad bowl, drizzle with balsamic vinegar and serve with the pizzas.

197 STEAK CIABATTA

SERVES 4
PREPARATION
10 minutes + marinating
COOKING
16 minutes

STORAGE
Leftovers will keep in the fridge for up to 1 day.

4 sirloin steaks, 115g/4oz each
1 red onion, sliced
1 clove garlic, crushed
2 thyme sprigs
4 tbsp olive oil, plus extra for drizzling
2 ciabatta loaves, halved lengthways
1 avocado
1 tomato, diced
1 tbsp lemon juice
handful of baby spinach leaves

1. Put the steaks in a shallow dish. Add the onion, garlic, thyme and oil to coat evenly. Cover and marinate for 2–3 hours, or preferably overnight, in the fridge.

2. Preheat the oven to 180°C/350°F/gas mark 4. Heat a frying pan (skillet). Reserving the marinade, sear the steaks in the pan for 3 minutes each side. Transfer to a plate and cover with foil.

3. Pour the marinade into the pan and cook gently for 5 minutes, or until thick and the onion has caramelized.

4. Heat the ciabatta in the oven for 5 minutes. Dice the avocado and mix it with the tomato and lemon juice.

5. Cut the steaks into thin strips. Drizzle each ciabatta with a little oil, then fill with the spinach, steak, caramelized onion and avocado. Cut in half and serve with coleslaw.

198 ORIENTAL BEEF WRAP

SERVES 4
PREPARATION 10 minutes
COOKING 2 minutes

STORAGE
Make the stir-fry the day before and keep in the fridge overnight. Strain off any liquid and assemble on the day.

2 tbsp sesame oil
4 cloves garlic, chopped
few slivers fresh ginger
400g/14oz lean beef, cut into strips
2 tbsp tamari
4 tbsp orange juice
8 iceberg lettuce leaves
4 spring onions (scallions), shredded
20cm/8in cucumber, cut into batons
1 red (bell) pepper, sliced
fresh coriander (cilantro) (optional)

1. Heat a wok over a high heat and add the oil, garlic, ginger and beef, then stir-fry for 1 minute. Add the tamari and orange juice and stir-fry for another minute until the liquid has thickened. Leave to cool.

2. Open out the lettuce leaves and divide the beef between them, spooning it down one half of each leaf. Top with the spring onion (scallions), cucumber, (bell) pepper and coriander (cilantro), if using.

3. Roll each leaf up to make a parcel. Cut each roll in half to serve..

199 LAMB AND PEA SAMOSAS

MAKES 16
PREPARATION 20 minutes
COOKING 40 minutes

STORAGE
Leftovers will keep in the fridge for up to 2 days.

1 tbsp olive oil, plus extra
1 spring onion (scallion), chopped
½ tsp ground cinnamon
pinch of paprika
pinch of cayenne pepper
250g/9oz minced lamb
1 tbsp chopped mint
60g/2¼oz/½ cup frozen peas
75g/2½oz feta cheese, crumbled
16 sheets of filo (phyllo) pastry, about 16 x 12cm/6¼ x 4½in each

1. Heat the oil in a frying pan (skillet). Add the spring onion (scallion), cinnamon, paprika and cayenne pepper, and cook for 1 minute. Add the lamb and cook until golden brown, stirring. Add the mint and peas; stir to mix. Transfer to a bowl and add the feta.

2. Preheat the oven to 190°C/375°F/gas mark 5. Brush a sheet of filo (phyllo) with oil and fold it in half lengthways. Put a spoonful of meat at one end of the pastry. Carefully fold the pastry corner over the filling to form a triangle. Continue folding the triangle along the length of the strip to make a neat samosa. Repeat.

3. Brush with olive oil and bake for 20 minutes, until golden brown.

200 EGG AND BACON ROLL

SERVES 4
PREPARATION
10 minutes
COOKING
7 minutes

STORAGE
Make the filling the day before and keep in the fridge overnight. Assemble on the day. Keep chilled until ready to eat.

4 slices bacon
4 eggs
4 ciabatta rolls
1 tomato, quartered and seeded
handful of alfalfa sprouts or cress
freshly ground black pepper

1. Preheat the grill (broiler) to medium-high and line the grill pan with foil. Grill (broil) the bacon until crisp, then leave to cool.

2. Meanwhile, boil the eggs for about 6 minutes until the yolks are still very slightly runny. Hold the eggs under cold running water until they are cool enough to handle.

3. Peel the eggs, place in a bowl and roughly chop. Cut the bacon into small pieces and stir into the egg. Season.

4. Cut the ciabatta rolls in half. Squeeze a tomato quarter and rub it into one half of one of the ciabattas. Spoon the egg and bacon mixture over the top and sprinkle with a few alfalfa sprouts or cress. Put the other half of the ciabatta on top. Repeat with the remaining rolls.

201 PORK AND EGG-FRIED RICE

SERVES 4
PREPARATION
15 minutes
COOKING
40 minutes

STORAGE
Leftovers will keep in the fridge for up to 1 day. If reheating, ensure that the rice is piping hot before serving.

200g/7oz/1 cup brown basmati rice
3 tbsp olive oil
250g/9oz minced (ground) pork
2 eggs, beaten
2 tsp sesame oil
2 spring onions (scallions), sliced
2 tomatoes, chopped
75g/2½oz/½ cup frozen peas
½ red (bell) pepper, diced
2 tbsp tamari
freshly ground black pepper
handful of fresh coriander (cilantro)

1. Cook the rice according to the package instructions until tender. Drain and cool.

2. Heat a wok and add 1 tablespoon of the olive oil. Add the pork and stir-fry for 5 minutes until browned. Set aside in a bowl.

3. Heat half the remaining olive oil in the wok. Beat the eggs with half the sesame oil, then cook, stirring, until scrambled. Set aside.

4. Heat the remaining oil in the wok. Stir-fry the rice, spring onions (scallions), tomatoes, peas and (bell) pepper for 1-2 minutes. Stir in the pork, egg and tamari until hot. Season with pepper, sprinkle with the coriander (cilantro) and serve.

202 HAM AND EGG "PIES"

MAKES 4
PREPARATION
15 minutes
COOKING
10–12 minutes

STORAGE
Make in advance and keep in the fridge for up to 3 days. Keep chilled until ready to eat.

olive oil, for brushing
4 thin slices good-quality ham
4 eggs

① Preheat the oven to 190°C/375°F/gas mark 5. Lightly brush four holes of a deep muffin tin (pan) with oil.

② Arrange a slice of ham in each hole, overlapping the sides where necessary. Carefully trim the top of the ham slices to make them even but leaving the ham slightly above the edge of the tin (pan).

③ Crack an egg into a bowl, then drop it into a ham-lined hollow; repeat with the remaining eggs. Bake for 10–12 minutes until the eggs are set.

④ Leave to cool slightly then lift out the "pies" with a palette knife. Leave to cool completely.

203 OMELETTE SANDWICH

MAKES 4
PREPARATION
10 minutes
COOKING
10 minutes

STORAGE
Best eaten immediately.

OMELETTE BATTER
8 eggs
a little milk or water
sea salt and black pepper to taste
oil, for frying

FILLING
2 small red onions, finely chopped
2 small red (bell) peppers, chopped
200g/7oz bacon, diced
2 tbsp hazelnut butter
4 tbsp fresh parsley, chopped
2 cloves garlic, crushed

① Mix your batter ingredients in a bowl and add the red onion and red (bell) pepper to the batter.

② Heat a little oil in a frying pan (skillet) over a medium heat and pour in a quarter of the batter. Fry for a minute or so on each side to make a thin omelette. Repeat to make four omelettes.

③ Meanwhile, in a separate pan, fry the bacon in a little oil until crisp and drain on paper towels.

④ Place two omelettes on a warmed serving plate, top with half the hot, fried bacon and cover with the other two omelettes. Spread the hazelnut butter on top, then mix the chopped parsley and garlic and sprinkle over. Serve hot with ketchup.

204 BASQUE PEPPERS with HAM and EGGS

SERVES 4
PREPARATION
5 minutes
COOKING
22 minutes

STORAGE
Best eaten immediately.

2 tbsp olive oil
500g/1lb 2oz tomatoes, chopped
1 red (bell) pepper, sliced
1 green (bell) pepper, sliced
75g/2¾oz ham, diced
200g/7oz/1⅓ cups peas
4 eggs, beaten
sea salt and black pepper to taste

1. Heat the oil in a large heavy frying pan (skillet) and gently fry the tomatoes and the (bell) peppers for 15 minutes. Add the ham and peas, cover and cook for a further 5 minutes. Add the beaten eggs to the vegetables and cook until they are scrambled (but still quite soft), and season.

2. Serve hot with toast.

205 COOL DOGS

SERVES 4
PREPARATION
10 minutes
COOKING
20 minutes

STORAGE
Cook in advance and keep in the fridge for up to 3 days. Assemble on the day. Keep chilled until ready to eat.

8 good-quality chipolata sausages or vegetarian alternative
8 tsp olive oil
2 onions, thinly sliced
4 tsp balsamic vinegar
mild mustard, for spreading
4 soft wholemeal tortillas

1. Preheat the grill (broiler) to medium–high and line the grill pan with foil. Grill (broil) the sausages for about 20 minutes, turning occasionally, until cooked through and golden.

2. Meanwhile, heat the oil in a frying pan (skillet) and fry the onion over a medium–low heat for about 10 minutes, stirring frequently. Pour in the balsamic vinegar and cook the onions for another 5–8 minutes until golden and glossy.

3. Spread a little mustard over the tortillas, then cut it in half. Divide the onions between the tortilla halves and top each one with a sausage. Fold in the rounded end of each tortilla half and roll up to encase the sausage.

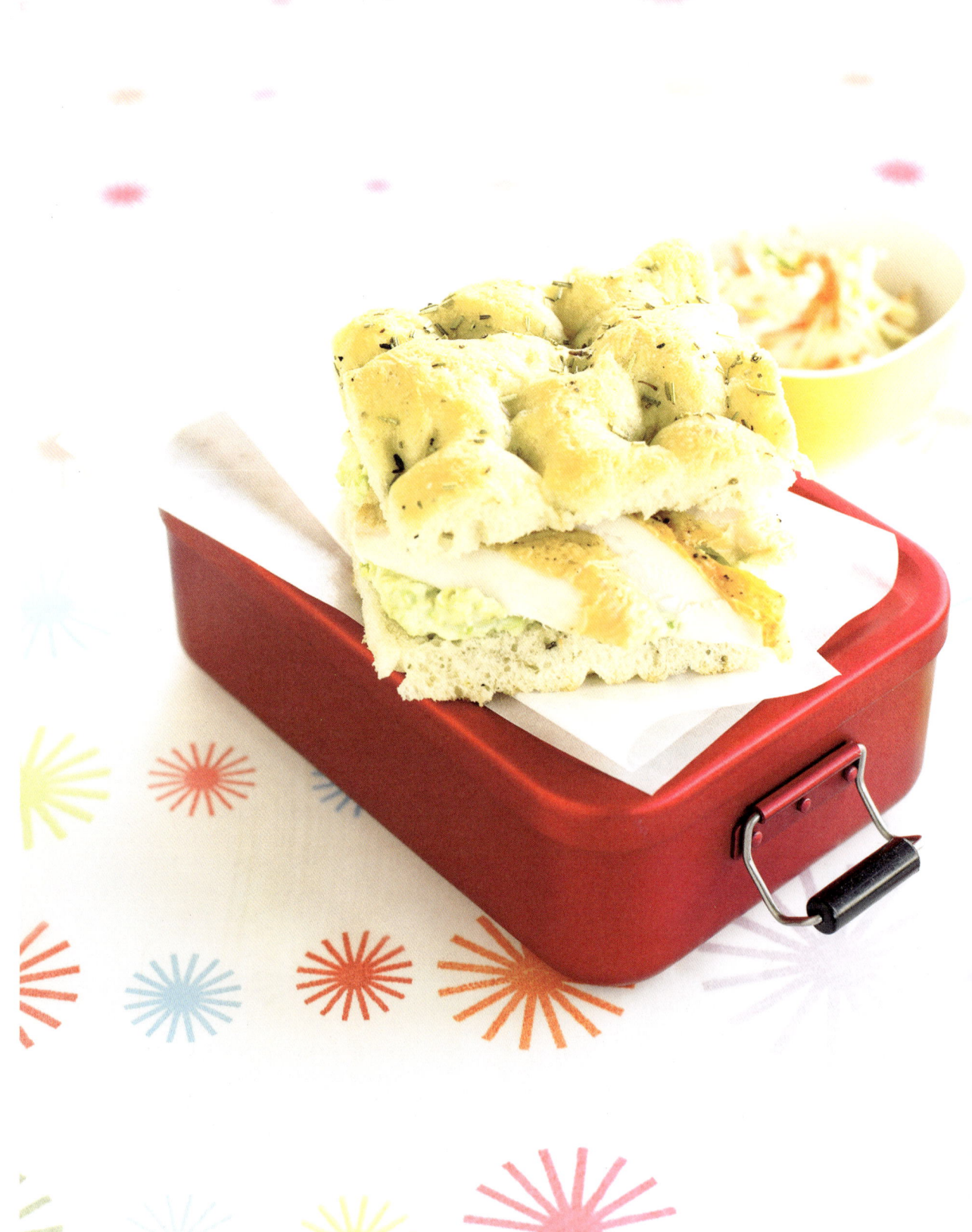

206 RICE PAPER ROLLS

MAKES 10
PREPARATION
20 minutes
COOKING
2 minutes

STORAGE
Make in advance and keep in the fridge for up to 3 days or freeze for up to 1 month. Keep chilled until ready to eat.

1-cm/½-in piece fresh ginger, peeled and grated
1 tbsp tamari, plus extra for dipping
1 tsp sesame oil
4 spring onions (scallions), shredded
1 carrot, cut into matchsticks
½ yellow (bell) pepper, sliced
20 medium rice paper wrappers
5 tbsp gluten-free hoisin sauce
55g/2oz rice vermicelli noodles, cooked
400g/14oz roast pork, sliced

1. Mix together the ginger, tamari and sesame oil in a bowl. Add the spring onions (scallions), carrot and (bell) pepper and turn to coat.

2. Fill a bowl with just-boiled water. Put two rice paper wrappers on top of one another and soak for 20 seconds or until pliable and opaque. Carefully remove using a spatula, drain for a second and place flat on a plate.

3. Spread a teaspoonful of hoisin sauce over a wrapper, then top with a bundle of noodles, a few strips of pork and a few strips of spring onion (scallion), carrot and (bell) pepper.

4. Roll the wrapper around the filling, folding in the edges to seal. Repeat using the remaining wrappers and filling ingredients. Serve with a little pot of tamari to dip into.

207 ROAST CHICKEN AND AVOCADO FOCACCIA

SERVES 4
PREPARATION
10 minutes

STORAGE
Prepare the avocado the day before and keep in the fridge overnight. Assemble on the day.

2 small avocados, pitted
4 tsp lemon juice
3 tbsp mayonnaise
salt and freshly ground black pepper
4 pieces of focaccia, about 10cm/4in square (preferably the roasted red (bell) pepper variety)
few slices roast chicken

1. Scoop the avocado out of its skin into a bowl. Mash with the lemon juice and mayonnaise. Season to taste.

2. Cut the focaccia pieces in half crossways. Spread the avocado over one half of the focaccia pieces. Top with a few slices of chicken, then the other half of the focaccia pieces.

208 GRIDDLED CHICKEN AND GUACAMOLE BAPS

SERVES 4
PREPARATION
10 minutes
COOKING
8 minutes

STORAGE
Leftovers will keep in the fridge for up to 1 day.

3 skinless, boneless chicken breast fillets
3 tbsp olive oil
1 clove garlic, crushed
$1/2$ tsp jerk seasoning
4 wholemeal baps, halved
2 tbsp soured cream

GUACAMOLE
1 avocado
$1/2$ red onion, finely chopped
1 tbsp chopped coriander (cilantro) leaves
1 tbsp lime juice
1 small tomato, deseeded and diced

1. Put the chicken between two sheets of clingfilm (plastic wrap) and flatten with a rolling pin until very thin. Remove the clingfilm (plastic wrap) and put the chicken in a dish. Mix together 2 tbsp of the oil, the garlic and jerk seasoning and pour it over the chicken. Cover and marinate in the fridge for 30 minutes.

2. To make the guacamole, halve the avocado, remove the stone and scoop the flesh into a bowl. Mash, using a fork, then mix in the remaining ingredients, cover and chill.

3. Heat the remaining oil in a griddle pan. Sear the chicken for 3–4 minutes on each side until charred and cooked through. Cool for 5 minutes, then slice thinly. Spread the guacamole on each bap base. Top with the chicken and sour cream. Replace the tops and serve.

209 CHICKEN SPRING ROLLS

SERVES 4
PREPARATION 10 minutes
COOKING 25 minutes

STORAGE Leftovers will keep in the fridge for up to 1 day.

1 tbsp olive oil, plus extra for brushing
4 spring onions (scallions), sliced
1 clove garlic, crushed
150ml/5fl oz tomato ketchup
1 tbsp honey
2 tsp molasses
2 tsp Worcestershire sauce
16 sheets of filo (phyllo) pastry, each 20cm/8in square
225g/8oz cooked chicken, shredded
2 tbsp chopped coriander (cilantro)

1. Heat the oil in a pan. Add the spring onions (scallions) and garlic and cook for 2 minutes. Stir in the ketchup, honey, molasses and Worcestershire sauce. Simmer for 2 minutes until thickened, then remove from the heat. Set aside.

2. Preheat the oven to 200°C/400°F/gas mark 6. Lay a sheet of filo (phyllo) on a board with a corner facing you. Brush all over with oil, lay another sheet on top and brush again with oil.

3. Lay a few strips of chicken towards the corner of the pastry, top with a little sauce and coriander (cilantro) and fold the corner over the filling. Brush the sides with oil and fold them over the filling, then roll up. Repeat with the remaining pastry and filling and put them on a baking sheet.

4. Brush with oil and bake for 15–20 minutes until golden and crisp. Serve hot or cold.

210 CHICKEN DIPPERS WITH PEANUT SAUCE

SERVES 4
PREPARATION 5 minutes
COOKING 10 minutes

STORAGE You can refrigerate the satay sauce for up to a month.

220g/8oz/1⅓ cups basmati rice
2 tsp turmeric
100g/4oz/1⅓ cups raisins
4 chicken breasts, cubed
220g/8oz/1 cup peanut butter
4 tbsp olive oil

1. Half fill a small pan with boiling water, then add the rice, turmeric and raisins. Simmer, covered, for 10 minutes until the rice is cooked. Drain and let cool.

2. Preheat the grill (broiler). Spear the chicken onto eight skewers and grill (broil) for 8–10 minutes, turning frequently until golden.

3. Mix the peanut butter and olive oil with a fork. Serve the rice topped with the chicken skewers, and with the sauce on the side for dipping.

211 CHICKEN NOODLE NEST

SERVES 4
PREPARATION
10 minutes
COOKING
5 minutes

STORAGE
You can refrigerate for up to a day and then reheat.

1 tbsp olive oil
2 chicken breasts, sliced
1 tsp chopped fresh ginger
115g/4oz/½ cup mangetout (snow peas)
115g/4oz/½ cup chopped cabbage
115g/4oz udon noodles
1 lemongrass stalk, sliced
6 spring onions (scallions), sliced
2 star anise, chopped
3 tbsp sweet chilli sauce
3 tbsp tamari
25g/1oz/⅓ cup chopped coriander (cilantro)

1. Heat the oil in a wok, add the chicken and fry lightly until cooked. Then add the ginger, mangetout (snow peas), cabbage greens, noodles and lemongrass and stir-fry for 2–3 minutes.

2. Add the spring onions (scallions), star anise and sauces and fry for another minute. If the mixture is too dry, add extra tamari.

3. Remove from the heat and serve on plates garnished with the chopped coriander (cilantro).

212 CHICKEN TIKKA NAAN

SERVES 2–4
PREPARATION
15 minutes + marinating
COOKING
4 minutes

STORAGE
Prepare the chicken and keep in the fridge for up to 3 days or freeze for up to 1 month. Assemble on the day. Keep chilled until ready to eat.

4 small chicken breasts, sliced
olive oil, for brushing
4 small naan breads
crisp salad leaves

MARINADE
175g/6oz/¾ cup thick plain yogurt
4 cloves garlic, crushed
4 tbsp tikka curry paste

YOGURT SAUCE
4 tbsp thick plain yogurt
4 tsp chopped fresh mint

1. Mix together the ingredients for the marinade in a shallow dish. Add the chicken strips and spoon over the marinade to coat. Leave in the fridge for 1 hour, or overnight.

2. Preheat the grill (broiler) to medium-high and line a grill pan with foil. Brush the foil with olive oil and place the chicken on top. Grill (broil) for 3–4 minutes on each side until cooked through. Leave to cool.

3. Mix together the yogurt and mint. Split the naan in half, leaving one side attached. Place the chicken in the naan, followed by a few lettuce leaves, then spoon over the yogurt sauce and close up.

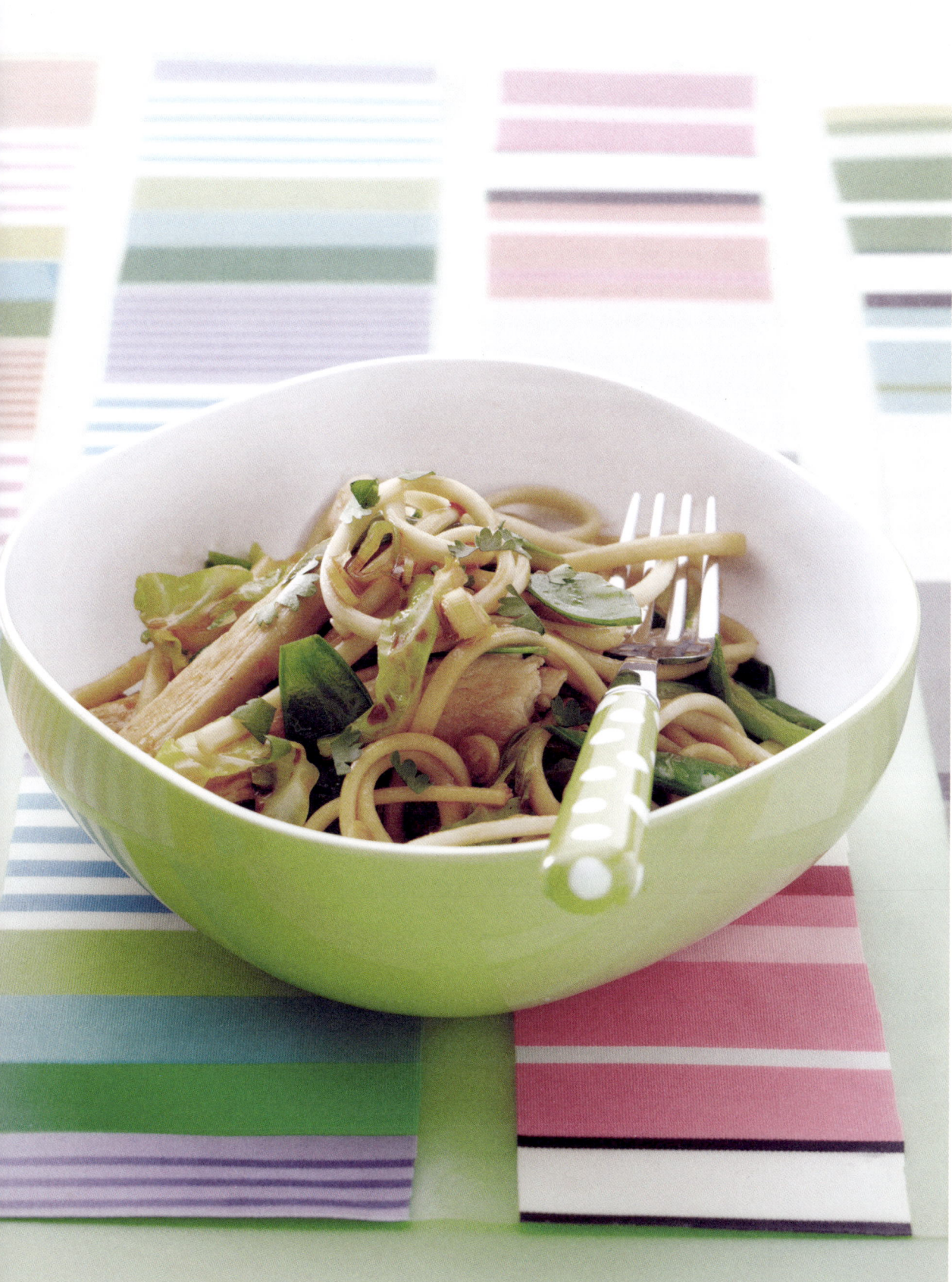

213 CHICKEN STRIPS with SATAY DIP

SERVES 4
PREPARATION 10 minutes
COOKING 6 minutes

STORAGE Make in advance, and keep the dip in the fridge for up to 1 week and the chicken for up to 3 days.

4 tbsp olive oil
4 tsp paprika
540g/19oz chicken breasts, sliced

SATAY DIP
110g/4oz/½ cup peanut butter
4 tsp olive oil
4 tsp tamari
2 tsp soft light brown sugar
4 tbsp reduced-fat coconut milk

1. Put the oil in a shallow dish; add the paprika and then the chicken. Turn the chicken in the oil to coat.

2. To make the satay dip, mix together all the ingredients with 1 tbsp hot water in a bowl. Set aside.

3. Heat a large frying pan (skillet) and fry the chicken for about 2–3 minutes on each side until golden and cooked through. Leave to cool.

4. Serve the strips dipped into the satay sauce.

214 MOROCCAN TURKEY WRAPS

SERVES 2-4
PREPARATION 15 minutes + marinating
COOKING 11 minutes

STORAGE Leftovers will keep in the fridge for up to 1 day.

400g/14oz turkey breast, sliced
juice and zest of 1 lemon
¼ tsp turmeric
½ tsp each ground cumin, paprika, ground coriander
3 tbsp olive oil
100g/3½oz cherry tomatoes, quartered
1 roasted red (bell) pepper in oil, drained and sliced
4 large soft tortilla wraps
150ml/5fl oz/⅔ cup plain yogurt
2 tbsp chopped coriander (cilantro)
½ Cos lettuce, shredded

1. Put the turkey in a shallow bowl. Mix together the lemon juice, zest, spices and 2 tbsp of the oil. Pour over the turkey, cover and marinate for at least 20 minutes.

2. Heat the remaining oil in a non-stick frying pan (skillet) and cook the turkey for 6–8 minutes, stirring until golden brown. Add the tomatoes; cook for a further 1–2 minutes to soften. Remove from the heat; stir in the (bell) pepper.

3. Heat the wraps according to the package instructions. Mix the yogurt and coriander (cilantro) in a bowl. Divide the turkey and lettuce among the wraps and add a little of the yogurt. Fold over the wraps and roll up. Serve with the remaining yogurt alongside.

215 FESTIVE TURKEY BALLS

MAKES 16
PREPARATION
10 minutes
COOKING
20 minutes

STORAGE
Make in advance and keep in the fridge for up to 3 days or freeze for up to 1 month (unless the turkey was frozen). Keep chilled until ready to eat.

140g/5oz good-quality organic stuffing mix
40g/1½oz unsalted butter
400g/14oz turkey breast, diced
olive oil, for brushing

1. Preheat the oven to 200°C/400°F/Gas 6. Make up the stuffing mix with 300ml/10fl oz/1⅓ cups just-boiled water and the butter, following the package instructions. Put the turkey in a food processor and process until very finely chopped. Add the stuffing mix and blend until combined.

2. Roll the mixture into eight balls slightly larger than a walnut and place in an oiled baking tin (pan). Brush the balls with oil, then bake in the oven for about 20 minutes, turning occasionally, until golden and cooked through.

216 TOWERING TURKEY BAGELS

MAKES 16
PREPARATION
10 minutes
COOKING
10 minutes

STORAGE
Refrigerate for up to 1 day.

2 turkey breasts, about 230g/8oz
4 sesame or wholemeal bagels
4 tbsp cranberry sauce
4 handfuls rocket (arugula)
4 sprigs coriander (cilantro)
4 tbsp mayonnaise
4 spring onions (scallions)

1. Preheat the grill (broiler) to high. Place the turkey breasts on a grill pan and grill (broil) for 10 minutes, turning occasionally. Remove from the heat, cool and slice thinly. Cut the bagels in half and toast lightly.

2. Spread one half of each bagel liberally with cranberry sauce. Place the turkey on top and cover with a handful of rocket (arugula) and a sprig of coriander (cilantro). Spread mayonnaise on the other four halves.

3. Cut the spring onions (scallions) into four pieces, then again in half lengthways. Lay these on top of the rocket (arugula). Sandwich the bagel slices together, cut in half and serve.

217 SMOKED SALMON PATE

SERVES 6
PREPARATION
10 minutes

STORAGE
Make in advance and keep in the fridge for up to 3 days.

175g/6oz smoked salmon pieces
juice of ½ lemon, or to taste
100g/3½oz low-fat cream cheese
½ tsp paprika
freshly ground black pepper

1. Put the salmon, lemon juice, cream cheese and paprika into a blender or food processor. Process until smooth and creamy. Season with pepper to taste.

2. Transfer to a bowl, cover and put in the fridge until ready to serve.

218 SUSHI CONES

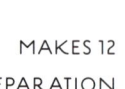

MAKES 12
PREPARATION
25 minutes
COOKING
15 minutes

STORAGE
Make the day before and keep in the fridge overnight.

200g/7oz/1 cup sushi rice
3 tbsp rice vinegar
1 tsp caster (superfine) sugar
½ tsp salt
6 sheets nori
4 tbsp mayonnaise
8 pea-sized amounts wasabi
160g/5½oz hot-smoked trout or salmon, in large flakes
large handful rocket (arugula)
12 thin sticks cucumber, deseeded, 5cm/2in long
tamari and pickled ginger, to serve (optional)

1. Put the rice and 340ml/12fl oz/1½ cups water in a saucepan. Bring to the boil, reduce to a simmer, cover and cook for 12–15 minutes until the water is absorbed. Leave for 5 minutes, covered.

2. Meanwhile, mix together the rice vinegar, sugar and salt. Transfer the rice to a bowl to cool, then gently stir in the rice vinegar mixture using a wooden spoon. Leave to cool.

3. Cut the nori sheets into twelve 10-cm/4-in squares. Mix the mayonnaise and wasabi and smear over each square.

4. Place 2 teaspoons of rice diagonally down the middle of each square. On top lay a few flakes of trout or salmon, a few rocket (arugula) leaves and a stick of cucumber. Wet one edge of the nori and roll into a cone shape; press the edge to seal.

5. Serve with tamari and pickled ginger, if liked.

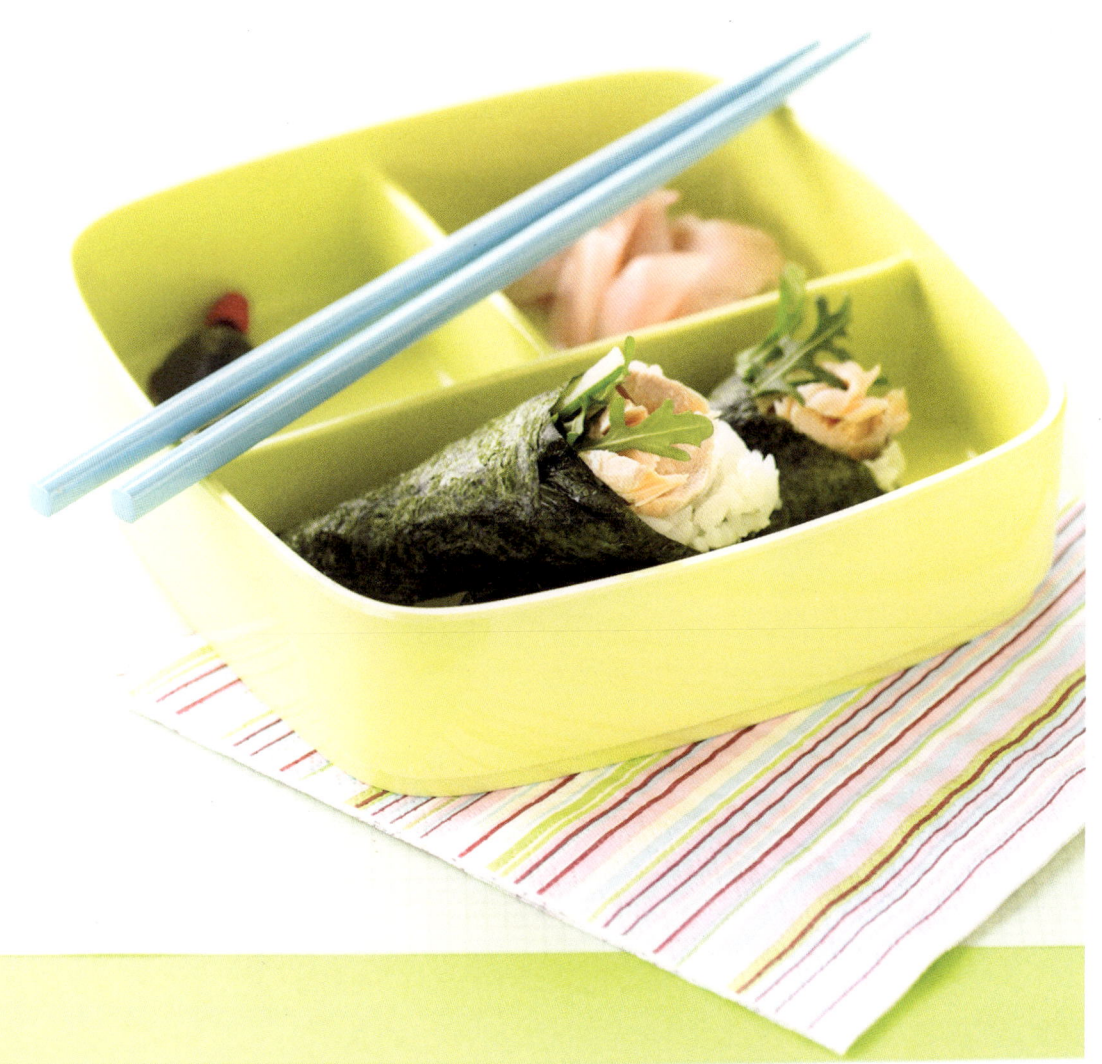

219 SALMON AND CORIANDER FISHCAKES

SERVES 2-4
PREPARATION 5 minutes
COOKING 50 minutes

STORAGE
You can freeze the raw mixture and use it within a month.

500g/1lb 2oz potatoes, peeled and chopped
4 salmon steaks, about 85g/3oz each
1 tbsp olive oil
4 spring onions (scallions), chopped
1 leek, trimmed and sliced
3 tbsp wholegrain mustard
1 tbsp sweet chilli sauce, plus extra for serving

1 Half fill a saucepan with water, bring to the boil and add the potatoes. Cover and let simmer for 15–20 minutes, until soft. Drain and mash. Cook the salmon steaks under a medium grill (broiler) for 10 minutes, turning frequently. When cooked, remove any skin and break into flakes.

2 Preheat the oven to 220°C/425°F/gas mark 7. Heat the oil in a frying pan (skillet), add the spring onions (scallions) and leek and sauté for 3 minutes until soft. Add these to the mash, together with the salmon flakes, mustard and sweet chilli sauce and stir.

3 Use your hands to mould the mixture into 8 fishcakes and place on a non-stick baking sheet. Put in the oven and cook for 20 minutes or until golden brown. Remove and serve with extra-sweet chilli sauce.

220 CREAMY SALMON AND ALFALFA PITTAS

SERVES 2–4
PREPARATION
10 minutes

STORAGE
The filling can be made in advance and stored in the fridge for up to 2 days.

6 small gherkins, finely chopped
175ml/5½fl oz/scant ¾ cup crème fraîche
2 tbsp chopped parsley
2 tbsp chopped dill
2 tsp lemon juice
210g/7½oz canned skinless, boneless salmon, drained
4 wholemeal pitta breads, halved crossways
large handful of alfalfa sprouts
freshly ground black pepper

1. Mix the gherkins, crème fraîche, parsley, dill and lemon juice in a bowl and season with black pepper to taste.

2. Flake the salmon into the herb mixture and mix well.

3. Spoon the salmon mixture into the pitta bread halves, top with alfalfa sprouts and serve.

221 SARDINES AND TOMATO ON BROWN

SERVES 2–4
PREPARATION
10 minutes

STORAGE
Make on the day. Keep chilled until ready to eat.

480g/12oz canned sardines in olive oil, drained
4 tomatoes, seeded and finely chopped
4 tsp mayonnaise
2 tsp grain or mild mustard
8 slices wholemeal bread (toasted if preferred)

1. Put the sardines in a bowl and mash with a fork. Add the tomato and mix with the sardines.

2. Mix together the mayonnaise and mustard and spread over half the bread slices. Spoon on the sardines and tomato, and place the other slices of bread on top. Cut into triangles.

222 FIGHTING FIT FAJITAS

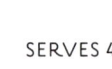

SERVES 4
PREPARATION 10 minutes

STORAGE You can store the mixture in the fridge for up to 3 days.

- 150g/5½oz canned tuna (in olive oil), drained
- 200-g/7-oz can kidney beans
- 110g/4oz sweetcorn
- 4 spring onions (scallions), chopped
- 1 red (bell) pepper, deseeded and chopped
- 4 tbsp mayonnaise
- pinch of chilli powder
- 230g/8oz/⅔ cup rocket (arugula)
- 4 tortilla wraps

1. Place the tuna into a small bowl and mash.

2. Add all the remaining ingredients except the rocket (arugula) and tortillas and stir together well.

3. Lay out the tortillas and place half the rocket (arugula) in the middle of each one and spoon 3 tablespoons of the mixture on top of the rocket (arugula). Roll tightly into wraps.

223 TUNA MELTS

SERVES 2–4
PREPARATION 10 minutes
COOKING 5 minutes

STORAGE Refrigerate and eat cold later the same day if you wish.

- 4 wholemeal pitta breads
- 2 x 150-g/5½-oz cans tuna (in olive oil), drained
- 6 spring onions (scallions), chopped
- ½ tsp cayenne pepper
- 25g/1oz/⅓ cup chopped parsley
- 115g/4oz/⅔ cup goat's cheese

1. Preheat the grill (broiler) to medium. Cut the pittas in half, then place under the grill (broiler) for a minute until lightly toasted.

2. In a mixing bowl, add the tuna, spring onions (scallions), cayenne pepper and parsley. Mix together well with a fork and then spoon the tuna mixture equally into each pitta bread.

3. Crumble the goat's cheese into a small bowl and fill each pitta with an equal amount. Place the pittas on the grill pan, cook until the cheese has melted, and serve.

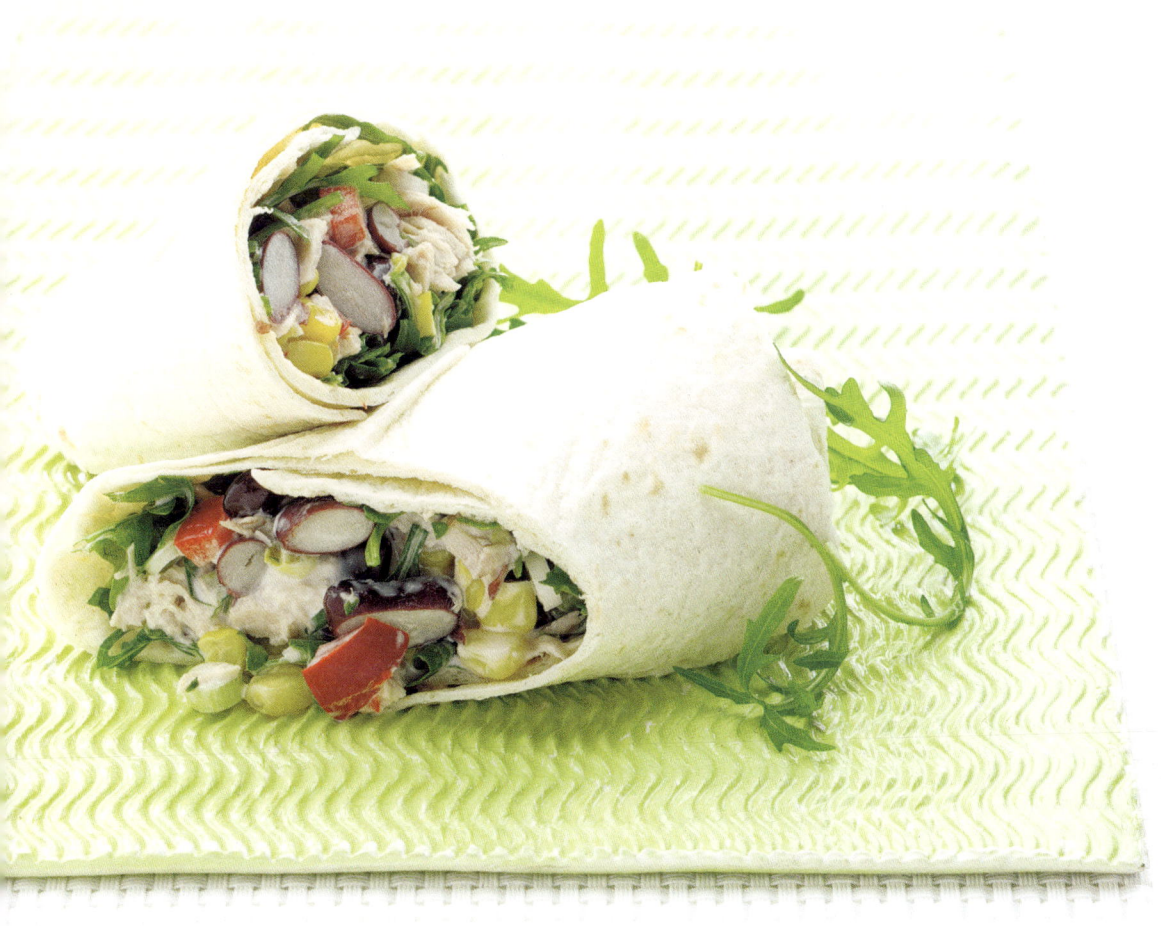

224 SARDINE BRUSCHETTA with HERB DRESSING

SERVES 4
PREPARATION 15 minutes
COOKING 12 minutes

STORAGE
Prepare the dressing in advance and keep it in an airtight container in the fridge for up to 2 days. The bruschetta are best eaten immediately.

400g/14oz canned sardines in olive oil
12 cherry tomatoes, halved
8 slices ciabatta

HERB DRESSING
1 clove garlic, crushed
grated zest of 1 lemon
3 tbsp lemon juice
15g/½oz parsley, chopped
5 tbsp omega oil or flaxseed oil
freshly ground black pepper

1. Preheat the oven to 200°C/400°F/gas mark 6. Drain the sardines, reserving 1 tablespoon of the oil, and put in a bowl. Put the tomatoes on a baking sheet, drizzle with the reserved oil and bake for 10 minutes until slightly softened.

2. Mix the dressing ingredients in a bowl and season with black pepper. Reserve 2 tablespoons of the dressing, then pour the rest over the sardines and break them up with a fork.

3. Add the tomatoes to the sardines and mix gently.

4. Lightly toast the ciabatta. Drizzle with the reserved dressing, spoon on the sardine mixture and serve immediately.

225 SARDINE SOLDIERS

SERVES 4
PREPARATION 5 minutes
COOKING 5 minutes

STORAGE
Refrigerate for up to 12 hours in airtight container.

8 slices wholegrain bread
100g/3½oz canned sardines in tomato sauce
50g/2oz/⅔ cup chopped parsley and 8 whole sprigs parsley

1. Preheat the grill (broiler) to medium and lightly toast the bread. Butter one side and cut each slice into two triangles.

2. In a small bowl, add the sardines and chopped parsley and mash together with a fork. Spread the sardine mixture equally onto the pieces of toast.

3. Return the toast to the grill pan and cook under the grill (broiler) for 5 minutes until the tops brown. Serve on individual plates garnished with the parsley sprigs.

226 TUNA PATTIES

MAKES 6
PREPARATION 10 minutes + chilling
COOKING 12 minutes

STORAGE Make in advance and keep in the fridge for up to 3 days or freeze for up to 1 month. Keep chilled until ready to eat.

2 slices day-old wholemeal bread
200g/7oz canned tuna
1 small onion, grated
1 tsp dried oregano
1 tbsp plain (all-purpose) flour, plus extra for dusting
1 small egg, beaten
salt and freshly ground black pepper
2 tbsp sunflower oil

1. Place the bread in a food processor and process to crumbs. Transfer to a mixing bowl with the tuna, onion, oregano, flour and egg. Season and chill for 1 hour.

2. Lightly cover a plate and your hands in flour. Divide the tuna mixture into six and form into pattie shapes, then dust with more flour.

3. Heat half of the oil in a frying pan (skillet) and cook three of the patties for about 3 minutes on each side until golden, then drain on paper towels. Repeat with the remaining patties, adding more oil if necessary. Serve immediately or leave to cool before packing in an airtight container, placing a sheet of baking paper between each pattie.

227 TUNA AND ONION TORTILLA

SERVES 4-6
PREPARATION 10 minutes
COOKING 17 minutes

STORAGE Make in advance and keep in the fridge for up to 3 days. Keep chilled until ready to eat.

1 tbsp olive oil
1 large onion, sliced
200g/7oz canned tuna, drained
450g/1lb cooked potatoes, peeled and diced
6 eggs, beaten
salt and freshly ground black pepper

1. Heat the oil in a medium frying pan (skillet) with a heatproof handle, then fry the onion for 8 minutes until softened and slightly golden. Stir in the tuna, retaining some chunks, then top with the potatoes, spreading the ingredients evenly.

2. Preheat the grill (broiler) to medium. Season the eggs and pour them into the pan. Cook for 5 minutes over a medium heat until the base is golden and set.

3. Place the pan under the grill (broiler) and cook the tortilla for about 3 minutes until set. Cool, then cut into wedges.

228 TUNA and CHEESE CALZONE

SERVES 4
PREPARATION 20 minutes + proving
COOKING 17 minutes
STORAGE Leftovers will keep in the fridge for up to 1 day.

125g/4½oz/scant 1 cup strong white bread flour
100g/3½oz/¾ cup strong wholemeal bread flour
1 tsp fast-acting dried yeast
125ml/4fl oz/½ cup warm milk
1 tbsp olive oil

FILLING
175g/6oz baby spinach leaves
225g/8oz ricotta cheese
200g/7oz canned tuna in oil or spring water, drained
pinch of freshly grated nutmeg
freshly ground black pepper

1. Put the flours in a bowl with the yeast. Add the milk and oil and mix to form a dough.

2. Knead for 10 minutes. Put in a clean bowl, cover and leave to rise for 1 hour.

3. Preheat the oven to 200°C/400°F/gas mark 6. Put the spinach in a pan with 1 tbsp water and cook for 2 minutes, or until wilted. Drain well, then put in a bowl with the rest of the filling ingredients.

4. Knock back the dough and divide it into 4 pieces. Roll each piece into a 16cm/6¼in round. Put a quarter of the mixture on half of each round, brush the edges with water and fold over to enclose. Pinch the dough together to seal. Brush the tops with oil.

5. Bake for 10–15 minutes until golden, then serve.

229 STUFFED AVOCADOS

SERVES 4
PREPARATION 15 minutes
STORAGE Best eaten immediately.

4 avocados, halved and pitted
1 banana, peeled and diced
4 tbsp lemon juice
½ small onion, finely chopped
1 green chilli, finely chopped
2 tomatoes, finely chopped
1 tsp paprika
sea salt and cayenne pepper to taste
200g/7oz cooked peeled prawns (shrimp), or 100g/3½oz Brazil nuts, chopped

1. Scoop out the avocado flesh and place it in a bowl. Add the banana, lemon juice, onion, chilli, tomato and paprika. Gently mix and season with salt and cayenne pepper.

2. Spoon the mixture back into the avocado shells, garnish with prawns (shrimp) or Brazil nuts and serve immediately.

230 PRAWN AND MANGO TARTS

MAKES 8
PREPARATION
15 minutes
COOKING
14 minutes

STORAGE
Prepare the prawn (shrimp) and mango mixture in advance and store it in the fridge to fill the tarts just before serving. Do not fill the tarts in advance.

4 tbsp olive oil, plus extra for greasing
8 sheets of filo (phyllo) pastry, each 20cm/8in square
150g/5½oz peeled raw prawns (shrimp)
2 tbsp macadamia nuts, toasted and chopped
1 small mango, peeled and diced
2 roasted red (bell) peppers in oil, drained
1 tbsp sweet chilli sauce
2 tsp tamari
1 tbsp omega or flaxseed oil
1 tsp lime juice

1. Preheat the oven to 200°C/400°F/gas mark 6 and grease eight cups in a muffin tin (pan) with oil. Reserve 1 tablespoon of the oil.

2. Brush 1 sheet of filo (phyllo) lightly with some of the remaining olive oil. Top with another sheet, brush again with oil and cut into 2 double-thick squares to line the muffin cups. Repeat with the remaining pastry and oil.

3. Bake the tarts for 8–10 minutes until crisp and golden. Turn out carefully onto a wire rack to cool.

4. Heat the reserved oil in a frying pan (skillet) and fry the prawns (shrimp) for 2 minutes on each side until pink. Put in a bowl with the nuts and mango.

5. Purée the remaining ingredients in a blender, then stir into the prawn (shrimp) mixture. Spoon the filling into the tarts and serve immediately.

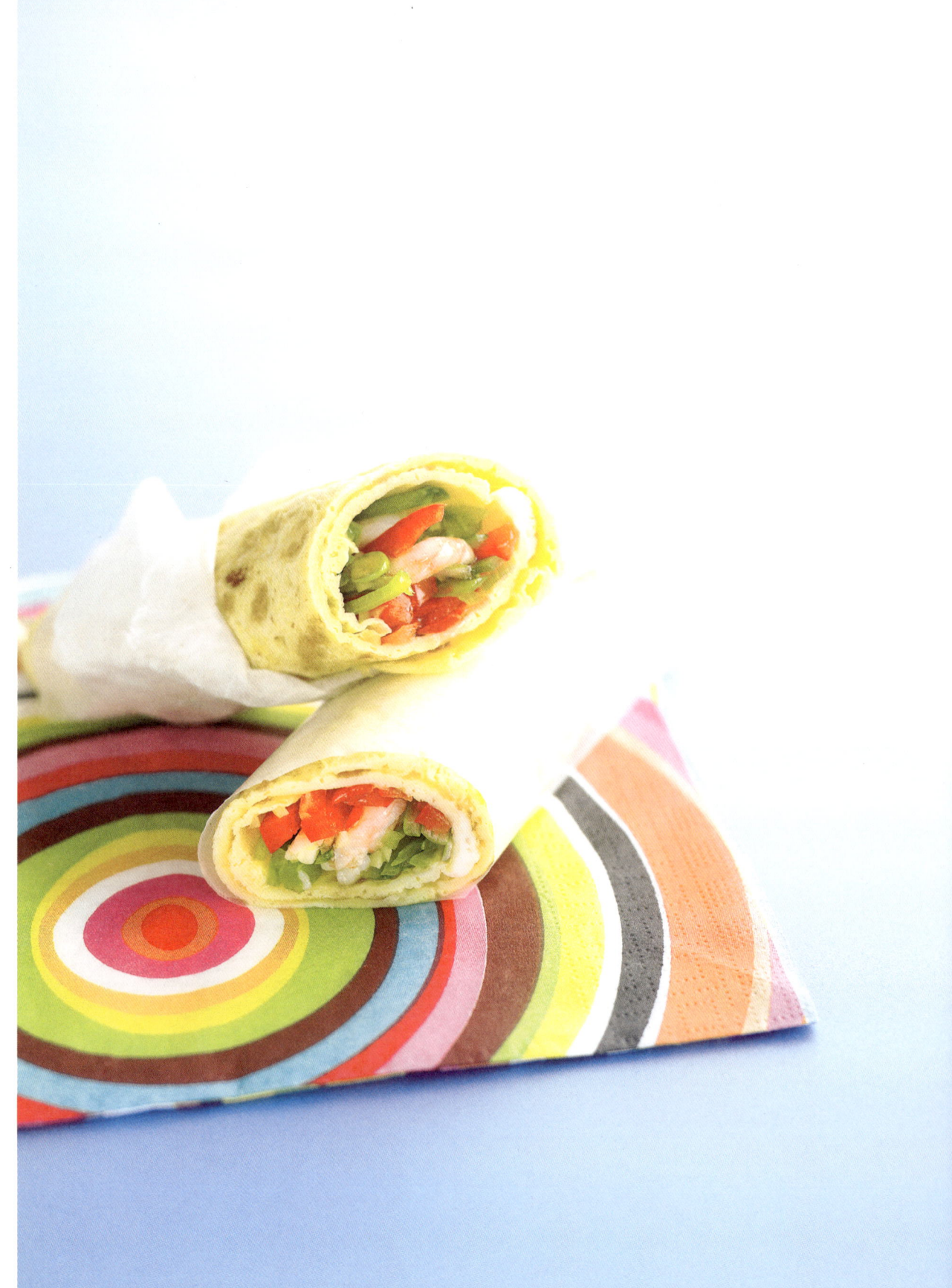

231 PRAWN OMELETTE WRAPS

SERVES 4
PREPARATION 10 minutes
COOKING 12 minutes

STORAGE Make the omelettes the day before, wrap and keep flat in the fridge overnight. Assemble on the day.

4 tsp sunflower oil
8 eggs, lightly beaten
4 spring onions (scallions), cut into long, thin strips
1 red (bell) pepper, seeded and cut into thin strips
8 sugar snap peas, sliced diagonally lengthways
220g/4oz small cooked prawns (shrimp) (optional)
4-cm/2-in piece fresh ginger, peeled and grated
1 tsp toasted sesame oil
4 tsp tamari

1. Heat 1 teaspoon of oil in a frying pan (skillet). Pour a quarter of the beaten egg into the pan and swirl around so that it covers the bottom. When the egg begins to set, draw the edges towards the middle using a wooden spoon, allowing the raw egg to run into the space. Cook for about 2 minutes until the egg is set. Slide the omelette on to a plate and leave to cool. Repeat to make 4 omelettes.

2. Put the spring onions (scallions), red (bell) pepper, sugar snap peas, prawns (shrimp), if using, and ginger in a bowl. Pour the sesame oil and tamari over them and toss until they are coated.

3. Arrange the vegetables and prawns (shrimp) down the middle of the omelettes, then roll up and cut in half.

232 HONG KONG PRAWNS

SERVES 4
PREPARATION 5 minutes
COOKING 6 minutes

STORAGE Leftovers will keep in the fridge for up to 1 day.

1 tbsp olive oil
1cm/½in fresh ginger, grated
1 clove garlic, crushed
1 carrot, cut into matchsticks
1 red (bell) pepper, cut into strips
20 king prawns (jumbo shrimp), peeled and deveined
3 tbsp tamarind
2 tbsp gluten-free oyster sauce
2 tbsp Chinese rice wine
2 tbsp chopped coriander (cilantro)

1. Heat a wok over a medium heat. Add the oil and stir-fry the ginger, garlic, carrot and pepper for 1 minute, then add the prawns (shrimp) and fry for 1 minute more.

2. Stir in the tamarind, oyster sauce and rice wine, and cook for 3-4 minutes until the prawns (shrimp) are cooked and turn pink.

3. Sprinkle with the coriander (cilantro) and serve.

233 NIÇOISE WRAPS

SERVES 4
PREPARATION
10 minutes
COOKING
10 minutes

STORAGE
You can refrigerate the wraps for up to a day.

3 eggs, boiled for 8 minutes, then peeled and sliced
1 red onion, peeled and sliced
175g/6oz/¾ cup alfalfa sprouts
2 x 150-g/5¾-oz cans tuna
200-g/7-oz can sweetcorn
2 Little Gem lettuces, chopped
3 tbsp olive oil
1 tbsp wholegrain mustard
1 tbsp runny honey
8 tortilla wraps

1) In a mixing bowl, place the egg slices, red onion, alfalfa sprouts, tuna, sweetcorn and lettuce and stir together well.

2) In a small bowl, whisk together the olive oil, mustard and honey. Pour over the tuna mixture and stir together. Lay out the tortillas and pile the mixture equally into the middle of each one and roll tightly into wraps.

234 VEGETABLE SAMOSAS

MAKES 10
PREPARATION
15 minutes + 6 hours soaking
COOKING
20 minutes

STORAGE
Make in advance and keep in the fridge for up to 3 days or freeze for up to 1 month.

1 tbsp vegetable oil, plus extra
1 onion, finely chopped
1 carrot, diced
2 large cloves garlic, finely chopped
1 tbsp grated fresh ginger
2 tsp garam masala
¼ tsp chilli powder (optional)
250g/9oz cooked new potatoes, diced
3 tbsp frozen petits pois
salt and freshly ground black pepper
6 sheets filo (phyllo) pastry

1) Heat the oil in a frying pan (skillet) and fry the onion for 3 minutes, then add the carrot and cook for another 4 minutes. Add the garlic, ginger and spices and cook for 1 more minute.

2) Stir in the potatoes, peas and 4 tablespoons of water, cover and simmer for 5 minutes. Place in a bowl to cool. Preheat the oven to 190°C/375°F/gas mark 5.

3) Grease two baking sheets. Take three sheets of filo (phyllo) pastry and place on top of one another. Cut five 15cm/6in rounds and place on a baking sheet. Repeat.

4) Place a tablespoon of filling in the middle of one round, wet the edge of the pastry and fold over to make a half-moon shape, sealing the edges well. Brush with oil.

5) Repeat to make 10 samosas. Bake for 15 minutes until golden.

235 SPANISH OMELETTE

SERVES 4
PREPARATION
10 minutes
COOKING
20 minutes

STORAGE
Best eaten immediately.

OMELETTE
8 eggs
2 small yellow courgettes (zucchini), grated

FILLING
olive oil for frying
2 red (bell) peppers, deseeded and diced
2 tomatoes, chopped
2 cloves garlic, crushed
1 large handful parsley, finely chopped
sea salt and black pepper to taste

1) Beat the eggs in a bowl and add the grated courgette (zucchini).

2) Stir-fry the filling ingredients in a large frying pan (skillet) with a little oil for 3 minutes, then add to the batter, and season.

3) Add a little more oil to the pan and pour in the mixture. Turn down the heat and leave the mixture to cook very slowly for 10 minutes. Turn and cook over a medium heat for a further 5–7 minutes. Serve with spicy tomato sauce.

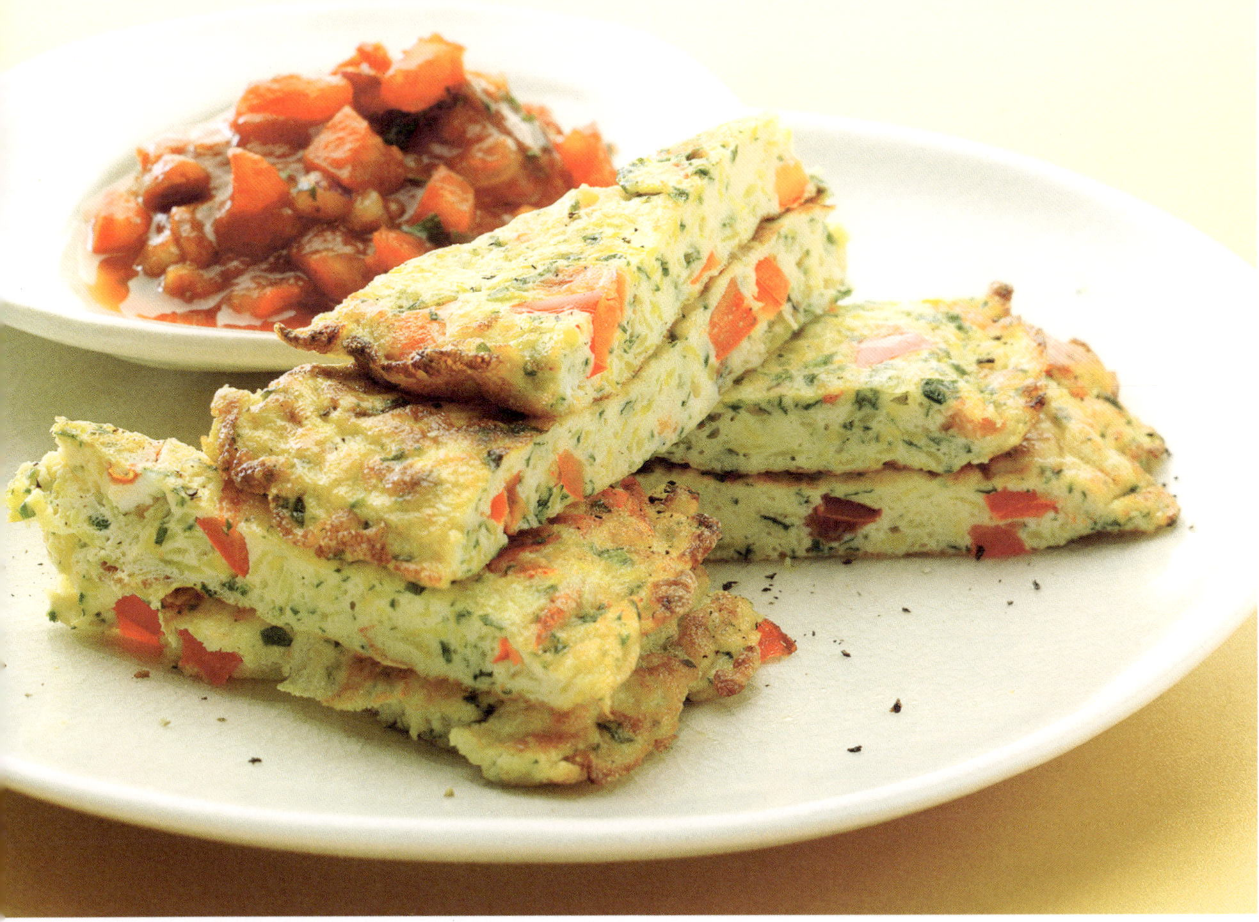

236 MYSTERY ROLL

SERVES 4
PREPARATION 15 minutes
STORAGE Make the day before and keep in the fridge overnight.

4 crusty rolls
olive oil, for brushing
4–8 tbsp pesto
4 small cloves garlic, crushed
12 slices mozzarella cheese
4 tomatoes, deseeded and sliced
4 handfuls baby spinach leaves

1. Slice off the top of the rolls to make lids and pull out the soft insides, leaving the crusts intact. Lightly brush the inside with oil.

2. Put the bread in a processor and pulse to crumbs. Transfer to a bowl and stir in sufficient pesto to flavour the breadcrumbs without making them soggy, and the garlic.

3. Spoon a layer of the breadcrumbs into the roll. Add a layer of mozzarella, tomato and spinach followed by the rest of the breadcrumbs and the remaining mozzarella, tomato and spinach. Place the lid on top and wrap tightly. Press down lightly.

237 SALMON, MANGO AND ASPARAGUS SALAD

SERVES 4
PREPARATION 10 minutes
COOKING 8 minutes
STORAGE Prepare and cook the tofu in advance and keep chilled for up to 3 days. Assemble on the day.

250g/9oz firm tofu, patted dry and cut into 8 long slices
olive oil, for brushing
4 small baguettes
4 lettuce leaves, shredded
4 tomatoes, seeded and thinly sliced

MARINADE
2 tbsp clear honey
2 tbsp tomato ketchup
2 tbsp soy sauce
1/2 tsp smoked paprika (optional)

1. In a shallow dish, mix together the ingredients for the marinade. Place the tofu slices in the dish with the marinade. Spoon the marinade over the tofu so it is well coated. Leave to marinate for at least 1 hour or overnight.

2. Generously brush a griddle pan with olive oil, then heat until hot. Carefully put the tofu slices in the pan and cook for 4 minutes on each side until golden, occasionally spooning over more of the marinade.

3. Slice the baguettes lengthways and open them out. Place two of the tofu slices in each baguette and top with the lettuce and tomato. Close up the baguettes and press down lightly.

LUNCH | 175

238 TOFU BITES

SERVES 4
PREPARATION
10 minutes + marinating
COOKING
20 minutes

STORAGE
Make in advance and keep in the fridge for up to 3 days.

4 tbsp black bean sauce
1 tbsp clear honey
1 tbsp soy sauce
2 tsp sesame oil
225g/8oz firm tofu, patted dry and cut into 2-cm/¾-in cubes
sunflower oil, for brushing

(1) Mix together the black bean sauce, honey, soy sauce and sesame oil in a shallow dish. Add the tofu and spoon the marinade over until the tofu is completely covered. Leave to marinate for 1 hour, turning the tofu occasionally.

(2) Preheat the oven to 180°C/350°F/gas mark 4. Lightly brush a roasting tin (pan) with oil. Arrange the tofu in the tin (pan) and roast for 20 minutes, turning halfway, until golden and slightly crisp all over.

239 KOFTA PITTA POCKETS

MAKES 12 KOFTA (SERVES 2-3)
PREPARATION
20 minutes
COOKING
10 minutes

STORAGE
Make the kofta in advance and keep in the fridge for up to 3 days or freeze for up to 1 month. Assemble on the day. Keep chilled until ready to eat.

4 wholemeal pittas
4 tbsp Roasted Aubergine (Eggplant) Dip (see page 51)
salad leaves and sliced tomato

KOFTA
225g/8oz minced (ground) lamb
1 shallot, grated
1 clove garlic, crushed
¼ tsp ground cinnamon
1 tsp ground cumin
½ tsp ground coriander
olive oil, for brushing
salt and freshly ground black pepper

(1) Put the lamb in a mixing bowl and break it up with a fork. Add the shallot, garlic and spices, season and mix well.

(2) Preheat the grill (broiler) to medium. Shape the lamb mixture into 12 walnut-sized balls. Line a grill pan with foil and lightly brush with oil. Grill (broil) the kofta for 8-10 minutes, until golden.

(3) Warm the pittas slightly, then cut in half to make two pockets. Spread a little Roasted Aubergine Dip inside each pocket.

(4) Place a few salad leaves and slices of tomato in each pocket, followed by one or two kofta, which can be left whole or cut in half for easier eating.

240 FALAFEL

MAKES 12
PREPARATION
15 minutes + chilling
COOKING
20 minutes

STORAGE
Make in advance and keep in the fridge for up to 5 days or freeze for up to 1 month.

400-g/14-oz can chickpeas (garbanzo beans), drained and rinsed
3 spring onions (scallions), finely chopped
2 cloves garlic, crushed
1 tsp ground cumin
1 tsp ground coriander
1-2 tbsp chopped mint (optional)
1 small egg, lightly beaten
salt and freshly ground black pepper
plain (all-purpose) flour, for dusting
sunflower oil, for frying

1. Put the chickpeas (garbanzo beans), spring onions (scallions), garlic, cumin, coriander and mint, if using, in a food processor and pulse until the chickpeas (garbanzo beans) are roughly chopped. Add the egg and seasoning and blend until the mixture forms a coarse paste. Chill for 1 hour to allow the mixture to firm up.

2. Form the chickpea mixture into 12 walnut-sized balls using floured hands, then lightly dust each ball in flour.

3. Heat 1 tablespoon sunflower oil in a non-stick frying pan (skillet) and cook the falafel four at a time (adding more oil when necessary) for 6 minutes, turning them occasionally, until golden all over. Drain on paper towels.

241 ROASTED VEG and HALLOUMI PITTA

SERVES 4
PREPARATION 15 minutes
COOKING 35 minutes

STORAGE Cook the vegetables and halloumi in advance and keep in the fridge for up to 3 days. Assemble on the day.

5 tbsp olive oil
2 tbsp balsamic vinegar
2 small red (bell) peppers, seeded and cut into 8 slices
2 small courgettes (zucchini), sliced lengthways
2 small onions, each cut into 8 wedges
4 tomatoes, halved
8 slices halloumi cheese, patted dry
4 wholemeal pitta breads

1. Preheat the oven to 200°C/400°F/gas mark 6. Mix together 4 tablespoons of the oil and the balsamic vinegar in a shallow dish. Add the red (bell) pepper, courgette (zucchini), onion and tomatoes and turn the vegetables to coat them in the oil mixture.

2. Put the vegetables, except the tomatoes, in a roasting tin (pan). Roast for 20 minutes, turning occasionally, then add the tomatoes. Return the tin (pan) to the oven and cook for another 10–15 minutes until the vegetables are tender and slightly blackened around the edges. Leave to cool.

3. Meanwhile, wipe the remaining oil over a griddle or frying pan (skillet) and heat until hot. Griddle or fry the halloumi for a few minutes, turning once, until beginning to turn golden.

4. Slice each pitta lengthways, leaving each end intact, and open out to make a large pocket. Divide the vegetables and halloumi between the pittas and close to encase the filling.

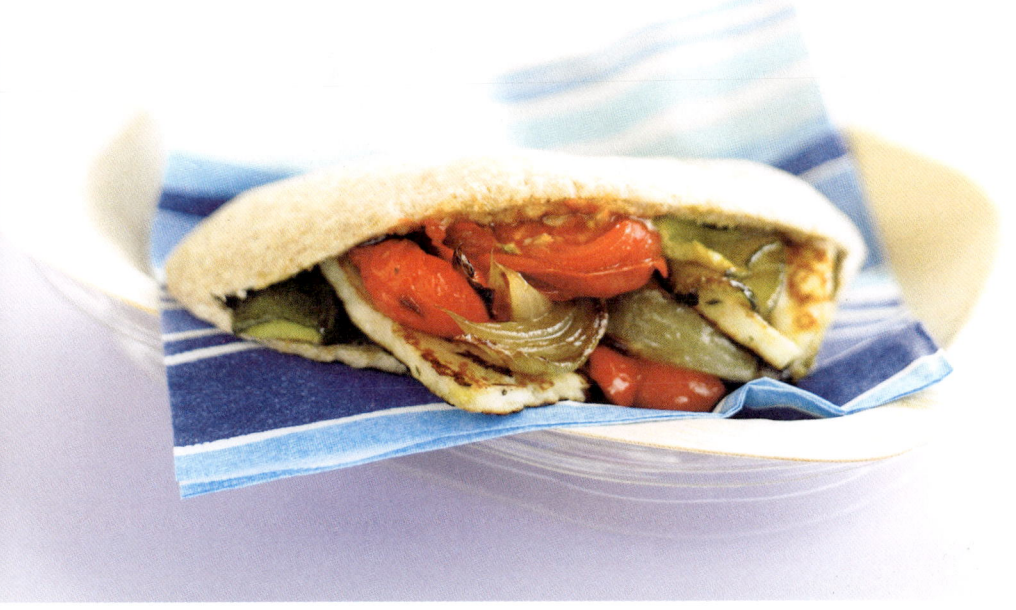

242 INDIAN PANCAKES

SERVES 4
PREPARATION 20 minutes
COOKING 20 minutes
STORAGE Best eaten immediately.

PANCAKES
200g/7oz/1½ cups plain (all-purpose) flour
2 tbsp desiccated (dried shredded) coconut
200ml/7fl oz/scant 1 cup plain yogurt
2 pinches of cayenne pepper
2 pinches of sea salt
oil, for frying

FILLING
2 radishes, chopped into thin sticks
1 large handful beansprouts
400g/14oz green beans, topped, tailed and blanched
2 tsp tamari
1 handful fresh coriander (cilantro)

1. Mix the flour, coconut, yogurt, , cayenne pepper, salt and 400ml/14fl oz/1⅔ cups of water to a smooth batter in a bowl, then cook approximately eight thin pancakes in a frying pan (skillet) with a little oil. Set aside (keep warm).

2. Stir-fry the radish, beansprouts and green beans in a separate pan with a little oil. Add the tamari just before removing from the heat and garnish with fresh coriander (cilantro). Fill and fold the pancakes, and serve with mango chutney.

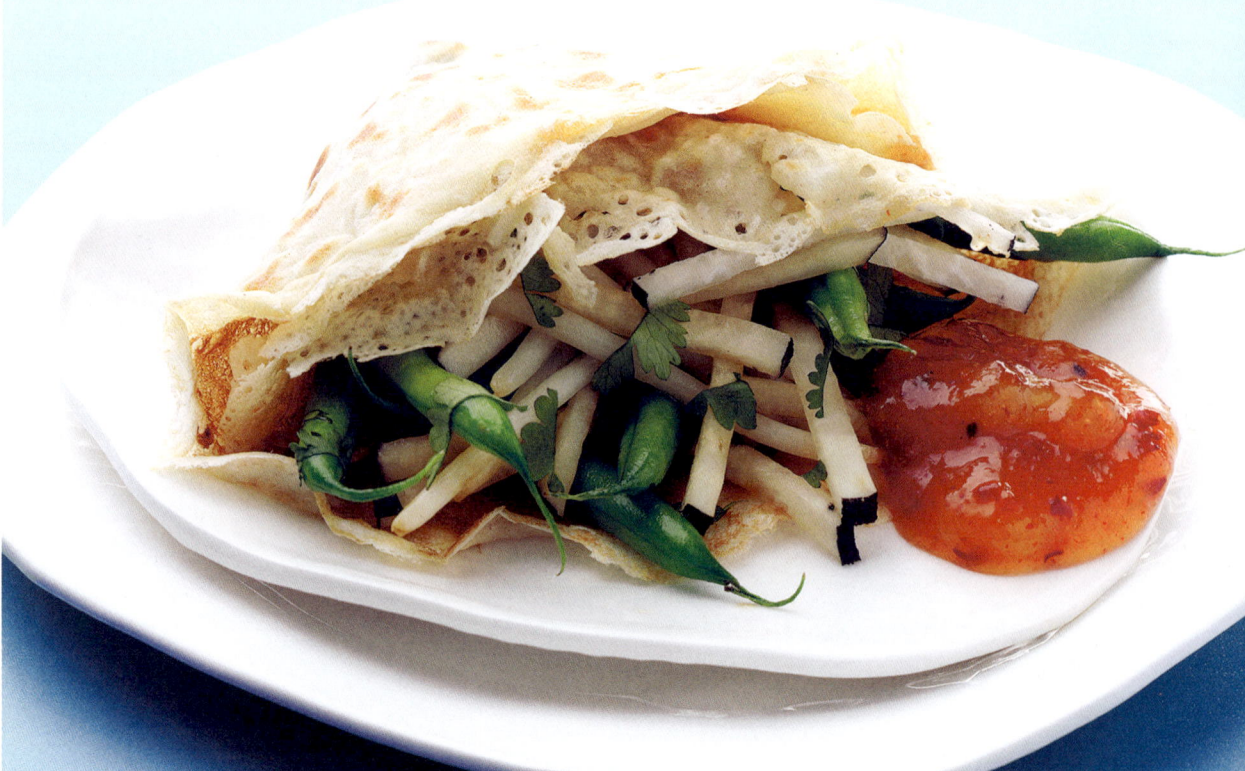

243 TUNA NIÇOISE

SERVES 4
PREPARATION 10 minutes
COOKING 15 minutes
STORAGE Best eaten immediately.

BATTER
200g/7oz/1½ cups chickpea (gram) flour
2 tsp finely chopped fresh ginger
2 pinches of sea salt
2 tsp baking powder
400ml/14fl oz/1⅔ cups water
olive oil, for frying

FILLING
1 large red onion, chopped
4 medium potatoes, finely diced
400g/14oz curly kale, chopped
½ tsp ground cardamom seeds
½ tsp hot chilli paste

1. Mix the batter ingredients in a bowl and pour into a large oiled frying pan (skillet). Turn down the heat and fry each side until golden.

2. Meanwhile, stir-fry the onion and potatoes in a separate pan with a little oil until they begin to soften. Add the curly kale, the cardamom seeds and a little water. Season and simmer until the potatoes are soft.

3. Place the filling on one half of the omelette, spread the chilli paste on the other half, fold and serve.

244 RICE NOODLES WITH MANGETOUT SAUCE

SERVES 4
PREPARATION 10 minutes
COOKING 10 minutes
STORAGE Best eaten immediately.

2 tbsp grapeseed oil
4 spring onions (scallions), finely sliced
2 tsp finely chopped fresh ginger
2 cloves garlic, finely chopped
700g/1lb 9oz mangetout (snow peas), sliced
200ml/7fl oz/scant 1 cup water
2 tbsp tamari
2 tsp cornflour (cornstarch) dissolved in a little cold water
2 tbsp toasted sesame oil
sea salt and black pepper to taste
400g/14oz vermicelli (rice noodles)

1. Gently heat the grapeseed oil in a large frying pan (skillet) or wok. Add the spring onions (scallions), ginger, garlic and mangetout (snow peas) and stir-fry for 2 minutes. Stir in the water and the tamari. Bring to the boil and cook for 2 minutes. Add the cornflour (cornstarch) mixture and the sesame oil, stir and cook until the sauce thickens. Season and set aside (keep warm).

2. Cook the rice noodles as instructed on the package. Drain and toss with the mangetout (snow pea) sauce. Serve hot.

245 COURGETTE AND PARMESAN FRITTERS

MAKES 12
PREPARATION
15 minutes
COOKING
18 minutes

STORAGE
Make in advance and keep in the fridge for up to 3 days or freeze for up to 1 month.

450g/1lb courgettes (zucchini), coarsely grated
6 tbsp finely grated Parmesan cheese
2 eggs, beaten
4 tbsp plain (all-purpose) flour
4 tbsp sunflower oil
salt and freshly ground black pepper

1. Squeeze the grated courgettes (zucchini) in a dishtowel to remove any moisture. Mix the courgettes (zucchini) with the Parmesan, egg and flour, then season.

2. Heat half the oil in a frying pan (skillet). Add 2 tablespoons of the courgette (zucchini) mixture for each fritter. Cook in three batches for 2–3 minutes on each side until set and golden. Drain on paper towels and leave to cool.

246 SPAGHETTI FRITTATA

SERVES 4–6
PREPARATION
10 minutes
COOKING
20 minutes

STORAGE
Make in advance and keep in the fridge for up to 3 days.

85g/3oz wholemeal or white spaghetti
olive oil, for stirring
5 eggs, beaten
60g/2¼oz Parmesan, grated
15g/½oz butter
salt and freshly ground black pepper

1. Cook the spaghetti in plenty of boiling water, following the package instructions, until al dente. Drain and refresh under cold running water. Tip the pasta into a bowl, stir in a little oil to stop it sticking together, then leave to cool.

2. Season the beaten eggs and mix in the Parmesan. Preheat the grill (broiler) to medium.

3. Melt the butter in a medium-sized frying pan (skillet) with a heatproof handle. Place the spaghetti in the pan in an even layer, then pour the egg mixture over the pasta. Cook for about 5 minutes until the base is set and slightly golden.

4. Place the pan under the grill (broiler) and cook the top of the frittata for about 3 minutes until set. Leave to cool, then cut into wedges.

247 FABULOUS FRITTATA

SERVES 4–6
PREPARATION
5 minutes
COOKING
10 minutes

STORAGE
Leftovers will keep in the fridge for up to 1 day.

6 eggs
2 tbsp olive oil
100g/3½oz chargrilled baby artichokes in oil, drained and sliced
8 pitted black olives, halved
1 roasted red (bell) pepper in oil, drained and sliced
75g/2½oz goat's cheese, crumbled
2 tbsp chopped basil leaves
freshly ground black pepper

1. Beat the eggs and season with a little black pepper.

2. Heat the oil in an ovenproof frying pan (skillet) and add the artichokes, olives and red (bell) pepper. Stir for 1 minute until heated through. Pour in the eggs and cook for 5–6 minutes, or until they are almost set.

3. Preheat the grill (broiler) to high. Scatter the goat's cheese and basil over the frittata and place the pan under the grill (broiler) for 2–3 minutes until golden. Cut into wedges and serve, or leave to cool before cutting.

248 MINTED PEA AND CHEESE OMELETTE

SERVES 4
PREPARATION
5 minutes
COOKING
6 minutes

STORAGE
Best eaten immediately.

8 large eggs
3 tbsp chopped mint leaves
2 tbsp olive oil
2 spring onions (scallions), chopped
175g/6oz/scant ¾ cup frozen peas, thawed
100g/3½oz goat's cheese, chopped
2 tbsp Parmesan cheese
freshly ground black pepper

1. Preheat the grill (broiler) to high. Beat the eggs with the mint and season with black pepper.

2. Heat the oil in an ovenproof frying pan (skillet). Add the spring onions (scallions) and cook for 1 minute, then add the peas and stir for 2 minutes. Pour in the eggs and cook for 1 minute until they begin to set.

3. Scatter the goat's cheese and Parmesan over the omelette and grill for 2 minutes until lightly browned.

4. Slide the omelette out onto a plate, cut it into wedges and serve.

249 BULGUR PILAF

SERVES 4
PREPARATION
10 minutes
COOKING
17 minutes

200g/7oz/1½ cups chickpeas (garbanzo beans), cooked or canned
2 tbsp grapeseed oil
2 tbsp tamari (optional)
200g/7oz/1¼ cups bulgur wheat
400ml/14fl oz/1⅔ cups hot water
200g/7oz/1½ cups green peas
sea salt and black pepper to taste
1 small red onion, finely chopped
1 lemon, peeled and chopped
20 small grape tomatoes, quartered
5–6 tbsp fresh mint, finely chopped

1. Gently sweat the chickpeas (garbanzo beans) in a frying pan (skillet) with 1 tablespoon of oil until they begin to brown. Add the tamari (if using), then the bulgur wheat and stir-fry for 2–3 minutes. Pour in the water and simmer at the lowest possible heat for 10–12 minutes, adding the peas after 5 minutes. Stir from time to time (adding a little more water if necessary).

2. Remove from the heat and season. Add the onion, lemon, tomatoes and mint, and sprinkle with the remaining tablespoon of oil. Serve immediately.

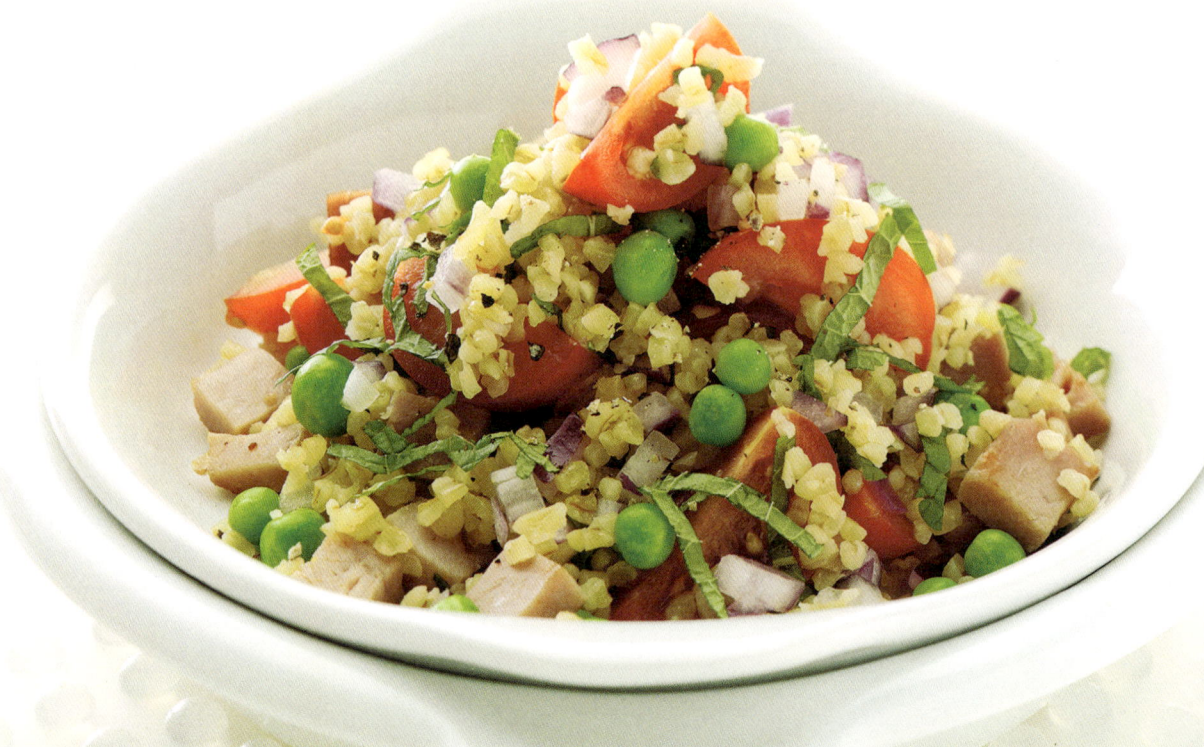

250 BEIJING-STYLE OMELETTE

SERVES 4
PREPARATION
10 minutes
COOKING
10 minutes

STORAGE
Best eaten immediately.

BATTER
8 eggs
a little milk or water
sea salt and black pepper, to taste

FILLING
2 pinches of ground Chinese five-spice powder
4 spring onions (scallions) or 2 small leeks, chopped
oil, for frying
handful of oyster mushrooms, sliced and fried, to garnish
beansprouts, to garnish

1. To make the batter, beat the eggs in a bowl, add the milk or water and season. Add the chopped spring onions (scallions) or leeks, together with the five-spice powder.

2. Pour the batter into an oiled frying pan (skillet) over a medium heat and fry each side until firm.

3. Serve, garnished with fried oyster mushrooms and beansprouts.

251 PITTA POCKETS

SERVES 4
PREPARATION
10 minutes
COOKING
2 minutes

STORAGE
You can prepare these the night before and refrigerate them.

4 wholemeal pittas
50g/2oz/½ cup spinach, chopped
2 carrots, peeled and grated
2 celery stalks, grated
2 tsp coriander seeds
4 tbsp sunflower seeds
8 tbsp hummus

1. Toast the pittas lightly under a grill (broiler), then slice along the edge of each to create large pockets.

2. Put the spinach, carrot, celery, seeds and hummus into a bowl and stir together. Spoon the mixture into the pockets.

252 MIDDLE EASTERN PUFFS

SERVES 4
PREPARATION
15 minutes
COOKING
10 minutes

200g/7oz/1⅓ cups shelled walnuts
4 tbsp breadcrumbs
4 cloves garlic, crushed
1 tsp pomegranate molasses
4 tbsp olive oil
1 package filo (phyllo) pastry sheets

1. Preheat the oven to 220°C/425°F/gas mark 7 and grease two baking sheets.

2. Roughly crush the walnuts in a mortar. Add the breadcrumbs, garlic, pomegranate molasses and oil, mix well and season.

3. Cut the pastry into 10cm/4in squares and use two layers of pastry for each puff. Place a spoonful of filling along one edge of each square and fold in the sides. Roll each square into a finger shape and firmly press together the edges. Place on the greased baking sheets and bake in the middle of the hot oven until golden (about 10 minutes). Serve with a green salad.

253 AVOCADO WITH SAVOURY CRUMBS

SERVES 4
PREPARATION
15 minutes
COOKING
18 minutes
STORAGE
Best eaten immediately.

1 tbsp olive oil, plus for greasing
2 rindless streaky bacon slices
1 slice of wholemeal bread
50g/1¾oz Cheddar cheese, grated
2 avocados, halved lengthways and pitted, shells reserved
175g/6oz canned refried beans
4 cherry tomatoes, quartered

1. Preheat the grill (broiler) to high and the oven to 200°C/400°F/gas mark 6. Grease a baking dish.

2. Grill (broil) the bacon for 2–3 minutes until crisp; crumble into a bowl when cool.

3. Process the bread to fine crumbs in a food processor. Put in a bowl and mix in the olive oil and half the cheese.

4. Dice the avocado flesh or mash it with a fork and mix with the beans, tomatoes, remaining cheese and bacon.

5. Spoon the bean mixture into the avocado shells and place them in the prepared dish. Sprinkle with the crumbs, press down lightly and bake for 10–15 minutes, or until golden. Serve immediately.

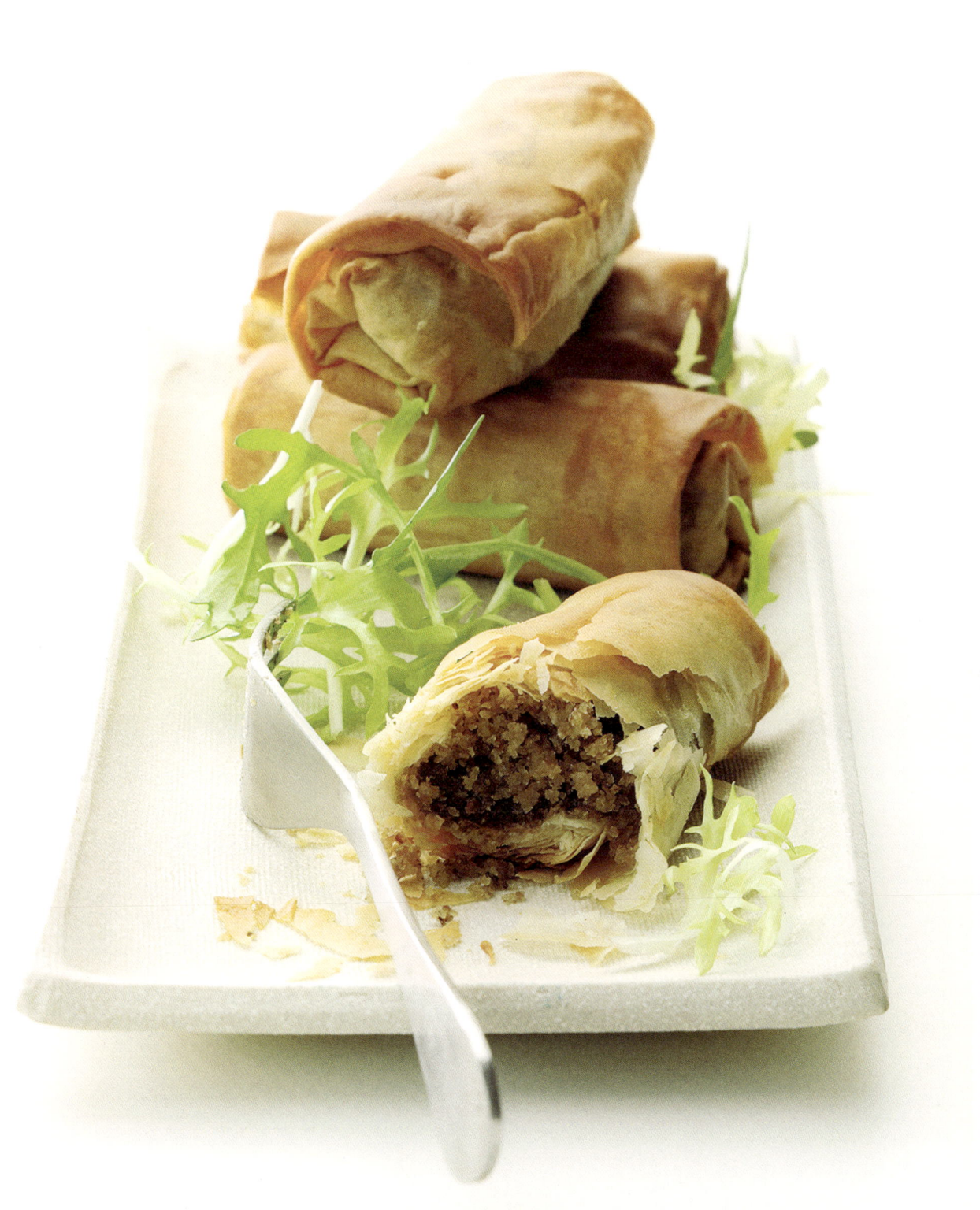

254 SUMMER KEBABS

SERVES 4
PREPARATION
10 minutes + 2 hours marinating
COOKING
12 minutes

STORAGE
The marinade can be prepared in advance. Once prepared, best eaten immediately.

20 cherry tomatoes
2 red (bell) peppers, cut into chunks
2 yellow courgettes (zucchini), cut into chunks
250g/9oz tofu, cut into cubes
2 aubergines (eggplant), cut into chunks
4 shallots, halved
32 button mushrooms, kept whole
8 bay leaves, halved

MARINADE
350ml/12fl oz tomato ketchup
juice of 2 lemons
2 tbsp raw cane sugar
12 cloves garlic, crushed
4 tsp thyme
4 tbsp olive oil
2 tbsp mustard

1. Mix all the marinade ingredients in a bowl. Add the kebab ingredients and mix. Cover and leave to marinate for 2 hours.

2. Thread the vegetables onto metal skewers and brush with the marinade. Place on a hot barbecue (or under a hot grill/broiler) for 10 minutes, turning from time to time.

255 BAKED STUFFED PEPPERS

SERVES 4
PREPARATION
15 minutes
COOKING
45 minutes

STORAGE
Leftovers will keep in the fridge for up to 2 days.

4 tbsp raisins
1 tbsp olive oil
1 red onion
1 clove garlic, crushed
3 sun-dried tomatoes, chopped
150g/5½oz cooked Puy lentils
4 tbsp pine nuts
2 tbsp chopped basil leaves
4 red (bell) peppers, halved
125g/4½oz mozzarella cheese, grated

1. Preheat the oven to 180°C/350°F/gas mark 4. Soak the raisins in boiling water for 5 minutes. Drain.

2. Heat the oil in a frying pan (skillet) and add the onion, garlic and sun-dried tomatoes. Cook for 2–3 minutes, stirring, until the onion is soft. Add the lentils, pine nuts, basil and raisins and cook, stirring, for a further 1 minute.

3. Put the (bell) peppers in a baking dish and spoon the lentil mixture into them. Top with the mozzarella cheese and bake for 30–40 minutes until the peppers are soft and the cheese is bubbling and golden. Serve immediately.

256 PISSALADIÈRE ONION TART

SERVES 2–4
PREPARATION
10 minutes
COOKING
20 minutes

STORAGE
Leftovers will keep in the fridge for up to 2 days.

- 1 package ready-made shortcrust pastry, rolled out very thinly
- 500g/1lb 2oz onions, halved and sliced
- 2 tbsp olive oil
- 1 clove garlic, chopped
- 1 tsp thyme
- 1 bay leaf
- sea salt and black pepper to taste
- 1 tbsp capers
- 12 anchovy fillets (optional)
- 12 black olives, pitted

1. Preheat the oven to 240°C/475°F/gas mark 9.

2. Place the rolled-out pastry on a baking sheet.

3. Gently sauté the onions in a saucepan with the oil until soft. Add the garlic, thyme and bay leaf, heat through and season. Pour the onion mixture onto the pastry, garnish with the capers, anchovies, if using, and olives. Bake for 15 minutes. Serve with a green salad.

257 BROCCOLI AND BRAZIL NUT STIR FRY

SERVES 2–4
PREPARATION
10 minutes
COOKING
10 minutes

STORAGE
Best eaten immediately.

- 2 tbsp olive oil
- 1 clove garlic, chopped
- 75g/2¾oz Brazil nuts, chopped
- 500g/1lb 2oz broccoli
- 2 tbsp tamari
- 100ml/3½fl oz/scant ½ cup vegetable stock
- 2 tbsp lemon juice
- 1 tbsp toasted sesame oil
- 2 tsp cornflour (cornstarch) dissolved in a little cold water
- black pepper to taste

1. Heat the olive oil in a wok and add the garlic and brazil nuts. Cut the broccoli into florets and add to the wok. Stir-fry for 1 minute, then add the tamari and the stock. Simmer for 5 minutes and add the lemon juice and sesame oil. Add the cornflour (cornstarch) mixture, stir and simmer for a few more minutes until the mixture thickens.

2. Season with black pepper and serve hot with rice noodles.

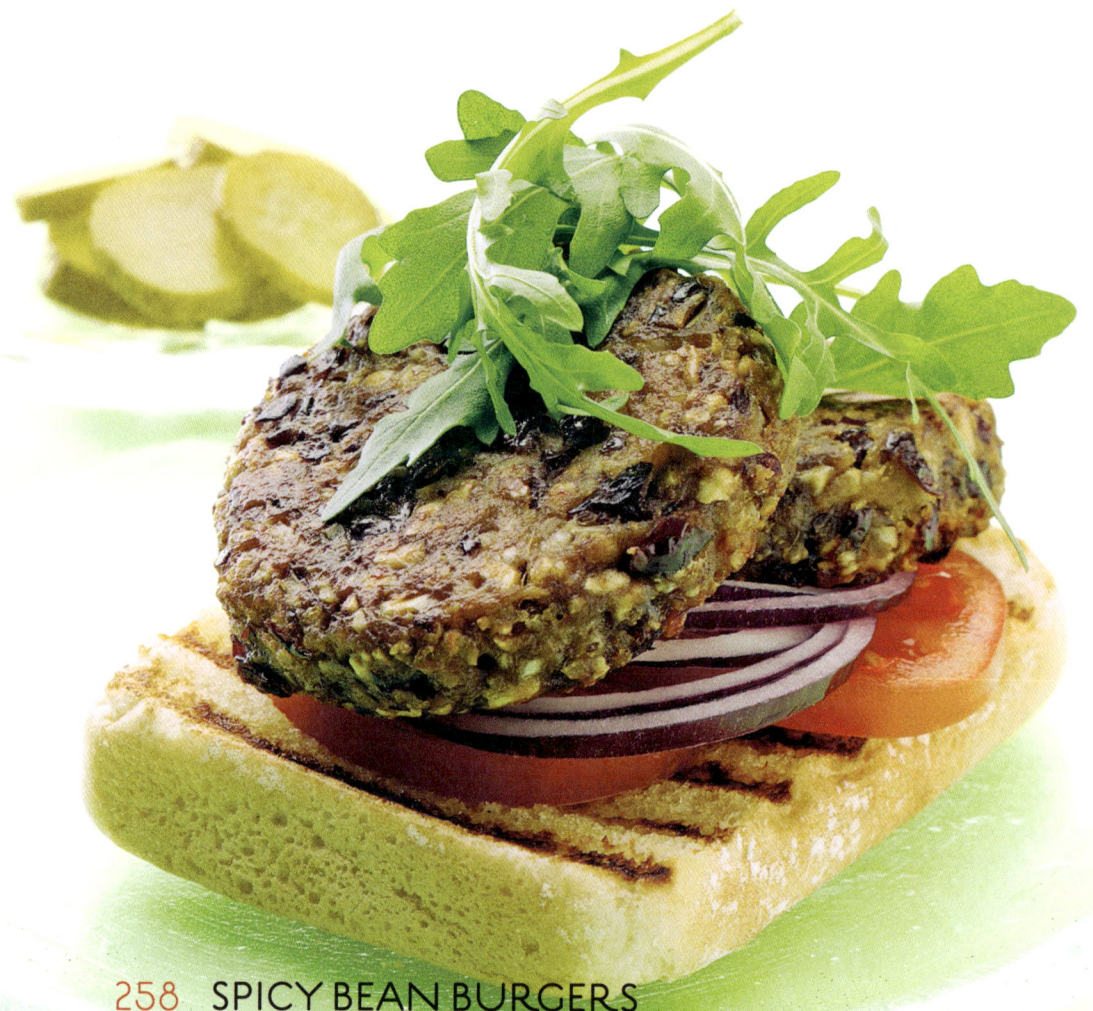

258 SPICY BEAN BURGERS

SERVES 4
PREPARATION 15 minutes
COOKING 10 minutes

STORAGE You can freeze the raw mixture and use it within a month.

- 200g/7oz red kidney beans, cooked or canned and drained
- 1 shallot, finely chopped
- 50g/1¾oz/scant ½ cup hazelnuts, finely chopped
- 1 tsp fresh ginger, finely chopped
- pinch of cayenne pepper
- 2 tsp tamari
- 2 tbsp breadcrumbs
- 2 tbsp soya flour
- sea salt to taste
- oil for grilling or frying

1. Mash or blend the kidney beans (with a little water if necessary) to a coarse paste, add the shallot, hazelnuts, ginger, cayenne pepper, tamari, breadcrumbs and soya flour, and mix well. Season and shape into approximately four 70g/2½oz flat burgers.

2. Brush the burgers with oil and grill over hot embers until cooked through (about 5 minutes on each side). Alternatively, fry the burgers in hot oil. Serve on a toasted bun with all the usual burger trimmings.

259 PUMPKIN HOTPOT with ROASTED VEGETABLES

SERVES 4
PREPARATION
20 minutes
COOKING
25 minutes

STORAGE
Leftovers will keep in the fridge for up to 2 days.

2 parsnips, cut into chunks
2 small beetroot (beets), quartered
8 potatoes, quartered
olive oil, for greasing and stir-frying
2 tbsp paprika
600g/1lb 5oz pumpkin, peeled, deseeded and chopped
2 red onions, halved and sliced
2 cloves garlic, crushed
2 tbsp fresh marjoram
400ml/14fl oz/1$^{2}/_{3}$ cups hot vegetable stock
2–4 tbsp almond butter
sea salt and black pepper to taste

1) Preheat the oven to 220°C/425°F/gas mark 7. Scatter the parsnips, beetroot (beets) and potatoes on an oiled baking sheet and sprinkle with paprika and a little salt and pepper. Roast in a hot oven for about 25 minutes until they begin to turn brown and soft. Check and turn from time to time.

2) Meanwhile, gently stir-fry the pumpkin with the onion and garlic in a heavy saucepan with a little oil for 5 minutes. Add the marjoram and the stock and bring to the boil. Cover and gently simmer for 10 minutes.

3) In a food processor, coarsely blend the pumpkin mixture and add the almond butter. Season and serve with the roasted vegetables.

260 POTATO AND LENTIL BURGERS

SERVES 4
PREPARATION
10 minutes
COOKING
40 minutes

STORAGE
You can freeze the raw mixture and use it within a month.

500g/1lb 2oz potatoes
115g/4oz/1 cup red lentils
1 tbsp olive oil
1 small onion, peeled and diced
1 clove garlic, peeled and crushed
1 egg, beaten
2 tbsp chives, finely chopped
55g/2oz/$^1/_3$ cup grated Cheddar cheese

1. Half fill a saucepan with water, bring to the boil and add the potatoes. Cover and let simmer for 15–20 minutes until soft. Drain and then mash. Meanwhile, in a separate pan, simmer the lentils for 10 minutes, until tender, then drain. Heat the oil in a small saucepan, add the onion and garlic and sauté.

2. Preheat the oven to 220°C/425°F/gas mark 7. In a large mixing bowl, mix the potato, lentils, onion mix, beaten egg, chives and cheese. Use your hands to mould the mixture into 12 burgers and place on a non-stick baking sheet.

3. Put the burgers in the oven and cook for 20 minutes or until golden and serve immediately.

261 BAGEL BURGER

SERVES 1
PREPARATION
10 minutes

STORAGE
You can prepare this the night before and refrigerate.

1 wholemeal bagel
25g/1oz/$^1/_3$ cup rocket (arugula)
1 Potato and Lentil Burger (see above)
1 tbsp hummus
1 tbsp Salsa (see page 68)
$^1/_2$ avocado, peeled and sliced

1. Cut the bagel in half and toast lightly. Place the rocket (arugula) on the base of the bagel and the burger on top of the rocket.

2. Spread the hummus and salsa on top of the burger and then add the avocado slices.

3. Place the other half of the bagel on top, sandwiching the burger.

262 CARROT AND COURGETTE LENTILS

SERVES 4
PREPARATION
10 minutes
COOKING
30 minutes

200g/7oz/1 cup Puy lentils
olive oil, for stir-frying
2 onions, finely chopped
4 carrots, finely chopped
4 cloves garlic, finely chopped
2 courgettes (zucchini), chopped
4 tomatoes, finely chopped
2 tbsp tamari
2 bay leaves
2 tsp thyme

1) Bring the lentils to the boil in a pan with twice their volume of water and simmer for 15 minutes.

2) Heat a little oil in a separate pan and stir-fry the onion, carrots, garlic, courgette (zucchini) and tomatoes (adding them one at a time). Then add the tamari, bay leaves and thyme, together with the lentils and enough water to cover. Heat through and simmer until the lentils are soft (10–15 minutes). Season and serve.

263 MEXICAN BEANFEAST

SERVES 4
PREPARATION
5 minutes
COOKING
20 minutes

STORAGE
You can refrigerate for up to 3 days or freeze and use within a month.

1 tbsp olive oil
1 small red onion, peeled and diced
2 tsp chilli powder
1 tsp cayenne pepper
2 tbsp Worcestershire sauce
200g/7oz/1 cup tomato purée (paste)
1/2 red (bell) pepper, sliced
200-g/7-oz can sweetcorn
400-g/14-oz can kidney beans
400-g/14-oz can chickpeas
2 x 400-g/14-oz cans chopped tomatoes
4 brown pitta breads
3 tbsp gravy granules
1 bunch spring onions (scallions), chopped
25g/1oz/1/3 cup chopped parsley

1) Heat the oil in a wok, add the onion and fry until slightly browned. Add the chilli, cayenne pepper, Worcestershire sauce and tomato purée and stir to mix.

2) Add the red (bell) pepper, sweetcorn, kidney beans, chickpeas and chopped tomatoes and simmer for 10 minutes. Toast the pittas lightly under the grill, then cut in half to make two pockets.

3) Add the gravy granules to the beanfeast, then simmer for 5 minutes. Add the spring onions (scallions) and parsley and serve with the pittas in a side dish.

264 SPRING ROLLS

MAKES 16
PREPARATION 25 minutes
COOKING 20 minutes

STORAGE Make in advance and keep in the fridge for up to 3 days or freeze for up to 1 month.

- 55g/2oz rice vermicelli noodles
- 2 tsp sunflower oil, plus extra
- 1 tsp toasted sesame oil
- 2 carrots, cut into thin strips
- 1 red (bell) pepper, cut into strips
- 85g/3oz mangetout (snow peas), sliced diagonally
- 2 cloves garlic, chopped
- 2 spring onions (scallions), finely sliced lengthways
- 2.5-cm/1-in piece ginger, grated
- 2 tsp soy sauce
- 85g/3oz beansprouts
- 16 small spring roll wrappers
- 1 egg white, beaten

1. Soak the noodles as instructed on the package, drain and refresh. Cut into short lengths.

2. Heat the oils in a wok and stir-fry the vegetables and ginger for 2 minutes. Add the soy sauce and cook for another minute. Add the beansprouts. Place in a bowl, stir and leave to cool.

3. Preheat the oven to 180°C/350°F/gas mark 4. Put one wrapper at a time on a work surface. Place a heaped tablespoon of filling on one corner, fold the corner over it, fold in the two sides and roll the wrapper. Brush the edge with egg white and fold to seal.

4. Place the spring rolls on a lightly oiled baking sheet. Brush each roll with oil and bake for 15 minutes until golden.

265 VEGGIE WRAPPERS

SERVES 4
PREPARATION 10 minutes

STORAGE You can prepare these the night before and refrigerate until the morning.

- 2 avocados, chopped
- 230g/8oz/1 cup spinach, chopped
- 230g/8oz/1 cup alfalfa sprouts
- 230g/8oz/1 cup beansprouts
- 50g/2oz/²/₃ cup pumpkin seeds
- 6 tbsp olive oil
- 2 tbsp wholegrain mustard
- 2 tbsp runny honey
- 4 tortilla wraps

1. Put the chopped avocado and spinach into a mixing bowl. Add the sprouts and seeds.

2. To make a dressing, whisk together the olive oil, mustard and runny honey with a fork. Pour into the vegetable mix and stir well.

3. Lay out the tortillas and pile a quarter of the mixture into the middle of each one. Roll into wraps.

266 MEXICAN BEAN TACOS

SERVES 4
PREPARATION
15 minutes
COOKING
7 minutes

STORAGE
You can prepare the bean mixture in advance, then warm through and add the avocado immediately before serving.

2 tbsp olive oil
1 red onion, chopped
1 clove garlic, crushed
1 small courgette (zucchini), diced
1 tsp Cajun spices
400-g/14-oz can kidney beans or mixed beans, drained and rinsed
3 tomatoes, deseeded and diced
8 corn taco shells
1 avocado, diced
2 tbsp chopped coriander (cilantro) leaves
100g/3½oz Cheddar cheese, grated

1. Heat the oil in a frying pan (skillet) and add the onion, garlic, courgette (zucchini) and Cajun spices. Sauté for 3–4 minutes, or until the onion is tender.

2. Stir in the kidney or mixed beans and diced tomatoes and cook gently for a further 3 minutes.

3. Warm the taco shells according to the package instructions.

4. Stir the avocado and coriander (cilantro) into the bean mixture, then spoon it into the taco shells, top with the grated cheese and serve.

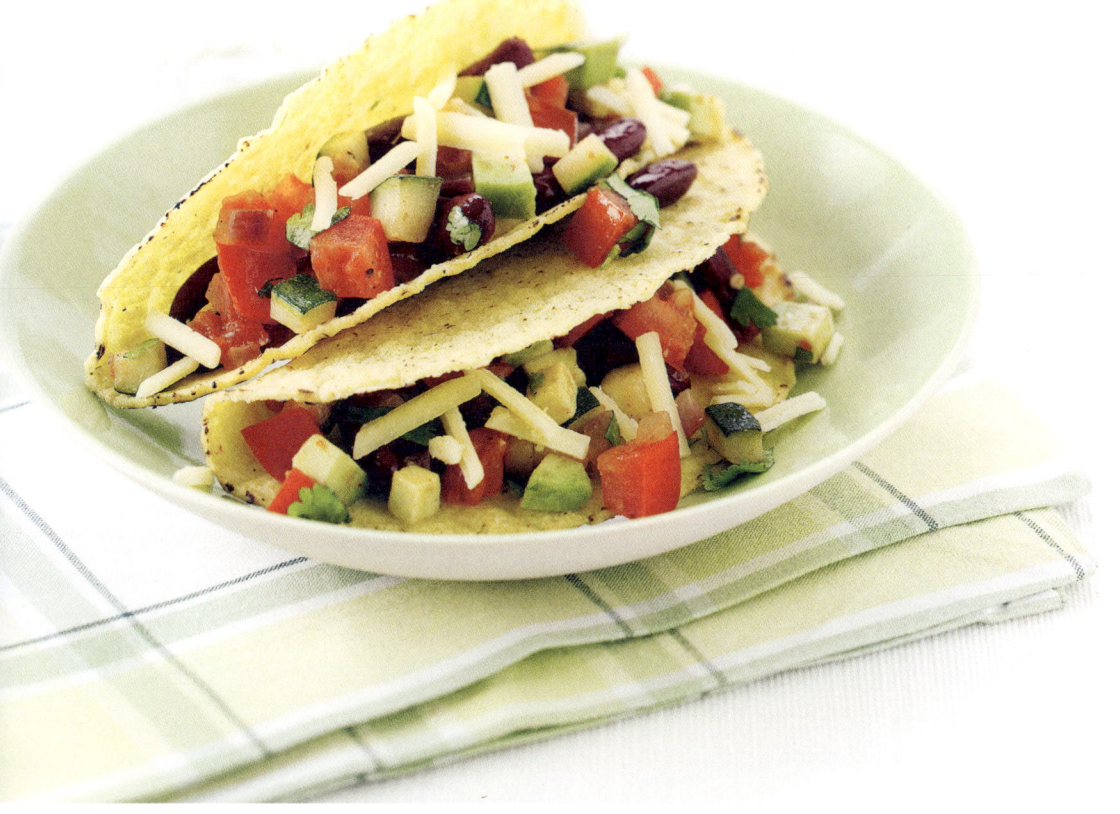

267 POTATO SKIN BATTALIONS

SERVES 4
PREPARATION
15 minutes
COOKING
1 hour or 10 minutes

STORAGE
You can refrigerate for up to 2 or 3 days.

6 medium potatoes, baked
16 spring onions (scallions), chopped
140g/5oz/²⁄₃ cup plain yogurt
200g/7oz tomato salsa
12 sprigs fresh coriander (cilantro)

1. Preheat the oven to 180°C/350°F/gas mark 4, or use the microwave. Bake the potatoes in the oven for 1 hour or in the microwave for 10 minutes, until soft.

2. Halve the potatoes. Scoop the soft potato out of the skins and into a bowl. Mix in the onions and yogurt, mashing together with a fork.

3. Put the mixture back into the potato skins, garnish with a dollop of salsa and a sprig of coriander (cilantro) and serve.

268 SWEET POTATO SCORCHERS

MAKES 12–15
PREPARATION
10 minutes
COOKING
25 minutes

STORAGE
You can refrigerate the raw mixture and use within 3 days, or freeze it for up to a month.

2 large sweet potatoes, peeled and chopped
200g/7oz/1 cup canned chickpeas
1 tbsp olive oil
1 tsp coriander seeds
2 tsp Dijon mustard
½ tbsp olive oil

1. Half fill a saucepan with water, bring to the boil and add the sweet potatoes. Cover and let simmer for 15–20 minutes, until soft.

2. Drain the sweet potatoes and put into a mixing bowl, add the chickpeas, olive oil, coriander seeds and Dijon mustard. Using a potato masher, mash together. Use your hands to mould the mixture into 12–15 balls.

3. Heat the olive oil in a griddle pan or in a frying pan (skillet) and add the potato balls, one at a time. Press down with a spatula until each one is slightly flattened and cook until lightly browned. Turn over and cook the other side, then serve.

269 INSTANT TORTILLAS AND PEPPER FILLING

SERVES 4
PREPARATION 10 minutes
COOKING 17 minutes

STORAGE You can refrigerate for up to 2 days.

oil, for frying
1 large red onion, halved and sliced
1 green chilli, deseeded and finely chopped
2 tsp ground coriander
1 each red, yellow and green (bell) peppers, deseeded and sliced
2 tbsp tamari
1 package ready-made corn tortillas
4 tbsp beansprouts
2 tbsp fresh coriander (cilantro) leaves, chopped

1. Heat a little oil in a wok or frying pan (skillet) and stir-fry the onion. Add the chilli and ground coriander, together with all the (bell) pepper slices, and stir-fry for 3 minutes. Add the tamari and a little water (if necessary). Turn down the heat and leave to simmer until soft.

2. Prepare eight ready-made tortillas as instructed on the package.

3. Add the beansprouts and coriander (cilantro) leaves to the wok or pan. Heat through, then divide the filling between the tortillas, roll and serve.

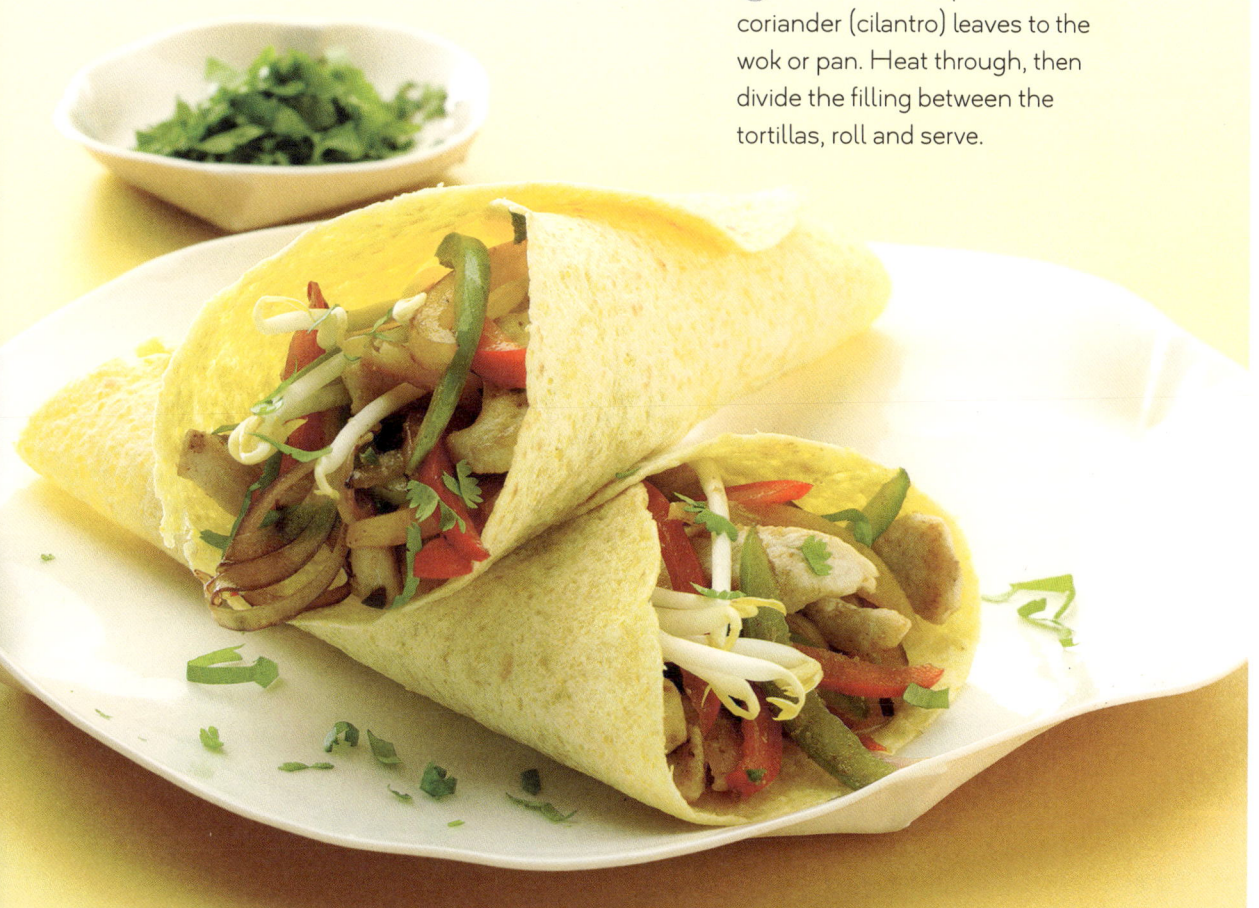

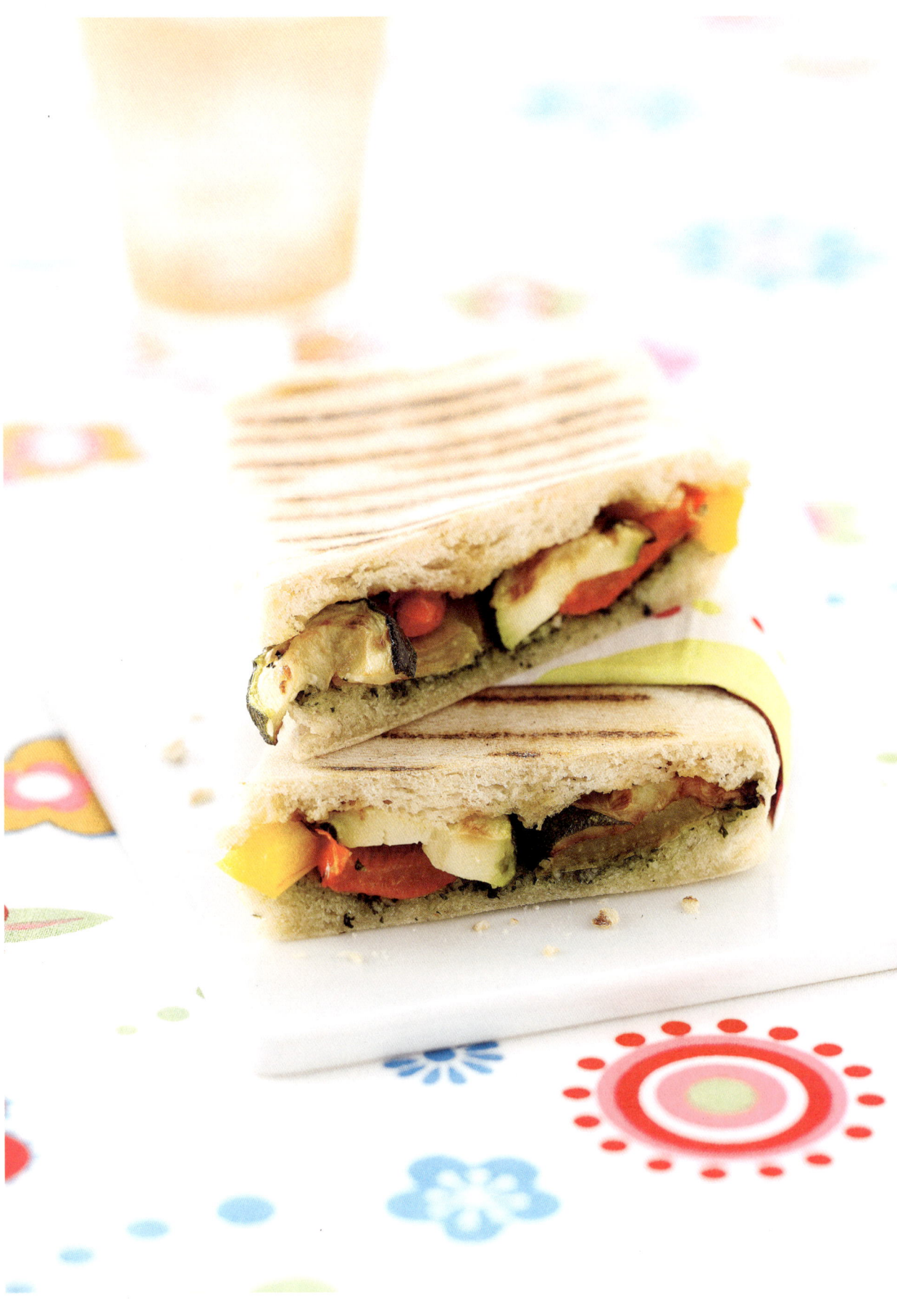

270 VEG AND PESTO PANINIS

SERVES 4
PREPARATION 15 minutes
COOKING 50 minutes

STORAGE
Prepare the vegetables in advance and chill them until required; leftovers will keep in the fridge for up to 1 day. The pesto can be stored in the fridge for up to 1 week.

1 red (bell) pepper, deseeded and quartered
1 yellow (bell) pepper, deseeded and quartered
1 courgette (zucchini), sliced
2 tbsp olive oil
2 thyme sprigs
6 cherry tomatoes, halved
4 paninis, cut in half horizontally

PESTO
1 clove garlic, chopped
25g/1oz basil leaves
3 tbsp pumpkin seeds
5 tbsp omega oil or flaxseed oil
15g/½oz Parmesan cheese, grated

1. Preheat the oven to 220°C/425°F/gas mark 7. In a roasting tin (pan), mix the (bell) peppers and courgette (zucchini) with the olive oil and thyme. Roast for 30 minutes, or until tender. Add the tomatoes and roast for a further 10 minutes.

2. To make the pesto, put the garlic, basil and pumpkin seeds in a food processor. Process to form a coarse paste, then add the oil with the motor running to create a smooth pesto. Stir in the cheese.

3. Preheat a sandwich toaster or grill (broiler). Spread the pesto on the panini halves. Divide the vegetables onto the panini bases and replace the tops, pesto-side down, pressing down firmly. Grill (broil) for 2–3 minutes until warmed through, then serve immediately.

271 FALAFEL AND HUMMUS LAVASH

SERVES 1
PREPARATION 5 minutes

STORAGE
Make the falafel in advance and keep in the fridge for up to 3 days or freeze for up to 1 month.

1 lavash
1–2 tbsp Roasted Red Pepper Hummus (see page 45) or Creamy Guacamole (see page 53)
1 Falafel (see page 176)
few sprigs of rocket (arugula) or watercress

1. Cut the lavash to the size of a small tortilla. Spread the hummus or guacamole over the lavash, then place the falafel in the middle.

2. Arrange the rocket (arugula) or watercress on top, then fold in the bottom and sides to make a pocket, leaving the top open.

272 PIZZA NAPOLETANA

SERVES 4
PREPARATION
10 minutes
COOKING
20 minutes

STORAGE
You can refrigerate for up to 2 days.

2 pizza bases
6 tbsp passata (sieved tomatoes)
200g/7oz mozzarella cheese, sliced
100g/3½oz black olives, pitted
200g/7oz mushrooms, sliced
2 tbsp capers
2 pinches of oregano
sea salt and black pepper to taste

1. Preheat the oven to 240°C/475°F/gas mark 9 and heat two baking sheets.

2. Cover the prepared bases with the passata (sieved tomatoes), followed by the cheese. Top with the olives, mushrooms, capers and oregano. Season and bake in the hot oven for approximately 20 minutes. Serve with a side salad.

273 FEISTY FIESTA PIZZA

SERVES 4
PREPARATION
15 minutes
COOKING
20 minutes

STORAGE
You can freeze the pizza dough for up to a month, or refrigerate the cooked pizza overnight and eat it cold for breakfast or lunch!

½ tsp dried yeast granules
250ml/9fl oz/1 cup warm water
1 tsp brown sugar
115g/4oz/1 cup chickpea (gram) flour
85g/3oz/½ cup cornflour (cornstarch)
1½ tbsp olive oil
1 tsp chilli powder
1 tsp celery salt
115g/4oz/½ cup passata (sieved tomatoes)
½ red (bell) pepper, sliced
½ yellow (bell) pepper, sliced
55g/2oz/½ cup mushrooms
85g/3oz/½ cup grated Cheddar

1. Preheat the oven to 220°C/425°F/gas mark 7. Dissolve the yeast in half the warm water, add the sugar, mix well and set aside for 15 minutes.

2. Meanwhile, place the chickpea (gram) flour in a bowl, add the yeast mixture, cornflour (cornstarch), olive oil, chilli powder and celery salt and beat with a wooden spoon. Add the remaining water, a little at a time, beating until thick. Remove the dough and knead.

3. Spread the dough out flat onto a non-stick baking sheet, then bake at the top of the oven for 5 minutes. Remove from the oven and add the passata (sieved tomatoes) and toppings, then return to the oven and cook for 20 minutes until browned.

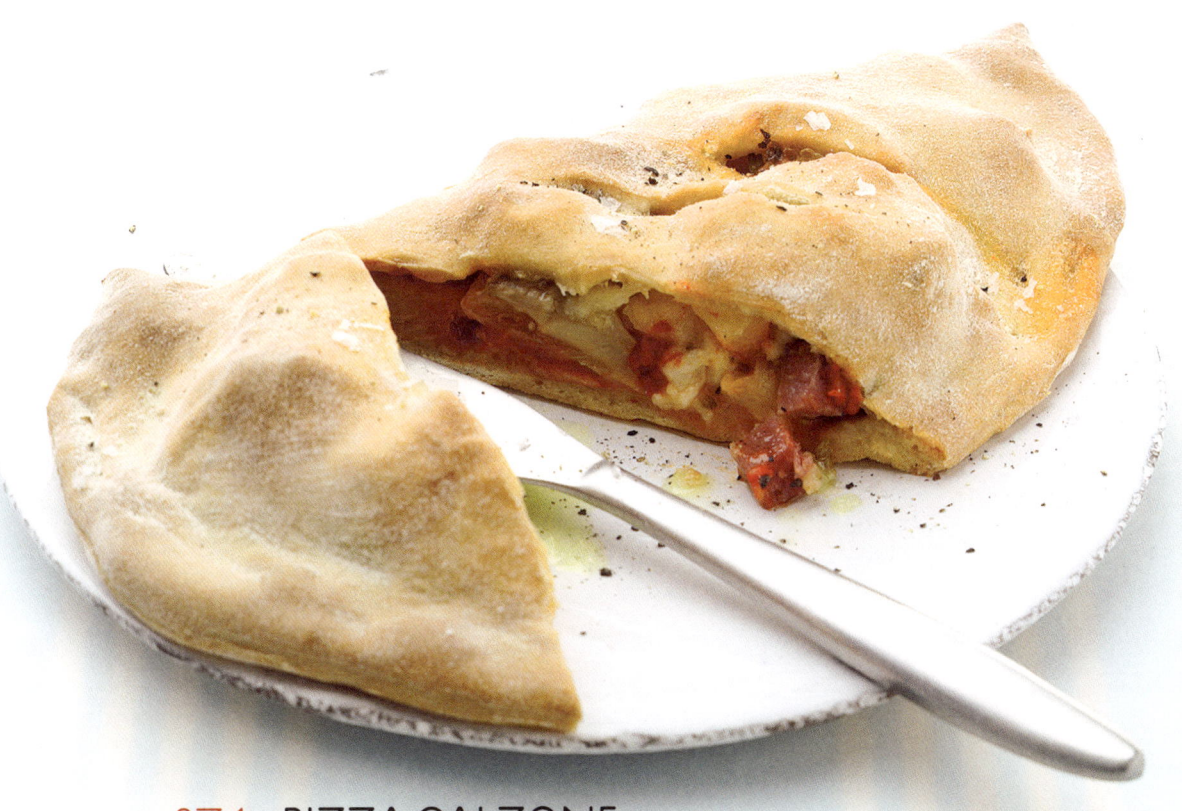

274 PIZZA CALZONE

SERVES 4
PREPARATION 15 minutes
COOKING 20 minutes

STORAGE You can refrigerate for up to 2 days.

- 2 dough pizza bases (see opposite)
- 2–3 tbsp passata (sieved tomatoes)
- 200g/7oz oyster mushrooms, sautéed
- 4 tbsp fresh pineapple chunks
- 2 pinches of oregano
- sea salt and black pepper
- 200g/7oz mozzarella cheese, grated

1. Preheat the oven to 220°C/425°F/gas mark 7 and heat a baking sheet.

2. Spread the passata over half of the prepared and rolled-out dough bases. Top with the mushrooms, pineapple chunks and oregano. Season to taste and sprinkle with grated cheese. Fold the bases over the fillings, press the edges together to seal and cut a couple of slits over the top of each.

2. Bake in the hot oven for approximately 20 minutes, or until the crusts are beginning to brown. Serve hot with a side salad.

275 SIMPLE MINI PIZZAS

MAKES 6
PREPARATION 20 minutes
COOKING 25 minutes

STORAGE Make the day before and keep in the fridge overnight. The dough and sauce can be frozen separately for up to 1 month.

1 tbsp olive oil
150ml/5fl oz/⅔ cup passata (sieved tomatoes)
2 tsp tomato purée (paste)
½ tsp dried oregano
175g/6oz/1½ cups white self-raising flour, plus extra for dusting
100g/3½oz/¾ cup wholemeal self-raising flour
½ tsp salt
150ml/5fl oz/⅔ cup milk
4 tbsp olive oil
150g/5½oz mozzarella, sliced
50g/2oz Cheddar cheese, grated

1. Preheat the oven to 200°C/400°F/gas mark 6.

2. Heat the oil in a pan and add the passata, tomato purée and oregano, stir and bring to the boil. Half-cover and simmer for 10 minutes, stirring, until reduced.

3. Sift the flours and salt into a bowl. Make a well in the middle and pour in the milk and oil. Mix with a fork until it starts to form a dough (adding a little more milk if dry). Tip out on to a floured work surface and knead to form a smooth ball.

4. Divide into six pieces, roll into balls, then flatten into rounds. Place on floured baking sheets. Divide the tomato sauce and cheeses between them. Bake for 10 minutes.

276 PENNE WITH BRAZIL NUT SAUCE

SERVES 4
PREPARATION 10 minutes
COOKING 13 minutes

STORAGE You can refrigerate leftovers for up to 2 days.

300g/10½oz penne pasta
4 tbsp olive oil
2 shallots, chopped
100g/3½oz Brazil nuts
4 tbsp breadcrumbs
2 red (bell) peppers, sliced
2 tbsp tamari
4 tomatoes, chopped
2 cloves garlic, crushed
2 tbsp fresh oregano, chopped

1. Cook the pasta according to the package instructions.

2. Heat the oil in a frying pan (skillet) and stir-fry the shallots for 30 seconds. Add the Brazil nuts and the breadcrumbs and stir-fry until they begin to turn brown. Add the (bell) peppers to the pan or wok with the tamari. Stir for a further few seconds, then add the tomatoes and the garlic. Heat through.

3. Drain the cooked pasta and mix with the Brazil nut sauce. Garnish with oregano and serve immediately.

277 GREEN TAGLIATELLE WITH RED HOT PEPPER SAUCE

SERVES 4
PREPARATION
10 minutes
COOKING
15 minutes

STORAGE
You can refrigerate leftovers for up to 2 days.

- 200ml/7fl oz/scant 1 cup hot vegetable stock
- 2 red (bell) peppers, deseeded and chopped
- 4 tbsp olive oil, plus extra for cooking and tossing
- sea salt to taste
- 2 pinches of cayenne pepper
- 400g/14oz green tagliatelle pasta
- 2 tbsp fresh basil, chopped
- black pepper to taste

1. Pour the stock into a small saucepan, add the red (bell) pepper, bring to the boil and simmer for 5 minutes. Use a hand-held stick blender to blend the (bell) peppers with the stock, while slowly adding the oil. Season with salt and cayenne pepper.

2. Cook the pasta in plenty of boiling water with a little salt and oil. Drain the pasta and return it to the pan. Toss with oil and fresh basil, and season with salt and black pepper. Serve with the sauce.

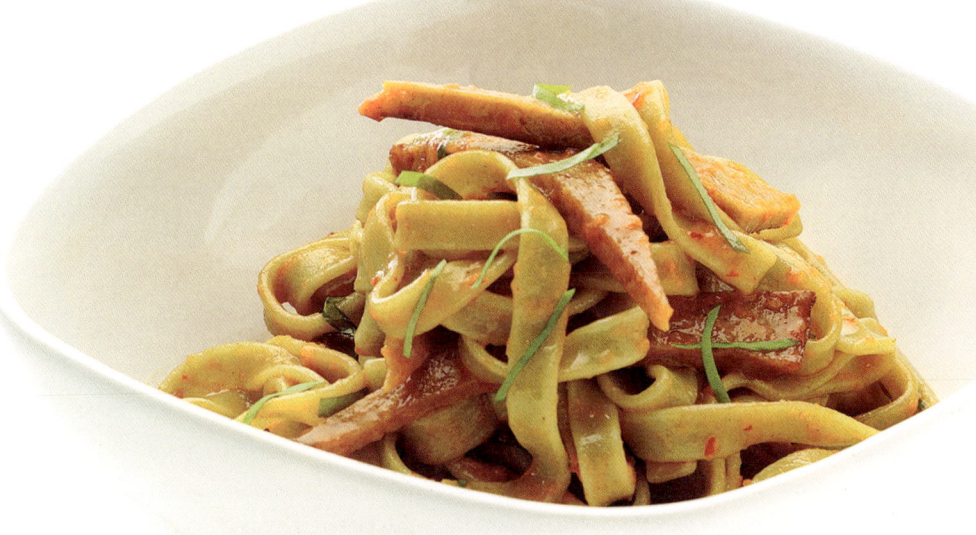

278 PENNE with PESTO and PEAS

SERVES 4
PREPARATION 10 minutes
COOKING 10 minutes
STORAGE You can refrigerate leftovers for up to 2 days.

400g/14oz penne pasta
6 tbsp pine kernels
1 tsp coarse sea salt
4 tbsp fresh basil, finely chopped
8 tbsp olive oil
2 cloves garlic, crushed
400g/14oz green peas, shelled

1. Cook the pasta in plenty of boiling water with a little salt and oil.

2. Grind the pine kernels and salt in a mortar. Add the basil, olive oil and garlic. Mix well.

3. Steam the peas in a vegetable steamer for 3–4 minutes. Drain the cooked pasta and place in a large (heated) serving bowl. Mix in the pesto, top with the steamed peas and serve immediately.

279 SPAGHETTI with BROCCOLI in YOGURT and BASIL SAUCE

SERVES 4
PREPARATION 10 minutes
COOKING 12 minutes
STORAGE You can refrigerate leftovers for up to 2 days.

400g/14oz spaghetti pasta
1 large head broccoli, cut into florets
2 tbsp Dijon mustard
200ml/7fl oz/scant 1 cup plain yogurt
1 tbsp vegetable margarine or butter
1 small red onion, finely chopped
2 cloves garlic, crushed
large handful fresh basil, finely chopped
sea salt and black pepper to taste

1. Cook the spaghetti in plenty of boiling water with a little salt and olive oil. Add the broccoli to the pan for the last 4–5 minutes of the cooking time.

2. Meanwhile, mix the mustard, yogurt and margarine or butter in a bowl. Add the onion, garlic and basil, season well and set aside.

3. Drain the spaghetti and broccoli in a colander. Put the sauce mixture into the pan and gently heat. Add the drained spaghetti and broccoli and mix. Serve with a side salad.

280 SPINACH FETTUCCINE with FRESH TOMATO SAUCE

SERVES 4
PREPARATION
5 minutes
COOKING
10 minutes

STORAGE
You can refrigerate leftovers for up to 2 days.

- 400g/14oz spinach fettuccine pasta
- 4 ripe beef tomatoes, blended
- 2 tbsp fresh basil, chopped
- 200g/7oz mozzarella cheese, cubed
- 2 tbsp sunflower oil
- sea salt and black pepper to taste

1. Cook the spinach pasta in plenty of boiling water with a little salt and oil.

2. Mix the blended tomatoes, chopped basil, cheese cubes and oil in a bowl, and season.

3. Drain the cooked pasta and toss with the sauce. Serve immediately with a green side salad.

281 CONCHIGLIE with CHUNKY SAUCE

SERVES 4
PREPARATION
10 minutes
COOKING
12 minutes

STORAGE
You can refrigerate leftovers for up to 2 days.

- 400g/14oz conchiglie pasta
- olive oil, for stir-frying
- 2 small red onions, halved and sliced
- 300g/10$\frac{1}{2}$oz vegetarian sausages, sliced
- 150g/5$\frac{1}{2}$oz shiitake mushrooms, sliced
- 2 cloves garlic, chopped
- 400ml/14fl oz/1$\frac{2}{3}$ cups vegetable stock
- 150g/5$\frac{1}{2}$oz green peas
- 4 tbsp tomato purée (paste)
- 2 tsp maple syrup
- 4 tsp dried oregano
- sea salt and black pepper to taste

1. Boil the pasta in plenty of water with a little salt and oil.

2. Gently stir-fry the onion in a frying pan (skillet) or a wok with a little oil until soft. Add the sausage, turn up the heat and sauté for 1 minute, then add the shiitake and continue to stir-fry until the sausage and mushrooms begin to brown. Add the garlic, stock and peas and heat through. Then add the tomato purée, maple syrup and oregano. Season and leave to simmer until the pasta is cooked.

3. Drain the pasta and serve immediately, topped with the sauce.

282 PASTA with CHEESY COURGETTES

SERVES 4
PREPARATION 10 minutes
COOKING 10 minutes
STORAGE You can refrigerate leftovers for up to 2 days.

- 400g/14oz rotini pasta
- 2 tbsp olive oil
- 4 cloves garlic, chopped
- 500g/1lb 2oz small courgettes (zucchini), sliced
- sea salt and black pepper to taste
- 300g/10½oz ricotta cheese, crumbled
- 1 large handful fresh basil, chopped

1. Cook the pasta in plenty of boiling water with a little salt and oil.

2. Meanwhile, heat the oil in a heavy-based saucepan and very gently fry the garlic until soft (don't let it brown). Add the sliced courgettes (zucchini) and gently stir-fry for 4–5 minutes. Season and set aside.

3. Drain the pasta and mix with the courgettes (zucchini). Add the cheese, check the seasoning, garnish with fresh basil and serve immediately.

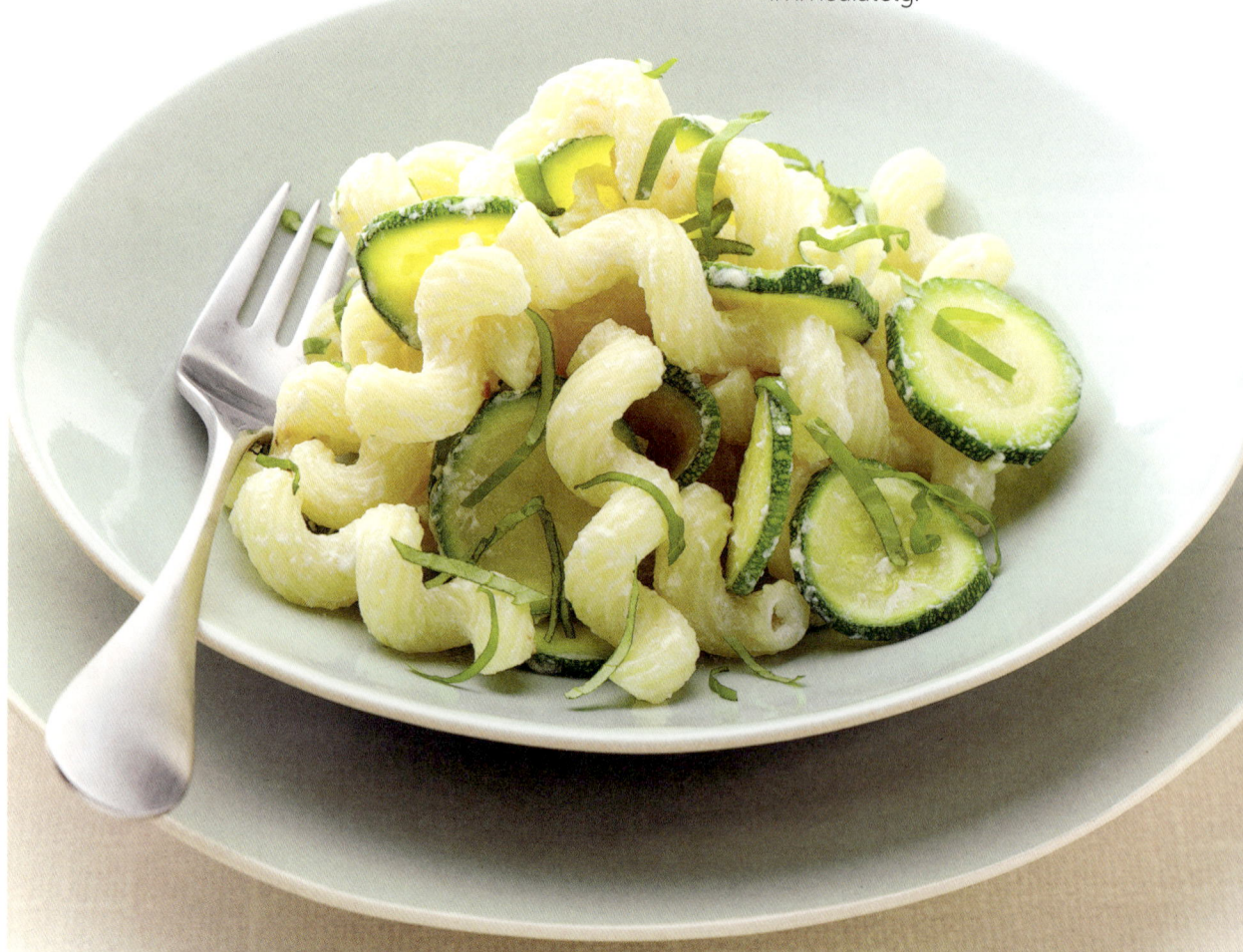

283 GREAT GREENS RISOTTO

SERVES 4
PREPARATION
10 minutes
COOKING
20 minutes

STORAGE
Ideally eat immediately, but you can store it overnight in the fridge and then reheat it.

1 litre/35fl oz/4 cups water
4 tsp vegetable bouillon powder
225g/8oz/1$\frac{1}{3}$ cups risotto rice
2 tbsp sesame oil
2 cloves garlic, peeled and sliced
175g/6oz broccoli florets
175g/6oz asparagus, chopped
175g/6oz/$\frac{2}{3}$ cup mangetout (snow peas), chopped
2 apples, grated
3 tbsp pumpkin seeds
1 sprig rosemary
115g/4oz/$\frac{2}{3}$ cup grated Cheddar cheese
freshly ground black pepper

1. Pour the water into a saucepan and add the bouillon powder and rice. Cover and simmer for 15 minutes, stirring occasionally, until the rice has absorbed all the water. Remove from the heat.

2. Heat the sesame oil in a wok, then add the garlic, broccoli, asparagus and mangetout (snow peas) and stir-fry for 2–3 minutes until tender. Add the apple, pumpkin seeds, rosemary and the risotto rice and mix.

3. If necessary, add a little more water for a smooth but sticky consistency. Serve on individual plates, garnished with the grated cheese and a sprinkle of black pepper.

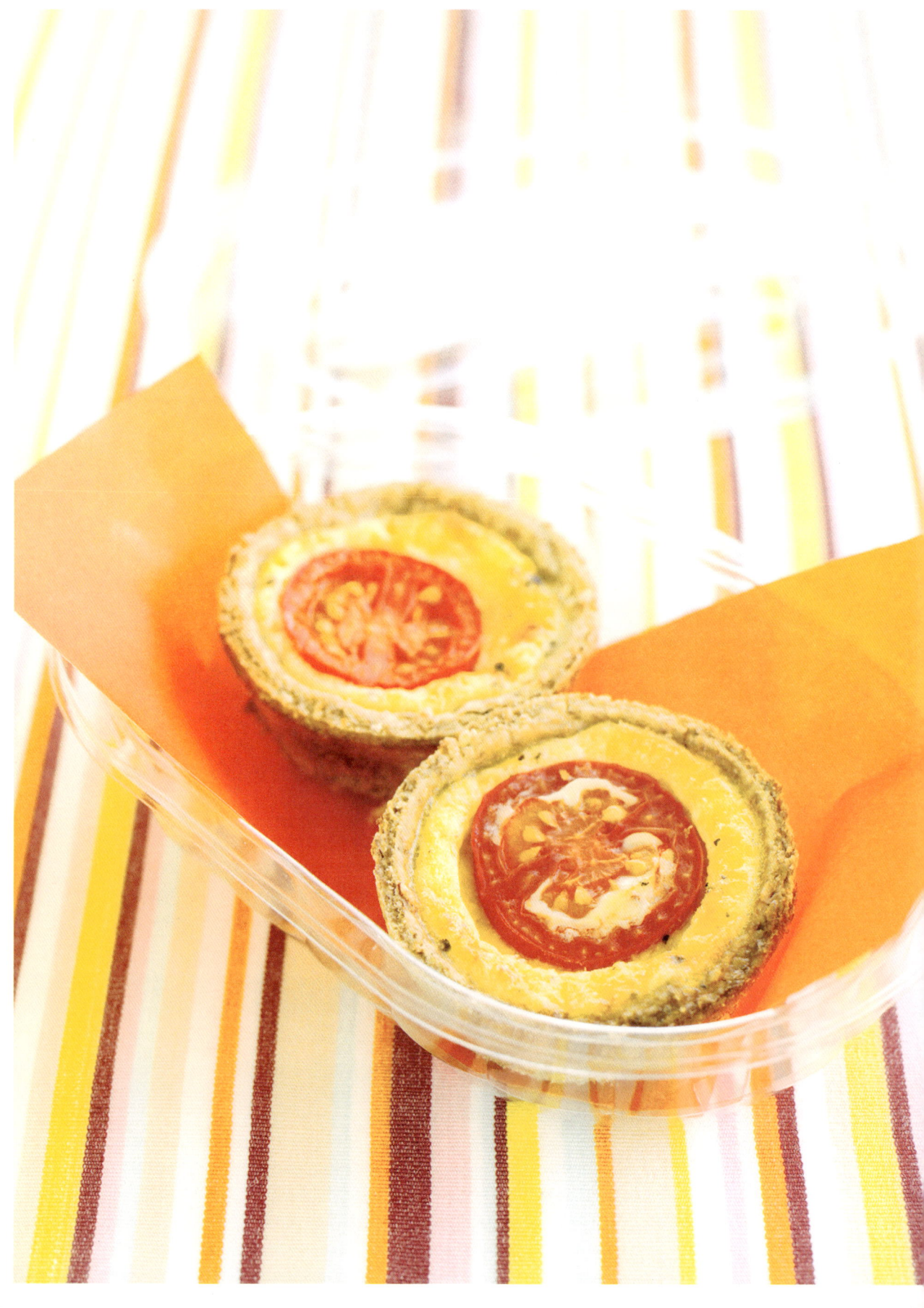

284 MINI TARTS

MAKES 8
PREPARATION
25 minutes + chilling
COOKING
22 minutes

STORAGE
Make in advance and keep in the fridge for up to 1 week or freeze for up to 1 month.

200g/7oz/1²/₃ cups wholemeal plain (all-purpose) flour
100g/3½oz cold unsalted butter, cut into small pieces
pinch of salt
150ml/5fl oz/²/₃ cup milk
4 eggs, lightly beaten
70g/2½oz Cheddar cheese, grated
1 tomato, sliced into 8 rounds
salt and freshly ground black pepper

1. Sift the flour into a mixing bowl. Rub the butter into the flour until it forms fine breadcrumbs. Pour in 2 tbsp iced water and bring together into a ball. Wrap in clingfilm (plastic wrap) and chill for 30 minutes.

2. Grease an eight-hole deep muffin tin (pan). Roll out the pastry on a floured surface and use to line the holes, leaving the pastry slightly proud at the top. Preheat the oven to 200°C/400°F/gas mark 6. Chill for 15 minutes.

3. Bake the pastry cases for 6 minutes, then remove from the oven. Whisk the milk and eggs together and season. Sprinkle the cheese into the cases, add the egg mixture, top with a slice of tomato and bake for 15 minutes until set.

4. Cool slightly before removing with a palette knife.

285 CRANBERRY AND ALMOND QUINOA

SERVES 4
PREPARATION
15 minutes
COOKING
25 minutes

STORAGE
Leftovers will keep in the fridge for up to 2 days.

175g/6oz/1 cup quinoa
500ml/17fl oz/2 cups stock
pinch of saffron strands
1 tbsp olive oil
1 red onion, chopped
1 clove garlic, crushed
50g/1¾oz/½ cup dried cranberries
50g/1¾oz/½ cup flaked almonds
½ cucumber, peeled and diced
½ red (bell) pepper, diced
2 tbsp lemon juice
2 tbsp chopped coriander (cilantro)
2 tbsp chopped mint leaves
1 preserved lemon, chopped
freshly ground black pepper

1. Bring the quinoa, stock and saffron to the boil. Reduce the heat, cover and simmer for 15–20 minutes. Set aside.

2. Heat the oil in a pan. Add the onion and garlic and fry for 2 minutes. Add to the quinoa with the remaining ingredients. Season, mix well and serve.

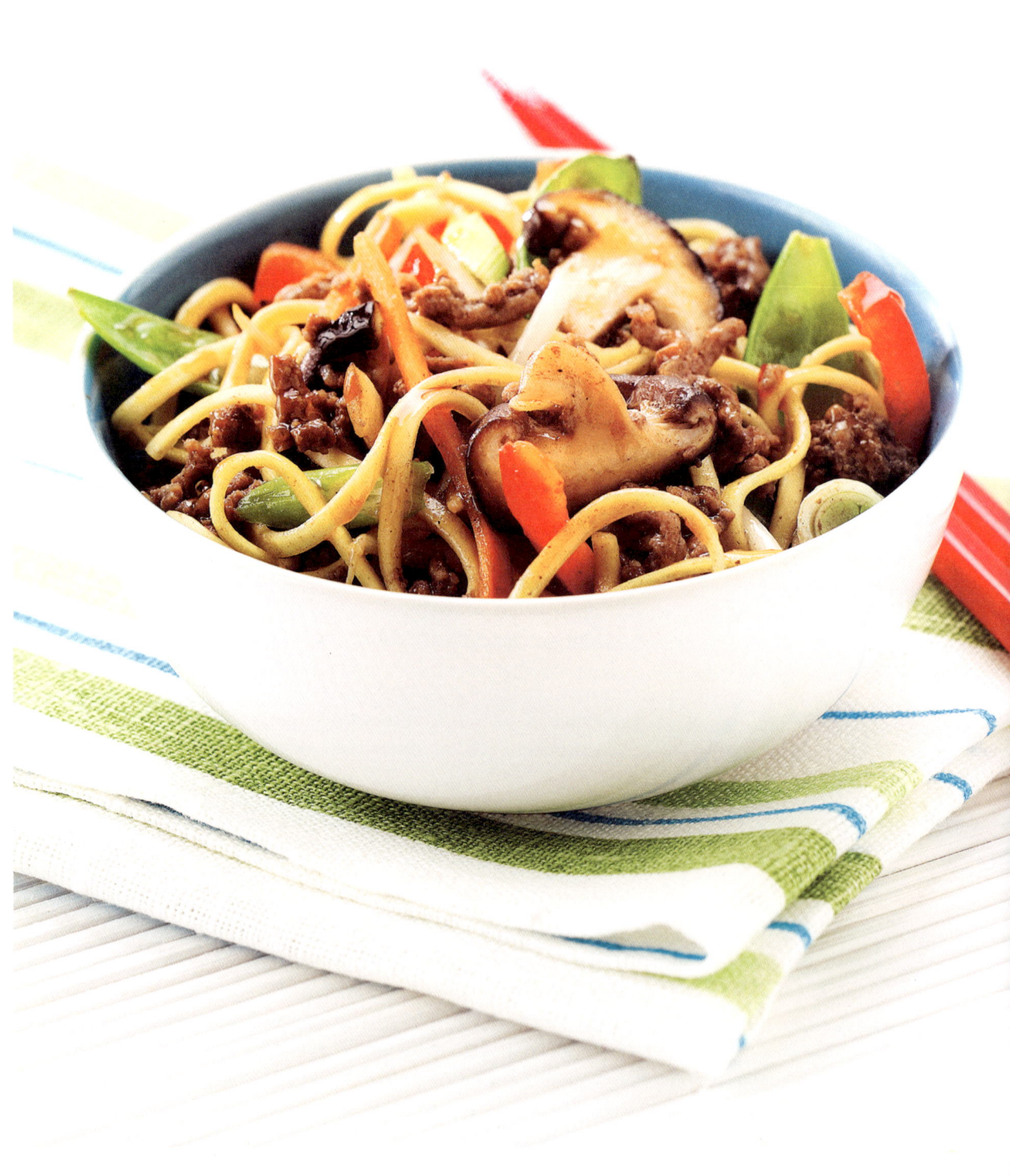

Dinners

Dinner need not be a struggle, even though it comes at the time of the day when everyone in the family is tired. Although we tend to think of dinner as our main meal of the day, it often suits children (and for that matter adults) better to have a substantial lunch and lighter evening meal. However, if lunch has been a snack, dinner should include all the essential nutrients needed to ensure that we maintain a healthy diet. Here are some simple, filling and nutritious options that will provide a superb end to the day.

This varied selection includes exciting international flavours, from Creamy Beef Korma (see page 212) to Mexican Casserole (see page 216) to Spanish Paella (see page 238) – what better way to educate your children about eating well than to try established favourites from cuisines the world over? Pastas, pilafs, vegetable kebabs, easy fishcakes ... all the essentials for fantastic family feasts are here.

286 CHOW MEIN

SERVES 4
PREPARATION
15 minutes
COOKING
20 minutes

STORAGE
Leftovers will keep in the fridge for up to 2 days.

- 270g/9½oz wholewheat egg noodles
- 1 tsp sesame oil
- 2 tsp olive oil
- 450g/1lb lean minced (ground) beef
- 1 tsp Chinese five-spice powder
- 1 clove garlic, crushed
- 1 tsp sweet chilli sauce
- 1 carrot, cut into thin strips or julienned
- 75g/2½oz shiitake or button mushrooms, sliced
- 50g/2oz mangetout (snow peas), trimmed
- 1 red (bell) pepper, deseeded and sliced
- 2 tbsp oyster sauce
- 2 tbsp tamari
- 1 tbsp rice wine or dry sherry
- 75g/2½oz beansprouts
- 1 spring onion (scallion), chopped

1. Cook the noodles according to the packet instructions. Drain and refresh under cold water. Put in a bowl and toss with the sesame oil.

2. Heat the olive oil in a wok or large frying pan (skillet). Add the beef, five-spice powder, garlic and sweet chilli sauce and stir-fry for 5 minutes, or until the meat is browned.

3. Add the vegetables and stir-fry for 2 minutes, or until they begin to soften.

4. Stir in the oyster sauce, tamari and rice wine and simmer for 4–5 minutes until the meat is cooked.

5. Add the noodles, beansprouts and spring onion (scallion) and stir-fry for 1–2 minutes until heated. Serve immediately.

287 BEEF TORTILLAS with BALSAMIC ONIONS

SERVES 4
PREPARATION
10 minutes
COOKING
25 minutes

STORAGE
Leftovers will keep in the fridge for up to 1 day.

2 tbsp olive oil
2 red onions, thinly sliced
1 tbsp soft brown sugar
3 tbsp balsamic vinegar
6 tbsp red wine (optional)
350g/12oz cold roast beef, sliced
4 wholemeal flour tortillas
handful of baby spinach leaves
freshly ground black pepper

1. Heat the oil in a pan. Add the onions and cook gently for 10–15 minutes, or until caramelized.

2. Add the sugar, vinegar and wine and cook for a further 10 minutes, stirring occasionally. Allow to cool, then season with black pepper.

3. Arrange the beef on the tortillas, top with the spinach leaves, then with the balsamic onions. Fold over the sides and roll up the tortillas. Slice in half diagonally and serve.

288 LAMB PROVENÇALE

SERVES 4
PREPARATION
20 minutes
COOKING
20 minutes

STORAGE
Leftovers will keep in the fridge for up to 1 day.

3 cloves garlic, finely chopped
2 tbsp parsley, finely chopped
6 tbsp breadcrumbs
4 tomatoes, halved and deseeded
10 large mushrooms, stalks removed and set aside
olive oil, for frying
2 shallots, finely chopped
8 lamb chops
2 tsp thyme
sea salt and black pepper to taste

1. Preheat the oven to 220°C/425°F/gas mark 7 and a grill (broiler) to hot.

2. Mix two cloves of garlic with the parsley and breadcrumbs to make a stuffing. Season the tomatoes and fill them with some of the stuffing. Set aside.

3. Finely chop the mushroom stalks and two of the mushrooms. Heat 2 tablespoons of oil in a heavy pan and fry the shallots, chopped mushrooms and remaining garlic. Mix with the remaining stuffing, then stuff the eight mushrooms and place on a greased baking sheet with the tomatoes. Bake for 15 minutes.

4. Sprinkle the lamb with thyme, then grill (broil) on both sides. Serve on large plates garnished with the stuffed tomatoes and mushrooms.

289 CREAMY BEEF KORMA

SERVES 4
PREPARATION 15 minutes
COOKING 40 minutes

STORAGE Leftovers will keep in the fridge for up to 2 days.

- 1-cm/½-in piece of root ginger, peeled
- 2 cloves garlic, crushed
- 1 red onion, chopped
- 1 tbsp olive oil
- ½ tsp turmeric
- 1 tsp ground coriander
- 1 tsp garam masala
- 400g/14oz lean beef fillet or braising steak, cubed
- 5 tbsp ground almonds
- 200ml/7fl oz/scant 1 cup lamb or chicken stock
- 6 tbsp low-fat crème fraîche
- 3 tomatoes, chopped
- handful of flaked (slivered) almonds, toasted
- handful of coriander (cilantro) leaves, chopped

1. Purée the ginger, garlic and onion to a paste in a blender.

2. Heat the oil in a large saucepan. Add the ginger paste, turmeric, ground coriander and garam masala and cook gently for 1 minute. Add the beef and cook, stirring, for 5 minutes until evenly browned.

3. Process the ground almonds, stock and crème fraîche in a blender until smooth, then stir this into the beef with the tomatoes. Bring to the boil, reduce the heat, cover and simmer for 20–30 minutes until the beef is cooked.

4. Scatter with the flaked (slivered) almonds and coriander (cilantro) and serve with rice.

290 TEX-MEX BURGERS

MAKES 8
PREPARATION
10 minutes +
chilling
COOKING
8 minutes

STORAGE
Leftovers will keep in the fridge for up to 1 day.

1 red onion, grated
½ tsp ground cumin
½ tsp paprika
400g/14oz lean minced (ground) beef
1 carrot, grated
2 tsp Worcestershire sauce
1 egg, beaten
8 wholemeal hamburger buns
2 tomatoes, sliced
handful of mixed salad leaves

1. Mix the onion, cumin, paprika, beef, carrot and Worcestershire sauce in a large bowl. Add the egg and mix well. Shape the mixture into 8 small burgers. Put on a plate, cover and chill for 30 minutes.

2. Preheat the grill (broiler) to high. Put the burgers on a baking sheet and grill (broil) for 4 minutes on each side, or until cooked through.

3. Cut the buns in half and toast lightly. Fill each one with 1 burger and some sliced tomato and salad leaves and serve.

291 GLAZED LAMB

SERVES 4
PREPARATION
10 minutes +
marinating
COOKING
17 minutes

STORAGE
Leftovers will keep in the fridge for up to 2 days.

1 tbsp tamari
1 clove garlic, crushed
5 tbsp pomegranate molasses
4 lamb fillets, about 125g/4½oz each
2 tsp olive oil
2 tbsp lemon juice
1 tbsp honey

1. Mix together the tamari, garlic and 3 tablespoons of the molasses. Pour over the lamb fillets, cover and marinate in the fridge for 1 hour or overnight.

2. Preheat the grill (broiler) to high. Put the lamb on a grill pan, reserving the marinade. Grill (broil) for 15 minutes, turning halfway through until cooked. Leave to rest for 5 minutes, then cut into thin slices.

3. Put the reserved marinade, oil, lemon juice, honey and remaining molasses in a pan. Simmer for 1–2 minutes until syrupy and serve with the lamb.

292 CHOPS with HONEY and THYME

SERVES 4
PREPARATION
10 minutes
COOKING
25 minutes

STORAGE
Leftovers will keep in the fridge for up to 2 days.

2 tbsp olive oil
8 lamb chops
sea salt and black pepper to taste
4 tsp honey
2 tsp thyme
juice of 1 lemon
200ml/7fl oz/scant 1 cup dry white wine
2 tbsp tamari

1. Preheat the oven to 250°C/500°F/gas mark 10.

2. Heat the oil in a large ovenproof frying pan (skillet) and sauté the lamb on both sides to seal, then remove from the pan, season, brush with 2 teaspoons of the honey and sprinkle with thyme. Return the lamb to the pan and bake in the oven for 10 minutes. Remove the lamb from the pan and set aside.

3. Make a sauce by browning the remaining honey in the pan and adding the lemon juice, white wine and tamari. Bring to the boil and reduce to half the volume. Place the lamb on serving plates and cover with the sauce. Serve with boiled potatoes and braised chicory (Belgian endive).

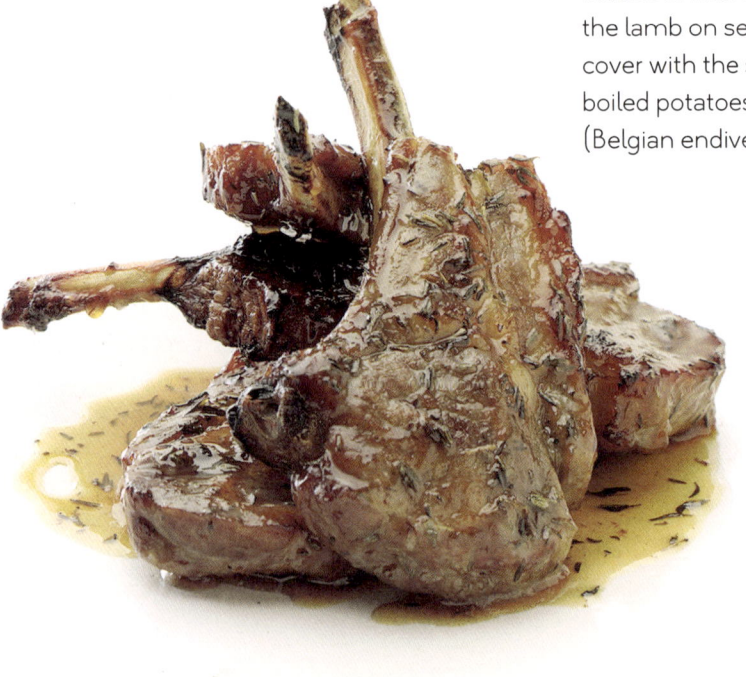

293 MOROCCAN LAMB

SERVES 4
PREPARATION
15 minutes
COOKING
1 hour 8 minutes

STORAGE
Leftovers will keep in the fridge for up to 2 days.

1 tbsp olive oil
400g/14oz lean boneless lamb, cut into chunks
1 tsp each ground coriander, ginger, cinnamon and paprika
1 onion, finely chopped
2 cloves garlic, crushed
juice and grated zest of 1 lemon
1 tbsp honey or agave nectar
1 red (bell) pepper, deseeded and cut into chunks
1 sweet potato, peeled and diced
10 cherry tomatoes
425ml/15fl oz/scant 1¾ cups chicken stock
16 dried apricots
25g/1oz flaked (slivered) almonds, lightly toasted

1. Preheat the oven to 190°C/375°F/gas mark 5. Heat the oil in a large flameproof casserole. Fry the lamb with the spices, onion and garlic for 3–4 minutes until the meat browns.

2. Add the lemon juice, zest, honey, red (bell) pepper, sweet potato, tomatoes and stock. Bring to the boil, then remove from the heat, cover and bake for 40 minutes.

3. Add the apricots and cook for a further 20 minutes until the lamb is very tender. Sprinkle with the almonds and serve with couscous.

294 ORANGE-ROASTED LAMB CHOPS

SERVES 4
PREPARATION
5 minutes
COOKING
30 minutes

STORAGE
Prepare the chops in advance and store them uncooked in the fridge for up to 12 hours.

10g/¼oz butter
8 lamb chops, about 55g/2oz each
4 cloves
2 oranges, the zest of 1 and juice of both
8 sprigs rosemary
25g/1oz/⅓ cup chopped mint

1. Preheat the oven to 200°C/400°F/gas mark 6. Spread the butter over the lamb chops on both sides and lay them in a shallow casserole dish.

2. Add the cloves, orange zest, juice and rosemary. Place in the oven for 30 minutes, turning the chops once during cooking.

3. Remove from the oven and serve on individual plates, garnished with the chopped mint.

295 ORIENTAL STIR-FRY

SERVES 4
PREPARATION
10 minutes + marinating
COOKING
15 minutes

STORAGE
Leftovers will keep in the fridge for up to 2 days.

4 tbsp tamari
4 tbsp dry sherry or rice wine
2 tsp cornflour (cornstarch) dissolved in a little cold water
2 tsp fresh ginger, finely chopped
500g/1lb 2oz lamb fillet, diced
4 tbsp olive oil
4 spring onions (scallions), chopped into strips
200g/7oz broccoli florets, cut into small pieces
200g/7oz sweetcorn kernels
1 large bunch watercress, chopped
sea salt and black pepper to taste
stock to taste (optional)

1 Mix the tamari, sherry or rice wine, cornflour (cornstarch) mixture and ginger in a bowl. Add the lamb cubes to the mixture. Leave to marinate while you prepare the rest of the ingredients.

2 Heat the oil in a wok and stir-fry the lamb with the marinade until all the liquid is absorbed. Remove from the pan and set aside. Add a little more oil to the pan and stir-fry the vegetables for 3 minutes. Add the fried lamb, mix and season, adding a little stock (if using). Serve with rice or noodles.

296 MEXICAN CASSEROLE

SERVES 4
PREPARATION
10 minutes
COOKING
40 minutes

STORAGE
Leftovers will keep in the fridge for up to 2 days.

oil, for frying
600g/1lb 5oz loin of lamb, diced
2 onions, sliced
1 red (bell) pepper, sliced
1 green (bell) pepper, sliced
2 cloves garlic, crushed
2 small hot chillies, kept whole
2 tomatoes, chopped
400ml/14fl oz/1$^{2}/_{3}$ cups white wine
large pinch of thyme
2 bay leaves
400g (14oz) canned kidney beans
sea salt and cayenne pepper to taste

1 Heat a little oil in a casserole dish and fry the lamb over a high heat. Set aside.

2 Fry the onions, red and green (bell) peppers and garlic in the same dish with a little more oil. Add the chillies, tomatoes, white wine, thyme and bay leaves. Bring to the boil, cover and simmer for 10 minutes. Add the beans and cook for 5 minutes. Add the cooked lamb, heat through and season. Serve with corn bread.

297 MAMMA'S MEATBALLS

SERVES 4
PREPARATION
10 minutes
COOKING
30 minutes

STORAGE
You can refrigerate the raw mixture for up to 3 days.

1 tbsp olive oil
1 onion, peeled and diced
1 leek, trimmed and sliced
2 cloves garlic, peeled and finely sliced
4 slices brown bread, crusts removed
1 tsp dried oregano
500g/1lb 2oz lean minced (ground) lamb
55g/2oz/⅓ cup sunflower seeds
25g/1oz/⅓ cup chopped fresh coriander (cilantro)
25g/1oz/⅓ cup chopped parsley
1 tbsp wholegrain mustard
2 eggs
400g/14oz/2⅓ cups brown rice
½ tsp ground cinnamon
200g/7oz/1 cup passata (sieved tomatoes)
115g/4oz/½ cup tomato purée (paste)
1 tbsp Worcestershire sauce
4 sprigs parsley

① Preheat the oven to 190°C/375°F/gas mark 5. In a wok, heat the oil and stir-fry the onion, leek and garlic until soft.

② Whiz the bread in a food processor to make breadcrumbs, transfer the crumbs to a mixing bowl and mix in the oregano, lamb, seeds, herbs, mustard and eggs. Using your hands, mould the mixture into small meatballs, place on a baking sheet and bake for 20–30 minutes. Meanwhile, add the rice to boiling water and simmer for 20 minutes.

③ Put the cinnamon, passata (sieved tomatoes), tomato purée and Worcestershire sauce into a separate small saucepan and stir over a low heat. Serve over the rice and meatballs. Garnish with parsley.

298 SPAGHETTI BOLOGNESE

SERVES 4
PREPARATION
10 minutes
COOKING
25 minutes

STORAGE
Leftovers will keep in the fridge for up to 2 days.

6 tbsp olive oil
2 onions, chopped
300g/10½oz minced (ground) pork
4 cloves garlic, crushed
2 carrots, diced
2 celery stalks, chopped
4 tsp thyme
2 sprigs each of rosemary and sage
2 tbsp fresh basil (or 2 tsp dried)
2 tbsp tamari
900g/2lb tomatoes, blended
2 tsp raw cane sugar
4 tbsp tomato purée (paste)
sea salt
400g/14oz spaghetti pasta
fresh parsley and black pepper, to garnish

1. Gently fry the onions in the oil until soft. Add the pork, together with the garlic and stir-fry until the meat browns. Add the carrot, celery, herbs and tamari. Heat through, then add the blended tomatoes, sugar and tomato purée. Bring to the boil and simmer for 10 minutes, stirring occasionally.

2. Meanwhile, boil the spaghetti in plenty of water with a little salt and oil, then drain.

3. Divide the cooked spaghetti between serving plates. Top with the bolognese sauce, garnish with plenty of fresh parsley and black pepper and serve immediately.

299 PASTA WITH SAUSAGE AND TOMATO SAUCE

SERVES 4
PREPARATION
10 minutes
COOKING
15 minutes

STORAGE
Leftovers will keep in the fridge for up to 2 days.

400g/14oz tricolor fusilli pasta
300g/10½oz sausages, chopped into chunks
4 tbsp olive oil
2 spring onions (scallions), chopped
400g/14oz fresh peas, shelled
2 small pickled peppers, sliced
400ml/14fl oz/1⅔ cups passata (sieved tomatoes)
sea salt and black pepper to taste
large handful fresh parsley, chopped
4 handfuls salad leaves, to serve

1. Cook the pasta according to the package instructions.

2. Heat the oil in a heavy-based frying pan (skillet), add the sausage and the spring onions (scallions). Stir-fry over a medium heat until browned. Add the peas, pickled peppers and passata, and simmer for 10 minutes.

3. Drain the pasta and divide between plates. Top with the sauce, season, garnish with parsley and serve with salad alongside.

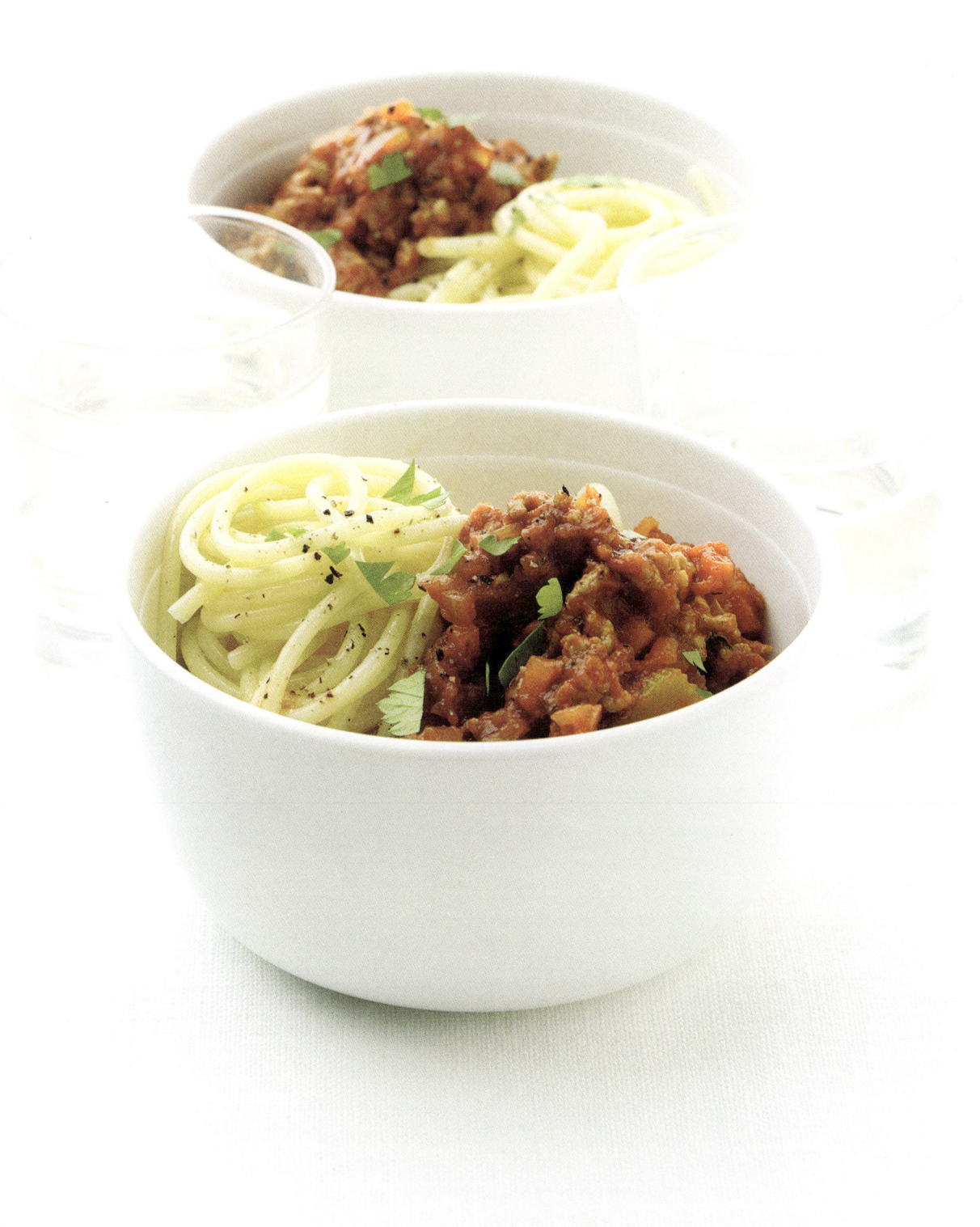

300 BRAZILIAN FEIJOADA

SERVES 4
PREPARATION
10 minutes
COOKING
15 minutes

STORAGE
Leftovers will keep in the fridge for up to 1 day.

4 cloves garlic, crushed
2 bay leaves
2 tsp paprika
2 tsp thyme
2 tsp cumin
2 leeks, sliced
2 sweet potatoes, cubed
about 400ml/14fl oz/1$^{2}/_{3}$ cups vegetable stock
oil for frying
250g/9oz bacon
400g/14oz black beans, cooked or canned
2 red (bell) peppers, deseeded and sliced
500g/1lb 2oz tomatoes, crushed
1 large bunch parsley and chives, finely chopped
sea salt and black pepper to taste
1 orange, thinly sliced

1. Place the garlic, bay leaves, paprika, thyme, cumin, leek and sweet potato in a medium casserole dish. Cover with the stock, bring to the boil and simmer over a medium heat for 10 minutes.

2. Meanwhile, heat a little oil in a frying pan (skillet) and fry the bacon and black beans for 2 minutes. Then add the red (bell) peppers, tomatoes, parsley and chives and stir-fry over a medium heat for a further 5 minutes.

3. Add the bean mixture to the vegetables and heat through. Season, garnish with orange slices and serve with rice.

301 AFRICAN CURRY

SERVES 4
PREPARATION
10 minutes
COOKING
25 minutes

STORAGE
Leftovers will keep in the fridge for up to 2 days

4 tbsp olive oil
800g/1lb 12oz pork fillet, cut into chunks
2 tbsp curry powder
2 onions, halved and sliced
1 red (bell) pepper, sliced
2 cloves garlic, crushed
400ml/14fl oz/1²⁄₃ cups coconut milk
2 apples, peeled, cored and diced
sea salt and cayenne pepper to taste

1. Heat the oil in a casserole dish. Add the pork chunks and half of the curry powder. Stir-fry over a medium-high heat until the pork chunks begin to brown. Remove from the pan and set aside.

2. Stir-fry the onion, red (bell) pepper and garlic in the same pan with the remaining curry powder (and a little more oil if necessary). Add the coconut milk, apple and cooked pork. Bring to the boil and simmer for 5 minutes. Season with salt and pepper and serve with rice.

302 LOUISIANA GUMBO

SERVES 4
PREPARATION
15 minutes
COOKING
25 minutes

STORAGE
Leftovers will keep in the fridge for up to 2 days

2 tbsp corn oil
2 red onions, halved and sliced
2 bay leaves
large pinch of cayenne pepper
2 tsp paprika
1 green (bell) pepper, sliced
1 red (bell) pepper, sliced
2 celery stalks, sliced
400g/14oz pumpkin, peeled, deseeded and chopped
2 tbsp plain (all-purpose) flour
500g/1lb 2oz tomatoes, chopped
400ml/14fl oz/1²⁄₃ cups vegetable stock
200g/7oz smoked sausages, sliced
sea salt and plenty of black pepper

1. Heat the oil in a heavy-based casserole dish and gently sweat the onion with the bay leaves, cayenne pepper and paprika. Add the (bell) pepper slices, followed by the celery and the pumpkin. Gently stir-fry for 3–5 minutes. Sprinkle with flour and stir for 1 minute to coat the vegetables. Add the tomatoes, stir, then add the stock. Bring to the boil, cover and simmer for 10 minutes. Add the sausage and heat through. Season and serve with rice.

303 BEAN and SAUSAGE HOTPOT

SERVES 4
PREPARATION
5 minutes
COOKING
22 minutes

STORAGE
Leftovers will keep in the fridge for up to 2 days.

2 tsp olive oil
8 good-quality sausages
2 cloves garlic, crushed
2 thyme sprigs
2 red (bell) peppers, deseeded and sliced
800g/1lb 12oz canned mixed beans, drained and rinsed
800g/1lb 12oz canned chopped tomatoes
freshly ground black pepper

1. Heat the oil in a large flameproof casserole. Add the sausages, garlic, thyme and (bell) peppers and fry for 3–4 minutes, turning occasionally, until the sausages are golden brown.

2. Add the beans and tomatoes and bring to a simmer, then cover and simmer for 15 minutes until the sausages are cooked through and the sauce has thickened.

3. Season with black pepper and then serve.

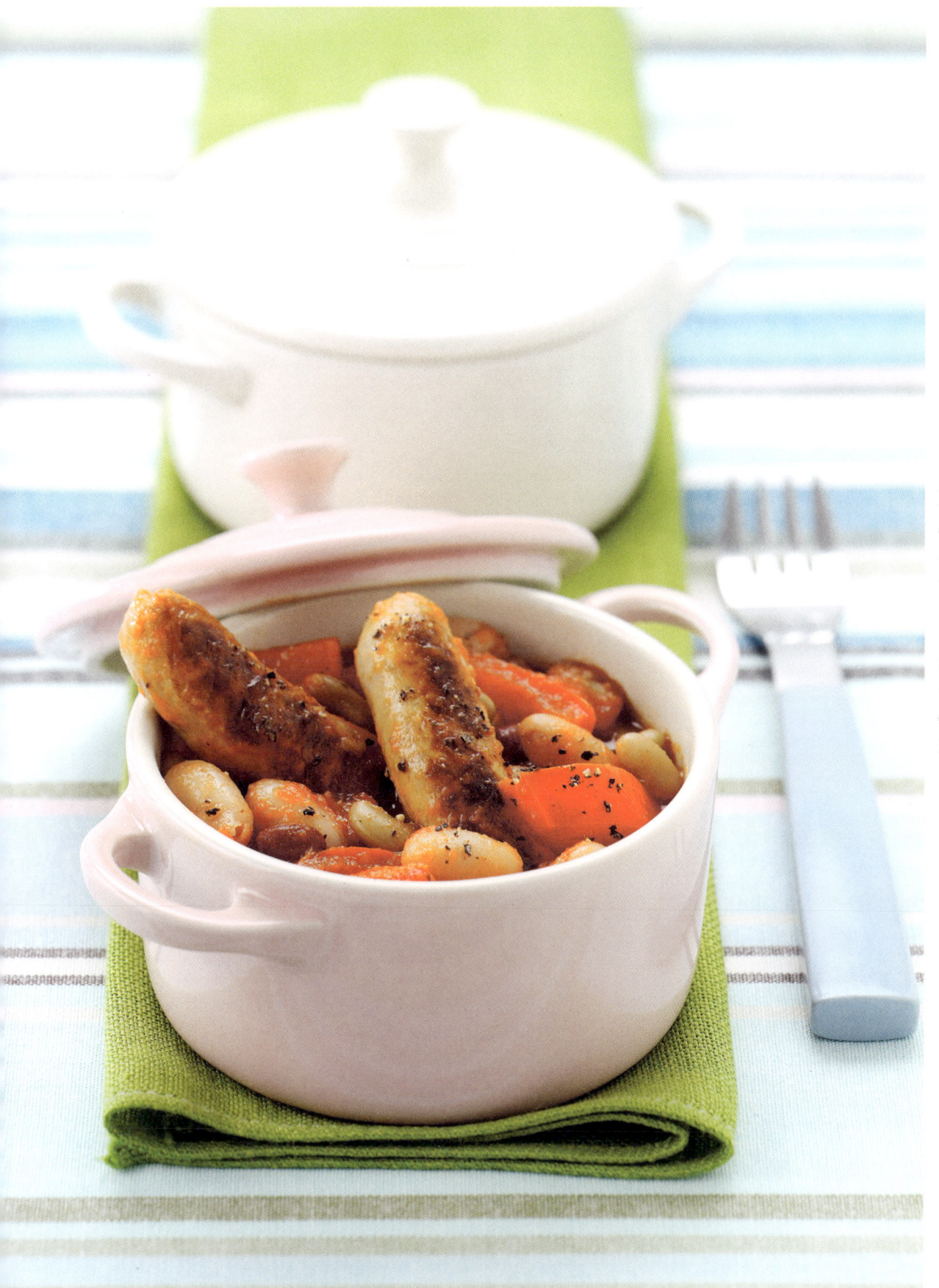

304 FARFALLE with CHANTERELLE and THYME SAUCE

SERVES 4
PREPARATION 10 minutes
COOKING 12 minutes
STORAGE Leftovers will keep in the fridge for up to 2 days.

- 400g/14oz farfalle pasta
- 4 tbsp olive oil
- 250g/9oz smoked ham, cubed
- 250g/9oz fresh chanterelle mushrooms, quartered
- 2 small red onions, finely chopped
- 2 cloves garlic, crushed
- 4 tbsp crème frâiche
- 2 tsp thyme
- sea salt and black pepper to taste

1. Cook the pasta according to the package instructions.

2. Meanwhile, heat the oil in a casserole dish and stir-fry the ham, chanterelles, onion and garlic over a medium heat for 5 minutes. Add the crème fraîche and the thyme, season and simmer for a further 5 minutes. Check the seasoning.

3. Place the drained, cooked pasta in a heated serving dish, top with the sauce and serve immediately.

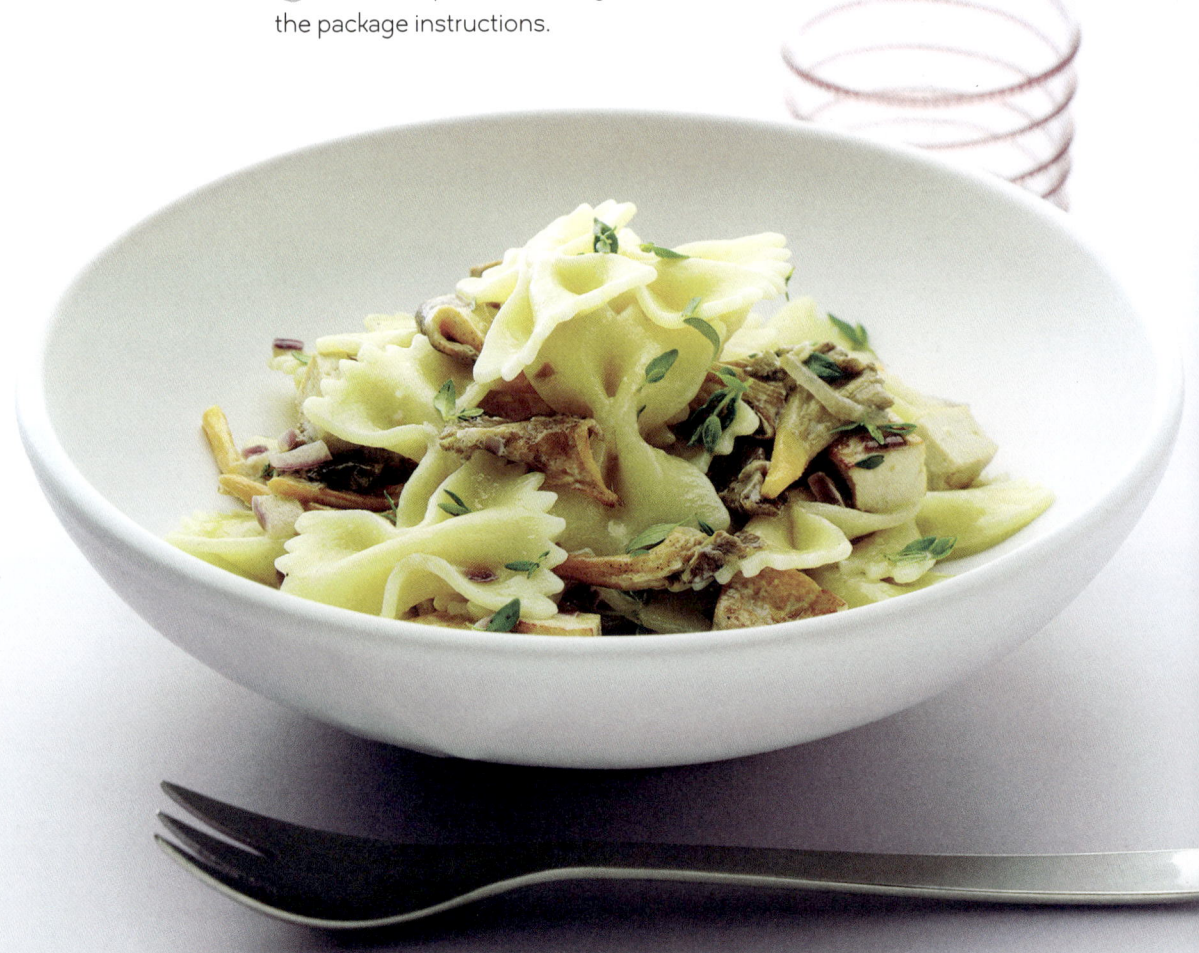

305 PENNE with SMOKY PESTO SAUCE

SERVES 4
PREPARATION
10 minutes
COOKING
15 minutes

STORAGE
Leftovers will keep in the fridge for up to 2 days.

- 4 tbsp pine kernels
- 6 tbsp fresh basil, finely chopped
- 6 tbsp olive oil, plus extra for frying
- 2–4 cloves garlic, crushed (optional)
- 400g/14oz penne pasta
- 350g/12oz green beans, chopped
- 200g/7oz smoked bacon, cubed
- 200ml/7fl oz/scant 1 cup plain yogurt
- 2 tbsp grated Parmesan

1. Crush the pine kernels in a mortar and mix in the basil, oil, garlic (if using) and a little salt to make the pesto.

2. Cook the pasta in boiling water according to the package instructions, for about 12 minutes or until al dente. After 4 minutes, add the beans to the water.

3. Sauté the bacon cubes in a frying pan (skillet) with oil until they begin to brown. Remove from the heat, add the pesto and the yogurt and mix well. Add the drained pasta and beans to the pan and gently mix. Sprinkle with Parmesan and serve.

306 PORK with APPLES and PEARS

SERVES 4
PREPARATION
10 minutes
COOKING
30 minutes

STORAGE
Leftovers will keep in the fridge for up to 2 days.

2 tbsp olive oil
15g/½oz butter
3 apples, peeled, cored and quartered
2 pears, peeled and quartered
150ml/5fl oz/scant ⅔ cup apple juice
1 cinnamon stick, broken in half
pinch of ground mixed spice
4 lean pork fillets, about 115g/4oz each
freshly ground black pepper
1 tbsp rosemary leaves
3 tbsp low-fat crème fraîche

1. Preheat the oven to 200°C/400°F/gas mark 6. Heat a small roasting tin (pan), add half the oil and the butter and swirl until the butter has melted. Add the fruit, apple juice, cinnamon and mixed spice. Turn to coat the fruit in the liquid. Bake for 20–25 minutes, or until tender and lightly browned.

2. Meanwhile, preheat the grill (broiler) to high. Rub the remaining oil over the pork fillets, put on a grill pan and sprinkle with black pepper and rosemary. Grill (broil) for 15 minutes, or until cooked through, turning once. Leave to rest for 5 minutes.

3. Stir the crème fraîche into the fruit and simmer for 1–2 minutes until thickened slightly. Arrange the fruit on a plate with the pork, spoon over the sauce and serve.

307 VIETNAMESE PORK

SERVES 4
PREPARATION 15 minutes + marinating
COOKING 10 minutes

STORAGE
Leftovers will keep in the fridge for up to 1 day.

2 tbsp fish sauce
1 lemongrass stalk, finely chopped
1 clove garlic, crushed
1 tbsp honey or agave nectar
1 tbsp sesame oil
400g/14oz pork tenderloin, cut into strips
1 tbsp olive oil
175g/6oz rice noodles
½ cucumber, peeled and cut into strips
2 carrots, cut into strips
1 red (bell) pepper, deseeded and cut into thin strips
3 tbsp chopped mint, chopped
25g/1oz/¼ cup roasted cashew nuts

DRESSING
2 tbsp tamari
1 tbsp balsamic vinegar
1 tsp sesame oil
2 tsp omega oil or flaxseed oil

1. Mix together the fish sauce, lemongrass, garlic, honey or agave nectar and sesame oil in a dish. Add the pork, mix well, then cover and marinate in the fridge for 30 minutes.

2. Heat the olive oil in a wok and stir-fry the pork for 5–6 minutes until golden brown and cooked through.

3. Cook the noodles according to the package instructions, drain and rinse. Toss in the cucumber, carrots, red (bell) pepper and mint.

4. Mix the dressing ingredients together and toss with the salad. Serve topped with the pork and cashew nuts.

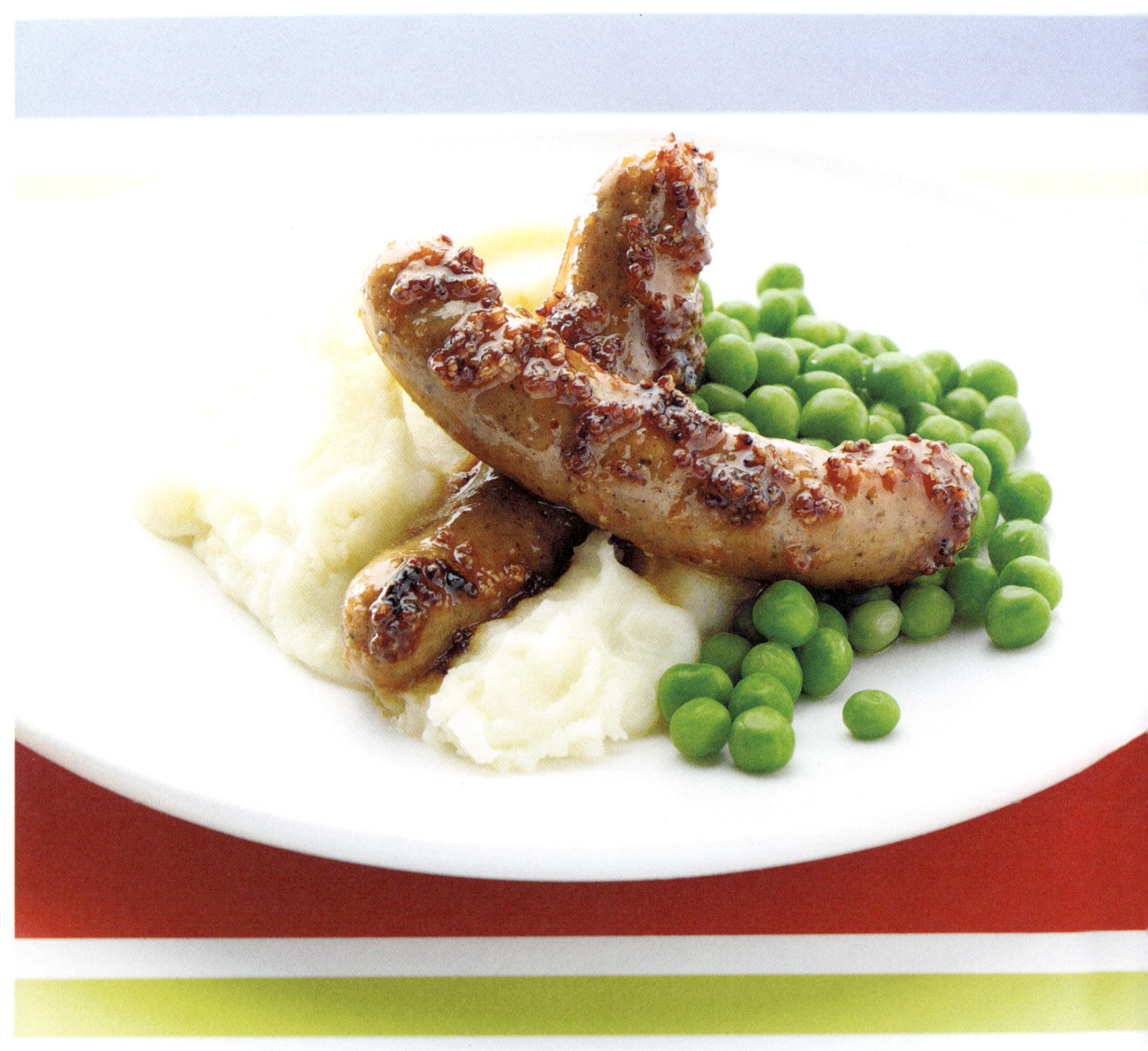

308 HONEY BANGERS AND MASH

SERVES 4
PREPARATION
10 minutes
COOKING
20 minutes

STORAGE
Once cooked, you can refrigerate the sausages and eat them within 24 hours.

- 500g/1lb 2oz potatoes, peeled and cut into chunks
- 4 tbsp honey
- 6 tbsp wholegrain mustard
- 8 sausages
- 115g/4oz/1 cup peas
- 80ml/2½fl oz/⅓ cup milk
- 15g/½oz butter

(1) Heat the oven to 190°C/375°F/gas mark 5. Half fill a saucepan with water, bring to the boil and add the potatoes. Cover and let simmer for 15–20 minutes, until soft.

(2) Meanwhile, mix the honey and mustard in a small bowl. Prick the sausages with a fork and place in an ovenproof dish. Pour the mustard and honey sauce on top and place in the oven for 20 minutes, until browned.

(3) Half fill a saucepan with water, bring to the boil and add the peas. Cover and let simmer for 5 minutes, until cooked. Add the milk and butter to the potatoes and mash. Remove the sausages from the oven, drain the peas and serve with the mash on individual plates

309 BACON-BAKED BRUSSELS

SERVES 4
PREPARATION
10 minutes
COOKING
30 minutes

STORAGE
You can refrigerate for up to a day and then reheat.

- 400g/14oz Brussels sprouts, trimmed and outer leaves removed
- 8 slices unsmoked bacon, finely chopped
- 100g/3½oz/½ cup cooked chestnuts, drained
- 55g/2oz/⅓ cup prunes, chopped
- 3 tbsp olive oil

(1) Preheat the oven to 200°C/400°F/gas mark 6. Half fill a saucepan with water, bring to the boil and add the sprouts. Cover and let simmer for 10 minutes, then drain.

(2) Pour the sprouts, bacon, chestnuts and prunes into a medium-sized oven-proof dish. Drizzle olive oil over the mixture and bake in the oven for 20 minutes.

310 AUBERGINE FARCIE

SERVES 4
PREPARATION
15 minutes
COOKING
40 minutes

STORAGE
Leftovers will keep in the fridge for up to 2 days.

2 aubergines (eggplant), sliced lengthways
olive oil, for frying
2 small courgettes (zucchini), halved and sliced lengthways
4 small potatoes, finely sliced
2 red (bell) peppers, finely sliced
300g/10½oz spicy sausages, crumbled
2 thick slices bread, soaked in milk or soya milk and grated
2 cloves garlic, grated
sea salt and black pepper to taste
500g/1lb 2oz tomatoes, blended
2–4 tsp paprika

1. Preheat the oven to 220°C/425°F/gas mark 7.

2. Fry the aubergines (eggplant) in a pan with oil until golden, then place in the bottom of an oiled baking dish. Add the courgette (zucchini), potatoes and pepper in layers. Mix the sausage, bread and garlic in a bowl, then season and spoon onto the vegetables. Pour the blended tomatoes over the mixture and make some holes with your finger, so that the liquid can run through each layer. Sprinkle with paprika and a little oil. Bake for 30 minutes, until it begins to brown. Serve hot or cold.

311 MUSHROOM AND HAM PIZZA

SERVES 4
PREPARATION
10 minutes
COOKING
15 minutes

STORAGE
Leftovers will keep in the fridge for up to 2 days.

4–5 tbsp passata (sieved tomatoes)
2 pizza bases
1 small hot chilli, finely chopped
8 mushrooms, sliced
200g/7oz ham, diced
2 spring onions (scallions), sliced
a little oregano
sea salt and black pepper to taste
200g/7oz mozzarella cheese, grated

1. Preheat the oven to 240°C/475°F/gas mark 9 and heat two baking sheets.

2. Spread the passata (sieved tomatoes) over the prepared bases. Top with the hot chilli, mushrooms, ham and spring onions (scallions), then add a sprinkling of oregano. Season, sprinkle with the grated cheese and bake in the hot oven for approximately 15 minutes. Serve hot with a side salad.

312 WILD MUSHROOM, SPINACH AND PANCETTA PIZZA

SERVES 4
PREPARATION
15 minutes
COOKING
20 minutes

STORAGE
Leftovers will keep in the fridge for up to 2 days.

4–5 tbsp passata (sieved tomatoes)
2 pizza bases
200g/7oz fresh spinach, sautéed
300g/10½oz wild mushrooms, chopped
4 cloves garlic, crushed
2 shallots, chopped
8 slices pancetta or bacon, fried
sea salt and black pepper to taste
200g/7oz mozzarella cheese, grated
1 tbsp grated Parmesan

1. Preheat the oven to 220°C/425°F/gas mark 7 and heat two baking sheets.

2. Spread the passata (sieved tomatoes) over the prepared bases. Cover with the sautéed spinach, wild mushrooms, garlic, shallots and pancetta or bacon. Season, sprinkle with the grated cheese and bake in the hot oven for approximately 20 minutes. Serve hot with a side salad.

313 TURKISH BOREG

SERVES 4
PREPARATION
10 minutes
COOKING
30 minutes

STORAGE
Leftovers will keep in the fridge for up to 2 days.

2 shallots, chopped
4 tbsp olive oil
200g/7oz minced (ground) pork
8 mushrooms, chopped
2 carrots, grated
50g/2oz couscous, soaked in boiling water for 10 minutes
4 tbsp fresh parsley, chopped
2 tsp thyme
zest of 1 lemon
sea salt and black pepper to taste
1 package ready-made shortcrust pastry, rolled out thinly

1. Preheat the oven to 220°C/425°F/gas mark 7.

2. Soften the shallots in a saucepan with the oil. Add the pork and the mushrooms and stir-fry for 5 minutes, then add the carrot, couscous, parsley, thyme and lemon zest. Pile the filling into the middle of the rolled-out pastry and fold in the edges to form a parcel. Turn upside down onto a greased baking sheet. Glaze with cold water and bake for 15–20 minutes.

3. Serve with steamed vegetables and plain yogurt mixed with fresh mint, cayenne pepper and celery salt.

314 TANDOORI CHICKEN DRUMSTICKS

SERVES 4
PREPARATION
15 minutes + marinating
COOKING
30 minutes

STORAGE
Make the day before and keep in the fridge overnight.

4 skinless chicken drumsticks
2 tbsp lemon juice
150ml/5fl oz/⅔ cup thick plain yogurt
4 tbsp tandoori spice blend
sunflower oil, for brushing

1. Pat the chicken dry with paper towels. Make three deep cuts in each drumstick and rub the lemon juice over them.

2. Put the yogurt and spice blend in a dish and mix. Add the chicken and cover with the marinade. Cover and chill for at least 1 hour.

3. Preheat the oven to 200°C/400°F/gas mark 6. Brush a baking sheet with oil and add the chicken. Cook for 15 minutes, then turn and spoon over some more of the marinade. Cook for 15 minutes more, until cooked through.

315 CHICKEN BURGERS

MAKES 6
PREPARATION
20 minutes + chilling
COOKING
16 minutes
STORAGE
Make in advance and keep in the fridge for up to 3 days or freeze for up to 1 month (unless the chicken was frozen).

1 small onion
2 tbsp chopped alfalfa sprouts
1 small carrot, finely grated
1 apple, cored and grated,
450g/1lb minced (ground) chicken
1 small free-range egg, lightly beaten
salt and freshly ground black pepper
plain (all-purpose) flour, for dusting
olive oil, for brushing

1. Put the onion, alfalfa sprouts, carrot, apple and chicken in a mixing bowl. Stir or use your hands to break up the minced (ground) chicken and mix together.

2. Add the egg and seasoning and mix again by hand.

3. Lightly cover a plate and your hands with flour. Divide the mixture into six portions and shape each into a round, flat burger. Place on a plate, cover with clingfilm (plastic wrap) and chill for 30 minutes.

4. Preheat the grill (broiler) to medium and line a baking sheet with foil. Lightly brush the foil with oil and place the burgers on top. Brush the top of the burgers with oil and grill (broil) for about 8 minutes on each side until golden. Serve with seeded burger buns, relish or tomato ketchup, lettuce and sliced tomatoes.

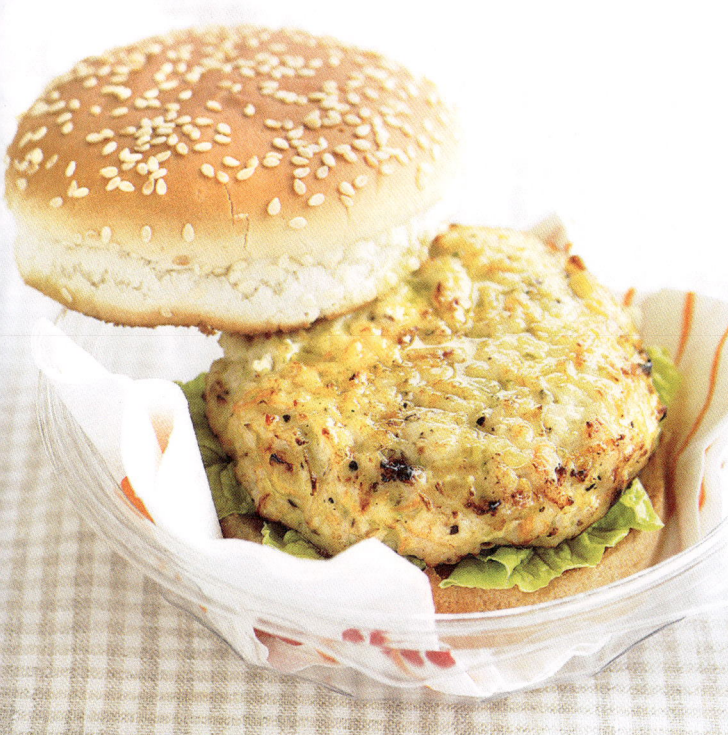

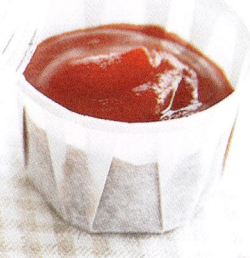

316 SESAME-POLENTA CHICKEN STRIPS

SERVES 4
PREPARATION 10 minutes
COOKING 20 minutes
STORAGE Leftovers will keep in the fridge for up to 2 days.

olive oil, for greasing
100g/3½oz/¾ cup polenta (cornmeal)
25g/1oz/¼ cup sesame seeds
25g/1oz/⅓ cup Parmesan, grated
450g/1lb skinless, boneless chicken breasts, cut into thin strips
2 eggs, beaten
1 lemon, cut into wedges, to serve

TOMATO DIP
4 tbsp mayonnaise
2 tbsp tomato purée

1. Preheat the oven to 200°C/400°F/gas mark 6 and grease a baking sheet with oil. To make the dip, mix the mayonnaise and tomato purée (paste) in a bowl, then cover and chill.

2. Mix the polenta, sesame seeds and Parmesan together in a bowl. Dip the chicken strips in the egg, then coat in the polenta and put them on the baking sheet. Bake for 15–20 minutes until golden.

3. Serve with the tomato dip and lemon wedges, if using.

317 SESAME AND HONEY GOUJONS

SERVES 4
PREPARATION 10 minutes + marinating
COOKING 13 minutes
STORAGE Leftovers will keep in the fridge for up to 2 days.

4 chicken breasts, sliced
6 tbsp tamari
2 tbsp honey
4 tbsp sesame seeds
olive oil, for frying
2 cloves garlic, chopped
1 tbsp red wine vinegar
black pepper to taste

1. Marinate the chicken strips in 2 tablespoons of the tamari and 1 tablespoon of the honey. Cover and chill for at least 1 hour.

2. Dip the chicken strips in the sesame seeds until they are coated

3. Heat a little oil in a heavy frying pan (skillet) over a medium heat, add the chicken strips and fry until browned, about 8 minutes. Set aside.

4. In the same pan, fry the garlic for 1 minute, then add the remaining honey and simmer for 2 minutes until the honey changes colour. Add the vinegar and the remaining tamari, heat through and season with black pepper.

5. Spoon the sauce over the goujons and serve with rice.

318 CARIBBEAN CHICKEN

SERVES 4
PREPARATION
20 minutes
COOKING
1 hour

STORAGE
Leftovers will keep in the fridge for up to 2 days.

4 tbsp plain (all-purpose) flour
8 chicken thighs
1 tbsp olive oil
½ tsp saffron strands
½ tsp turmeric
½ Scotch bonnet chilli, deseeded and finely chopped
2 cloves garlic, crushed
2 spring onions (scallions), chopped
4 tomatoes, quartered
200ml/7fl oz/scant 1 cup coconut milk
juice and grated zest of 1 lime
1 red (bell) pepper, deseeded and diced
1 yellow (bell) pepper, deseeded and diced
1 mango, peeled, pitted and chopped
freshly ground black pepper

1. Preheat the oven to 200°C/400°F/gas mark 6. Put the flour in a dish and season with black pepper. Turn the chicken thighs in the flour until evenly coated.

2. Heat the oil in a flameproof casserole and brown the chicken on both sides for 2–3 minutes. Remove from the pan. Add the saffron, turmeric, chilli, garlic and spring onions (scallions) and stir for 1 minute. Stir in the tomatoes, coconut milk, lime juice, zest, (bell) peppers and mango.

3. Add the chicken, cover and bake for 15 minutes, then remove the lid and cook for a further 30–35 minutes, or until the chicken is golden and cooked through – the juices will run clear when the thickest part of the chicken is pierced with a skewer. Serve hot.

319 SWEET AND SOUR CHICKEN

SERVES 4
PREPARATION
15 minutes
COOKING
7 minutes

STORAGE
Leftovers will keep in the fridge for up to 2 days. The sauce can be prepared in advance and kept in the fridge for up to 3 days or in the freezer for up to 1 month. Defrost in the fridge before using.

2 tbsp olive oil
400g/14oz skinless, boneless chicken breasts, cut into chunks
225g/8oz mixed stir-fry vegetables, such as carrots, (bell) peppers, mushrooms and mangetout (snow peas)
125g/4½oz canned pineapple pieces, drained
3 tbsp dry-roasted peanuts

SWEET & SOUR SAUCE
2 tomatoes
1 carrot
1 shallot
25g/1oz/¼ cup dates
3 sun-dried tomatoes in oil, drained
2 tbsp rice wine vinegar
2 tbsp tamari
1 clove garlic
1 tbsp tomato purée (paste)
125ml/4fl oz/½ cup pineapple juice

1) Purée all the sauce ingredients in a food processor or blender until smooth, then set aside.

2) Heat a wok and add the olive oil. Stir-fry the chicken pieces for 3–4 minutes until golden brown.

3) Add the vegetables, pineapple and sauce and cook, stirring, for 2–3 minutes, or until the vegetables are cooked but still crisp and the chicken is cooked through.

4) Sprinkle with the peanuts and serve hot.

320 POLENTA GRATIN

SERVES 4
PREPARATION
15 minutes
COOKING
20 minutes

STORAGE
Leftovers will keep in the fridge for up to 2 days.

olive oil, for stir-frying
2 red onions, chopped
300g/10½oz chicken breasts, diced
24 black olives, pitted and chopped
2 tbsp fresh coriander (cilantro)
sea salt and black pepper to taste
4 plum tomatoes, chopped
250g/9oz polenta (cornmeal)
2 celery stalks, sliced
200g/7oz green beans, topped and tailed and chopped
2 tbsp Parmesan cheese

1. Preheat the oven to 240°C/475°F/gas mark 9.

2. Heat the oil in a wok or a frying pan (skillet) over medium heat and gently stir-fry the red onion and the chicken until brown, about 6 minutes. Add the olives and coriander (cilantro), stir for 30 seconds, season and set aside.

3. Heat 2 tablespoons of oil in a separate frying pan (skillet), add the tomatoes and polenta (cornmeal) and stir-fry for 2 minutes, then add the celery and green beans. Simmer for 5 minutes.

4. Place half of the chicken in a roasting tin (pan), add half of the tomato and polenta (cornmeal) mixture, then add another layer of chicken, finishing with a layer of tomato and polenta (cornmeal). Sprinkle with Parmesan, then bake in the hot oven for 5 minutes and serve.

321 SPANISH PAELLA

SERVES 4
PREPARATION
15 minutes
COOKING
30 minutes

STORAGE
Leftovers will keep in the fridge for up to 2 days.

4 tbsp olive oil
1 Spanish onion
2 cloves garlic, crushed
200g/7oz chicken, cut into chunks
200g/7oz brown mushrooms, sliced
300g/10½oz/1½ cups long-grain rice
large pinch of saffron
2 bay leaves
2 small red (bell) peppers, quartered, deseeded and sliced
2 celery stalks (with leaves), sliced
800g/1lb 12oz tomatoes, blended
400ml/14fl oz/1⅔ cups vegetable stock
2 tbsp fresh oregano, chopped
1 lemon, cut into wedges

1. Gently heat the oil in a paella or deep frying pan (skillet). Add the onion and garlic and stir-fry for 1 minute. Add the chicken and the mushrooms and continue to stir-fry until they brown, about 6 minutes. Add the rice, saffron, bay leaves, (bell) peppers and celery. Stir-fry for 2 minutes, then add the tomatoes and stock. Bring to the boil and gently simmer until all the liquid is absorbed and the rice is cooked (about 20 minutes), adding more stock or water if necessary.

2. Garnish with oregano and lemon wedges, and serve hot.

322 CURRY WITH MANGO AND COCONUT

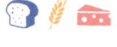

SERVES 4
PREPARATION
15 minutes
COOKING
20 minutes

STORAGE
Leftovers will keep in the fridge for up to 2 days.

4 tbsp olive oil
2 small onions, halved and sliced
2 cloves garlic, crushed
2 tsp fresh ginger, chopped
700g/1lb 9oz chicken breast, diced
2–3 tsp curry powder to taste
2 ripe mangoes, halved, pitted, peeled and diced
400ml/14fl oz/1⅔ cups coconut milk
2–3 tsp lemon juice (to taste)
sea salt and plenty of black pepper
water (optional)
large handful fresh coriander (cilantro) leaves, chopped

1. Heat the oil in a heavy-based pan or wok and gently stir-fry the onion and garlic until they begin to soften. Add the ginger and the chicken and fry until the chicken begins to brown. Add the curry powder and mix well before adding the mango, coconut milk and lemon juice. Season and very gently simmer for 5–7 minutes. (You may need to add a little water to prevent the curry from drying.)

2. Garnish with fresh coriander (cilantro) leaves and serve with rice and/or chapati bread.

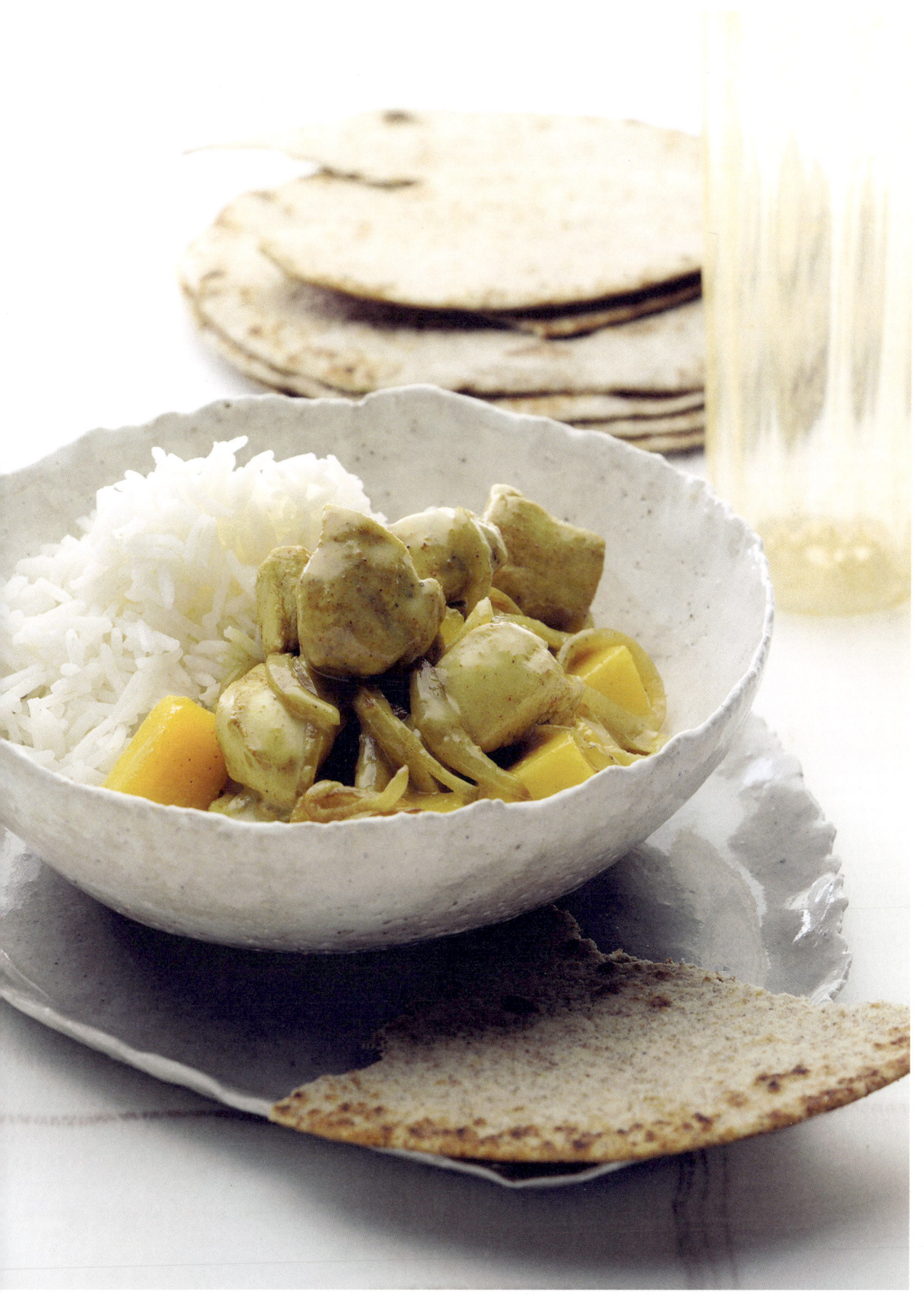

323 INDIAN CHICKEN KORMA

SERVES 4
PREPARATION 10 minutes
COOKING 20 minutes

STORAGE
Leftovers will keep in the fridge for up to 2 days.

4 tbsp olive oil
2 small onions, chopped
2 cloves garlic, chopped
700g/1lb 9oz chicken breasts, diced
4 tbsp plain (all-purpose) flour
2 tbsp mild curry powder
2 tbsp raisins
400ml/14fl oz/1²/₃ cups chicken or vegetable stock
4 tsp lemon juice
2 tbsp plain yogurt
2 tbsp almond butter
sea salt and black pepper to taste
2 tbsp flaked (slivered) almonds, toasted

1. Heat the oil in a heavy-based saucepan and gently stir-fry the onion and garlic until they begin to soften. Coat the chicken cubes with a mixture of flour and curry powder, add to the pan and fry until they begin to brown. Add the raisins and stock, bring to the boil and simmer for 10 minutes.

2. Remove from the heat, add the lemon juice, yogurt and almond butter. Season, garnish with the toasted flaked (slivered) almonds and serve with rice.

324 SENEGALESE YASSA

SERVES 4
PREPARATION 10 minutes
COOKING 25 minutes

STORAGE
Leftovers will keep in the fridge for up to 2 days.

2 tbsp groundnut (peanut) oil or grapeseed oil
2 large onions, grated
juice of 4 limes
2 tsp Tabasco sauce
500g/1lb 2oz chicken breasts, sliced
4 tbsp water
sea salt and black pepper to taste

1. Preheat a grill (broiler). Make a marinade of the oil, onion, lime juice and Tabasco sauce.

2. Brush the chicken with the marinade and grill (broil) on each side until well browned, about 10 minutes.

3. Pour the remaining marinade into a frying pan (skillet), heat through, add the cooked chicken and the water, cover and simmer until tender, about 15 minutes.

4. Season and serve with boiled rice and steamed spring greens, Swiss chard, curly kale or cabbage.

325 CHICKEN AND COCONUT CURRY

SERVES 4

PREPARATION
10 minutes

COOKING
40 minutes

STORAGE
You can refrigerate the curry for 2–3 days, or freeze it for up to a month.

300g/12oz/2 cups brown rice
25g/1oz butter
3 chicken breasts, about 150g/6oz each, sliced
2 small onions, sliced
2 cloves garlic, crushed
1 tbsp coriander seeds
55g/2oz/½ cup cashew nuts
55g/2oz/½ cup raisins
2 tbsp lime pickle
150g/6oz/1½ cups spinach
½ tsp chilli powder
500ml/17fl oz/2 cups water
3 tsp vegetable bouillon powder
2 tbsp mango chutney
250ml/9fl oz/1 cup coconut milk

1. Half fill a saucepan with water, bring to the boil and add the rice. Cover and simmer for 15–20 minutes, until soft.

2. Meanwhile, melt the butter in a saucepan. Add the chicken and brown gently over a low heat. Add the onions and garlic and sauté until soft.

3. Add the seeds, nuts, raisins, pickle, spinach, chilli powder, water and bouillon powder and let simmer for 15 minutes, stirring occasionally. Add the remaining mango chutney and coconut milk and simmer for another 3–5 minutes. Remove the rice from the heat, drain and serve on individual plates with the curry divided equally on top.

326 CHICKEN AND SWEET POTATO CASSEROLE

SERVES 4
PREPARATION
15 minutes + marinating
COOKING
25 minutes

STORAGE
Leftovers will keep in the fridge for up to 2 days.

500g/1lb 2oz chicken breasts, sliced
2 tbsp maple syrup
2 tbsp tomato purée (paste)
2 tsp paprika
2 tsp ground cumin
seeds from 4 cardamom pods
2 tbsp tamari
2 tbsp red wine vinegar
2 dashes Tabasco sauce
4 tbsp olive oil
4 shallots, quartered
8 cloves garlic, quartered
1 lemon, cut into wedges
700g/1lb 8oz sweet potatoes, sliced
sea salt and black pepper to taste
large handful of fresh parsley, chopped
2 tsp maple syrup or raw cane sugar (optional)

1. In a bowl, marinate the chicken chunks in the maple syrup, tomato purée (paste), paprika, cumin, cardamom seeds, tamari, vinegar, Tabasco sauce and 2 tablespoons of the oil. Cover and chill for at least 1 hour.

2. Gently heat the remaining 2 tablespoons of oil in a casserole dish and stir-fry the shallots for 3 minutes. Add the marinated chicken (with the marinade) and cook over a medium heat for 5 minutes. Then add the garlic, lemon and sweet potato. Cover and simmer for 15 minutes, or until the chicken is tender, adding a little water if necessary.

3. Season and garnish with fresh parsley and maple syrup or sugar (if using). Serve with rice.

327 SWEET and SOUR BUCKWHEAT PASTA

SERVES 4
PREPARATION
15 minutes
COOKING
15–20 minutes

STORAGE
Best eaten immediately.

olive oil for stir-frying
4 shallots, sliced
2 tsp ground coriander
350g/12oz chicken breasts, cut into chunks
2 red dessert apples, sliced
450g/1lb courgettes (zucchini), sliced
4 cloves garlic, crushed
2 tbsp cider vinegar
2 tsp maple syrup
2 tsp Tabasco sauce
2 tbsp tamari
400ml/14fl oz/1$^{2}/_{3}$ cups vegetable stock
400g/14oz buckwheat pasta
2 tsp cornflour (cornstarch) dissolved in a little cold water
sea salt and black pepper to taste

1. Heat a little oil in a casserole dish and stir-fry the shallots, ground coriander and chicken until golden, about 6 minutes. Add the apple, courgettes (zucchini) and garlic, turn up the heat a little and stir-fry for a further minute. Turn down the heat, add the vinegar, maple syrup, Tabasco sauce, tamari and stock. Bring to the boil and simmer for 5–10 minutes.

2. Meanwhile, cook the pasta in boiling water according to the package instructions.

3. Add the diluted cornflour to the sauce, stirring continuously, until the sauce thickens. Season and serve with the pasta.

328 TURKISH PILAF

SERVES 4
PREPARATION
10 minutes
COOKING
25 minutes

STORAGE
Leftovers will keep in the fridge for up to 2 days.

- 150g/5½oz/¾ cup Puy lentils
- 4 tbsp olive oil
- 1 tsp ground cinnamon
- 1 tsp ground coriander
- 2 tsp turmeric
- 2 leeks, sliced
- 300g/10½oz chicken breasts, cut into cubes
- 2 carrots, sliced
- 150g/5½oz/scant 1 cup bulgur wheat
- 2 tbsp raisins
- 300ml/10½fl oz/1¼ cups vegetable stock
- sea salt and black pepper to taste
- large handful fresh coriander (cilantro) leaves

1. Boil the lentils in a saucepan with three times their volume of water for 10 minutes.

2. Heat the oil in a heavy pan and add the spices, then the leek. Add the chicken and stir-fry for 5 minutes, until just golden. Add the carrot, bulgur wheat and raisins. Stir-fry for a further minute before adding the stock. Bring to the boil. Add the lentils (with their cooking water), cover and simmer for 15 minutes until the water is absorbed.

3. Season, garnish with coriander (cilantro) leaves and serve hot with plain yogurt.

329 WINTER KEBABS

SERVES 4
PREPARATION
15 minutes
COOKING
14 minutes

STORAGE
Best eaten immediately.

- 300g/10½oz turkey breast steaks, cut into cubes
- 8 cloves garlic, kept whole
- 2 sweet potatoes, cut into chunks
- 2 beetroot (beets), cut into chunks
- 12 Brussels sprouts, blanched
- 12 button mushrooms, kept whole
- 4–5 tbsp olive oil
- 50g/2oz/½ cup cup finely chopped walnuts
- 2 tsp dried basil
- sea salt to taste
- 2 tbsp tomato purée (paste)

1. Preheat the grill (broiler). Alternately spear the turkey cubes, garlic cloves and the vegetables onto four skewers.

2. Mix the oil with the chopped walnuts, basil, salt and tomato purée (paste) in a bowl, and brush the kebabs with the mixture. Place on a greased baking sheet and grill (broil) for 6–7 minutes on each side, or until golden and cooked through.

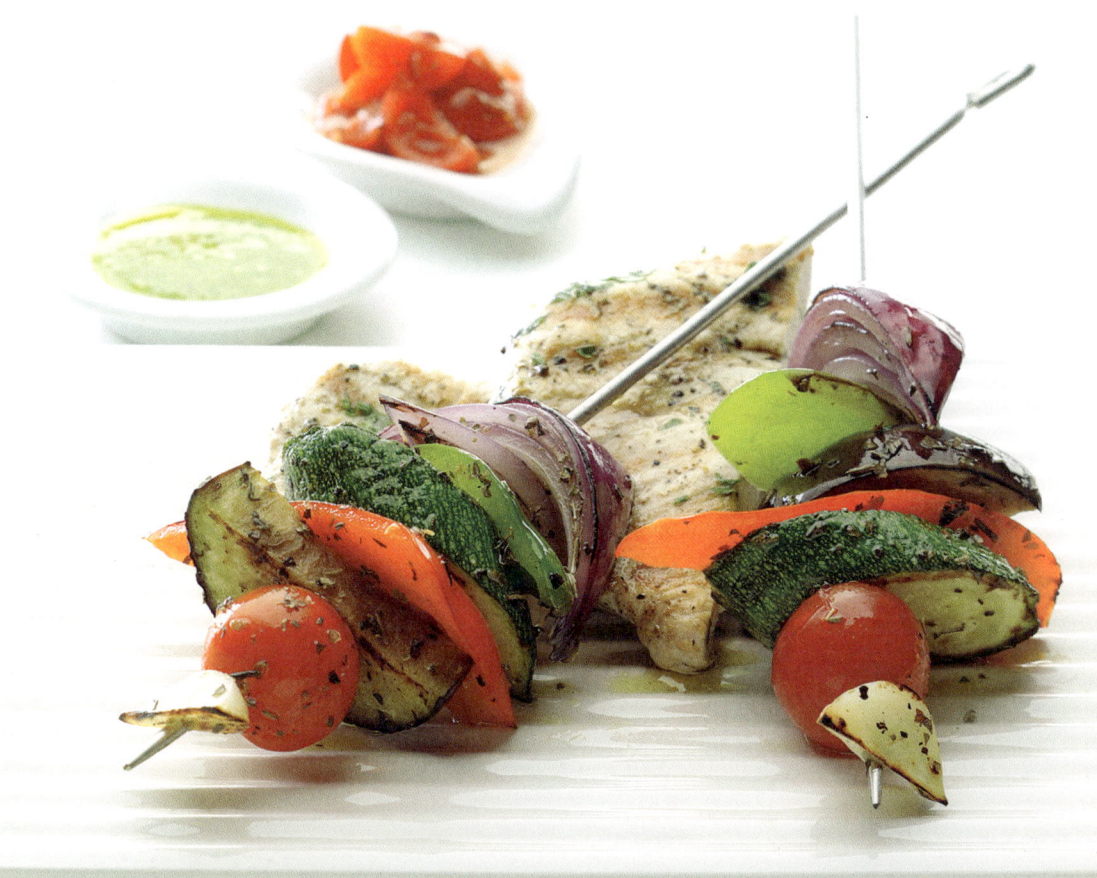

330 BARBECUED TURKEY AND RATATOUILLE KEBABS

SERVES 4

PREPARATION
15 minutes

COOKING
20 minutes

STORAGE
Best eaten immediately.

- 300g/10½oz turkey breast steaks, cut into cubes
- 2 red onions, quartered
- 1 aubergine (eggplant), cut into chunks
- 1 courgette (zucchini), cut into thick slices
- 1 red (bell) pepper, cut into triangles
- 1 green (bell) pepper, cut into triangles
- 4 cloves garlic, halved
- 20 cherry tomatoes
- 5 tbsp olive oil
- 4 tsp herbes de Provence
- sea salt and black pepper to taste

1. Alternately spear the turkey chunks, vegetable pieces, garlic halves and tomatoes onto four metal barbecue skewers, brush with oil, sprinkle with herbs and season.

2. Grill the kebabs over a hot barbecue or under a grill (broiler), turning frequently, until they are brown and the turkey is cooked through, about 15–20 minutes.

331 PAN-FRIED TURKEY

MAKES 12
PREPARATION
5 minutes
COOKING
10 minutes

STORAGE
Best eaten immediately.

110g/4oz butter
4 x 140-g/5-oz turkey breasts
230g/8oz/2 cups green beans
1 tbsp olive oil
8 spring onions (scallions), sliced
4 cloves garlic, peeled and sliced
juice of 2 limes
8 tbsp cranberry sauce
50g/2oz/²⁄₃ cup chopped parsley

1. Heat the butter in a frying pan (skillet), add the turkey breasts and cook until just golden on both sides.

2. Half fill a saucepan with water, bring to the boil, add the green beans and simmer for 5 minutes.

3. In a separate pan, add the olive oil and sauté the spring onions (scallions) and garlic for 30 seconds. Add the lime juice and cranberry sauce and stir over a low heat for 2 minutes.

4. Place the turkey breasts on plates, pour the sauce on top, garnish with the parsley and serve with the beans on the side.

332 INDONESIAN SATAY

SERVES 4–6
PREPARATION
15 minutes
COOKING
20 minutes

300g/10½oz chicken breasts, cut into cubes
16 cherry tomatoes
16 oyster mushrooms
16 pearl onions
2 small yellow courgettes (zucchini), cut into chunks
2 red (bell) peppers, deseeded and cut into triangles
juice of 2 limes
4 cloves garlic, chopped
4 fresh hot chillies, chopped
2 tsp tamarind paste dissolved in 2 tbsp water
tamari, to taste
grapeseed oil, for blending
6 tbsp peanut butter

1. Spear the chicken, tomatoes, mushrooms, onions, courgette (zucchini) chunks and (bell) pepper triangles onto four metal barbecue skewers. Prepare a barbecue or preheat the grill (broiler) to high.

2. Blend the lime juice, garlic, chillies, tamarind paste and tamari with oil to make a thick marinade.

3. Brush the kebabs with half the marinade and cook them on a medium barbecue or under the grill (broiler) until cooked through.

4. Mix the remaining marinade with the peanut butter to make a dip for the kebabs, and serve.

333 TURKEY SATAY

SERVES 4
PREPARATION 15 minutes + chilling
COOKING 10 minutes

STORAGE The sauce can be prepared in advance and chilled until required. Leftovers will keep in the fridge for up to 2 days.

450g/1lb skinless, boneless turkey breast, cut into strips
2 tsp olive oil
1 clove garlic, crushed
2 tbsp tamari
1 tbsp finely grated fresh ginger
zest of 1 lime
2 tbsp chopped coriander (cilantro) leaves

SATAY SAUCE
1 tbsp olive oil
2 shallots, finely chopped
1 clove garlic, crushed
2 tsp finely grated root ginger
175g/6oz/scant $3/4$ cup smooth peanut butter
150ml/5fl oz/scant $2/3$ cup coconut milk
1 tbsp lime juice
2 tbsp tamari
1 tsp sweet chilli sauce
freshly ground black pepper

1. Put the turkey in a dish. Mix the oil, garlic, tamari, ginger and lime; pour over the turkey. Cover and chill for 2 hours.

2. For the sauce, heat the oil in a pan and fry the shallots, garlic and ginger for 2 minutes until softened, then purée in a food processor with the remaining ingredients.

3. Preheat the grill (broiler) to high. Drain the turkey, reserving the marinade. Thread the strips onto 12 metal skewers, brush with the marinade and grill (broil) for 5–7 minutes until cooked through, turning once.

4. Heat the sauce until warm. Spoon a little over the skewers, sprinkle with the coriander (cilantro) and serve.

334 SESAME-LEMON TURKEY

SERVES 4
PREPARATION
10 minutes + chilling
COOKING
15 minutes

STORAGE
Leftovers will keep in the fridge for up to 2 days.

2 tbsp lemon juice
grated zest of 1 lemon
1 tbsp honey
1 tsp sesame oil
3 tbsp tamari
450g/1lb skinless, boneless turkey breast, cut into strips
2 tbsp sesame seeds
1 tbsp olive oil
2 shallots, finely chopped
100g/3½oz mangetout (snow peas), trimmed
2 small pak choi (bok choy), leaves separated
150g/5½oz shiitake mushrooms, sliced
4 spring onions (scallions), sliced
2 tbsp chopped coriander (cilantro) leaves

1. Mix the lemon juice, zest, honey, sesame oil and 2 tablespoons of the tamari in a bowl. Add the turkey and mix well, then cover and chill for 30 minutes.

2. Lightly toast the sesame seeds until golden brown in a large dry frying pan (skillet) or wok, shaking often. Remove from the pan and set aside.

3. Add the olive oil and shallots to the pan, and fry until softened. Add the turkey and marinade and cook for 5–7 minutes, tossing gently, until golden brown. Add the mangetout (snow peas), pak choi (bok choy), mushrooms and spring onions (scallions).

4. Stir-fry for 2–3 minutes, or until the pak choi (bok choy) begins to wilt. Stir in the sesame seeds and remaining tamari. Cook for 1–2 minutes, then sprinkle with the coriander (cilantro) and serve.

335 TURKEY MEATBALLS IN FIVE-VEG SAUCE

SERVES 4-6
PREPARATION
20 minutes
COOKING
1 hour

STORAGE
Leftovers will keep in the fridge for up to 2 days.

1 red onion, grated
1 clove garlic, crushed
450g/1lb minced (ground) turkey
1 egg, beaten
60g/2¼oz/¾ cup breadcrumbs
1 tbsp olive oil

FIVE-VEG SAUCE
1 tbsp olive oil
2 shallots, chopped
1 clove garlic, crushed
1 celery stalk, chopped
1 carrot, chopped
1 red (bell) pepper, chopped
400g/14oz canned tomatoes
1 tbsp tomato purée (paste)
1 tbsp balsamic vinegar
3 tbsp apple juice

1. Mix together the onion, garlic, turkey and egg, then stir in the breadcrumbs. Shape the mixture into 16 small balls.

2. Heat the oil in a frying pan (skillet) and fry the meatballs for 5 minutes until golden. Transfer to a baking dish.

3. Heat the oil for the sauce in a saucepan. Fry the shallots and garlic for 2 minutes. Add the celery, carrot and (bell) pepper and cook for 1-2 minutes. Stir in the remaining ingredients. Bring to the boil, then reduce the heat and simmer, covered, for 15 minutes.

4. Preheat the oven to 180°C/350°F/gas mark 4. Purée the sauce and pour it over the meatballs. Cover with foil and bake for 30 minutes until cooked through, then serve.

336 PASTA WITH GOUJONS IN A SPINACH SAUCE

SERVES 4
PREPARATION 10 minutes
COOKING 12 minutes
STORAGE Best eaten immediately.

320g/11oz penne pasta
300ml/10½fl oz/1¼ cups crème fraîche
2 pinches of freshly grated nutmeg
500g/1lb 2oz fresh spinach, cooked in boiling water, drained, rinsed and water pressed out
olive oil for frying
500g/1lb 2oz turkey breast, sliced

1. Cook the pasta in boiling water according to package instructions.

2. Heat the cream in a heavy pan with the nutmeg. When it boils, add the spinach. Mix well and set aside.

3. Heat a little oil in a frying pan (skillet) and sauté the turkey slices over a medium heat for 5 minutes.

4. Serve the pasta with the turkey slices on top and the spinach sauce poured over.

337 TURKEY ESCALOPES IN MUSHROOM SAUCE

SERVES 4
PREPARATION 10 minutes
COOKING 18 minutes
STORAGE Leftovers will keep in the fridge for up to 2 days.

4 turkey escalopes, flattened and seasoned
2 tsp paprika
olive oil, for frying
600g/1lb 5oz mushrooms, chopped
2 tbsp plain (all-purpose) flour
150ml/5fl oz/⅔ cup water
2 tbsp lemon juice
about 4 tbsp single (light) cream
sea salt to taste

1. Sprinkle the escalopes with paprika. Heat a little oil in a frying pan (skillet) over a medium heat and fry the escalopes until golden and cooked through, about 6 minutes. Set aside (keep warm).

2. Heat a little more oil in a small casserole dish, add the mushrooms and stir-fry until they give off their juices. Sprinkle with the flour and stir for a further minute. Add the water and the lemon juice, and enough cream to make a thick sauce. Gently simmer for 5 minutes, then season.

3. Place the fried escalopes on serving plates, cover with the mushroom sauce and serve with boiled potatoes and just-cooked artichoke hearts and carrots.

338 FIVE-SPICE DUCK

SERVES 4
PREPARATION
15 minutes
COOKING
17 minutes

STORAGE
Leftovers will keep in the fridge for up to 2 days.

4 boneless duck breasts, about 125g/4½oz each, skin on
1 tsp Chinese five-spice powder
2 tbsp olive oil
2 star anise, crushed
4 spring onions (scallions), chopped
2 tsp honey or agave nectar
1 tbsp tamari
3 tbsp orange juice

1. Preheat the oven to 190°C/375°F/gas mark 5. Cut a few slashes into each duck breast. Rub with the five-spice powder, put in a dish and drizzle with half the oil.

2. Heat a frying pan (skillet). Add the duck breasts, skin-side down, and brown the skin, then reduce the heat slightly and cook for 5 minutes.

3. Heat a roasting tin (pan) in the oven. Put the duck in the tin (pan). Add the star anise, spring onions (scallions), honey or agave syrup, tamari and orange juice. Roast for 10 minutes until the duck is cooked through.

4. Remove from the oven and leave to rest for 5 minutes. Slice thinly and serve topped with the onions and sauce.

339 MEDITERRANEAN FISH PARCELS

SERVES 4
PREPARATION 15 minutes
COOKING 25 minutes

STORAGE
Leftovers will keep in the fridge for up to 1 day.

- juice and zest of 1 lemon
- 1 roasted red (bell) pepper in oil, drained
- 3 tbsp olive oil
- 1 tsp sun-dried tomato paste
- 4 halibut fillets, 125g/4½oz each
- 8 pitted black olives, halved
- 1 tbsp capers, rinsed
- 8 cherry tomatoes, quartered
- 8 basil leaves

1. Preheat the oven to 180°C/350°F/gas mark 4. Cut squares of baking parchment and foil large enough to wrap up a portion of fish. Place a piece of parchment on top of each piece of foil.

2. Put the lemon juice, zest, red (bell) pepper, olive oil and sun-dried tomato paste in a blender and blend to make a thick purée.

3. Put 1 halibut fillet in the middle of each foil-and-parchment square. Scatter over the olives, capers, tomatoes and basil leaves and top with the (bell) pepper purée. Fold up the parchment to enclose the fish, folding the edges together to seal the parcels, and put on a baking sheet.

4. Bake for 25 minutes. Transfer the parcels to plates, unwrap carefully and serve.

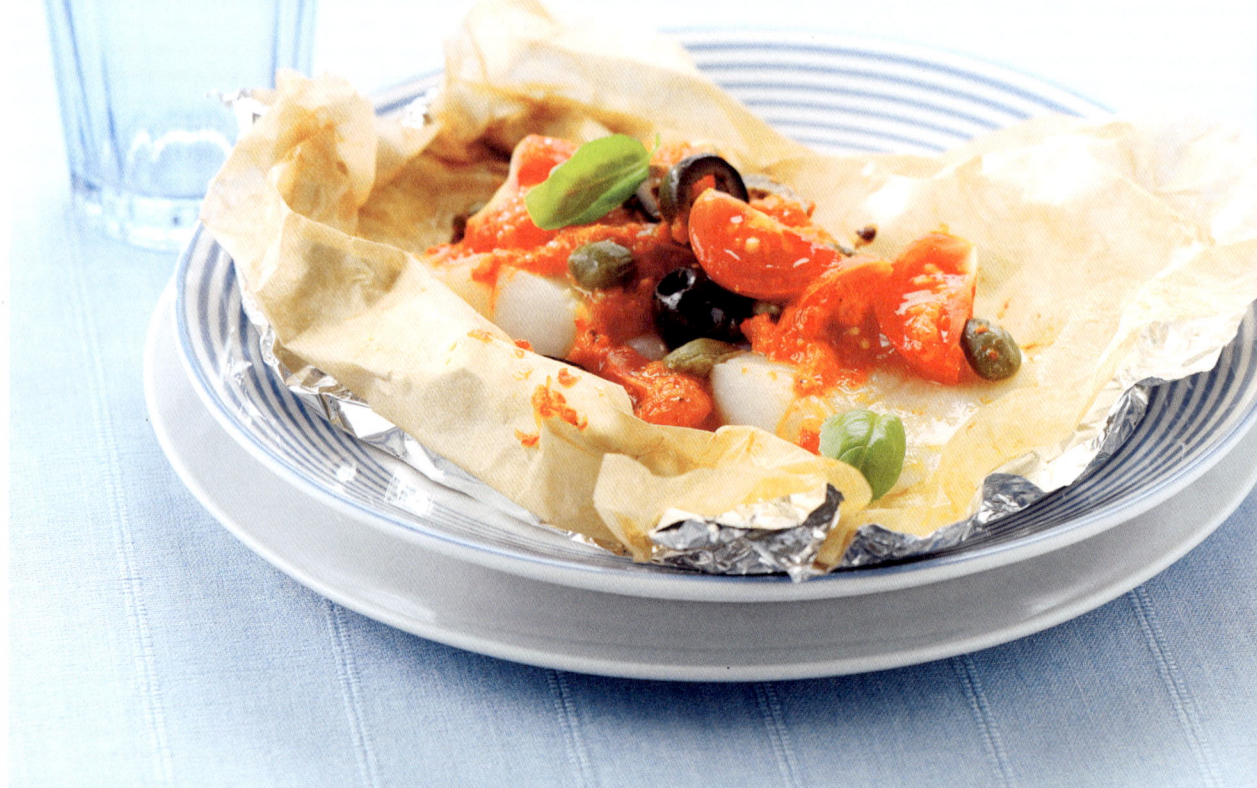

340 SPICY FISH TACOS

SERVES 4
PREPARATION
10 minutes
COOKING
7 minutes

STORAGE
Leftovers will keep in the fridge for up to 1 day.

1 avocado, diced
2 tsp lemon juice
400g/14oz skinless, boneless firm white fish fillets, such as halibut
25g/1oz/scant ¼ cup plain (all-purpose) flour
1 tbsp olive oil
3 tomatoes, deseeded and diced
200g/7oz canned kidney beans, drained and rinsed
1 tbsp sweet chilli sauce
1 tbsp tamari
1 tbsp rice wine
1 tsp caster (superfine) sugar
8 taco shells
freshly ground black pepper

1. Mix the avocado and lemon juice in a bowl. Cover and chill.

2. Cut the fish fillets into thick strips and dry on paper towels. Put the flour in a bowl, season with black pepper and toss the fish strips in the seasoned flour to coat.

3. Heat a large frying pan (skillet) and add the oil. Stir-fry the fish for 3–4 minutes until crisp and golden. Stir in the tomatoes, kidney beans, sweet chilli sauce, tamari, rice wine and sugar and simmer for 1–2 minutes until the tomatoes have softened.

4. Heat the taco shells according to the package instructions. Fill with the fish and beans and top with a spoonful of avocado, then serve.

341 SEAFOOD KEBABS

SERVES 4
PREPARATION 10 minutes + chilling
COOKING 10 minutes

STORAGE Leftovers will keep in the fridge for up to 1 day.

- 2 tbsp olive oil
- 2 tsp paprika
- 4 tbsp sun-dried tomato paste
- 4 tbsp lime juice
- 2 tbsp honey or agave nectar
- 12 raw king prawns (jumbo shrimp), peeled and deveined
- 225g/8oz monkfish fillet, cut into chunks
- 225g/8oz boneless trout fillets, cut into chunks
- 1 red and 1 yellow (bell) pepper, deseeded and cut into chunks

1. Mix the olive oil, paprika, tomato paste, lime juice and honey in a shallow dish. Add the prawns (shrimp), fish and peppers and mix. Cover and chill for 30 minutes.

2. Preheat the grill (boiler) to high. Thread the seafood and peppers onto 8 skewers, alternating the ingredients. Grill (broil) for 5 minutes on each side until cooked and browned.

3. Meanwhile, heat the marinade in a pan until boiling. Serve the kebabs drizzled with the marinade.

342 TERIYAKI SALMON

SERVES 4
PREPARATION 15 minutes
COOKING 8 minutes

STORAGE Leftovers will keep in the fridge for up to 1 day.

- 2 tbsp olive oil
- 1-cm/½-in piece root ginger, peeled and grated
- 1 garlic clove, crushed
- juice and grated zest of 1 lime
- 4 tbsp tamari
- 2 tbsp honey
- 3 tbsp mirin (Japanese sweet rice wine)
- 350g/12oz skinless, boneless salmon fillet, cut into thick strips
- 225g/8oz mixed stir-fry vegetables, such as beansprouts, (bell) peppers, pak choi (bok choy) and mangetout (snow peas)
- 3 spring onions (scallions), finely sliced
- 2 tsp sesame oil
- handful of coriander (cilantro) leaves, chopped
- 1 tbsp sesame seeds

1. Heat half the oil in a small pan and fry the ginger and garlic for 1 minute. Add the lime juice, zest, tamari, honey and mirin (rice wine). Cook for 1 minute until thickened and syrupy. Set this sauce aside.

2 Heat the remaining oil in a non-stick frying pan (skillet) or wok and fry the salmon for 1–2 minutes. Add the stir-fry vegetables and spring onions (scallions) with a splash of water. Cover and cook for 1–2 minutes until the vegetables soften.

3 Pour in the sauce along with the sesame oil, coriander (cilantro) and sesame seeds and heat through. Serve immediately.

343 SALMON FISHCAKES

MAKES 10–12
PREPARATION
20 minutes + chilling
COOKING
1 hour 45 minutes

STORAGE
Leftovers will keep in the fridge for up to 2 days. Freeze uncooked for up to 1 month and thaw in the fridge before cooking.

300g/10½oz sweet potatoes
300g/10½oz salmon fillet
2 tbsp lemon juice
1 tbsp chopped dill
grated zest of 1 lemon
1 egg, beaten
100g/3½oz/1 cup wholemeal breadcrumbs
2 tsp olive oil
freshly ground black pepper

SUN-DRIED TOMATO MAYO
6 tbsp mayonnaise
1 tsp lemon juice
1 tsp sun-dried tomato paste
3 sun-dried tomatoes in oil, drained and finely chopped

1 Preheat the oven to 200°C/400°F/gas mark 6. Wrap the potatoes in foil and bake for 1 hour, or until soft. When cool, peel and mash. Mix all the mayo ingredients together, cover and chill.

2 Put the salmon in a baking dish with the lemon juice. Cover and bake in the oven for 20 minutes until the flesh is opaque and flakes easily. Cool, then discard the skin and flake the fish.

3 Mix the salmon, dill and lemon zest into the potatoes. Season with black pepper, cover and chill for 30 minutes.

4 Shape into small patties and coat in the beaten egg then the breadcrumbs. Put on a baking sheet and chill for 30 minutes.

5 Drizzle the olive oil over the fishcakes and bake for 20–25 minutes until crisp and golden. Serve with the tomato mayo.

344 SPRING MASALA

SERVES 4
PREPARATION 15 minutes
COOKING 18 minutes

STORAGE
Leftovers will keep in the fridge for up to 2 days.

2 tbsp grapeseed oil
2 small red onions, chopped
2 cloves garlic, chopped
2 tsp turmeric
2 small green chillies, chopped
2 tsp fresh ginger, chopped
4 medium carrots, chopped
300g/10½oz prawns (shrimp), cooked and peeled
about 400ml/14fl oz/1⅔ cups coconut milk
2 tsp garam masala
sea salt to taste
200g/7oz green peas, shelled
large handful fresh coriander (cilantro) leaves, chopped

① Heat the oil in a heavy-based pan and gently stir-fry the onion and garlic for a few minutes until they begin to soften. Add the turmeric, chilli, ginger and carrots and stir-fry for a further 2 minutes before adding the prawns (shrimp). Stir for a further minute, then add the coconut milk and the garam masala and simmer for 5–10 minutes until the carrots are cooked (adding more coconut milk if necessary). Season with salt, add the peas and heat through. Garnish with fresh coriander (cilantro) leaves and serve with rice.

345 ORANGE-GLAZED SARDINES

SERVES 2-4
PREPARATION 15 minutes
COOKING 7 minutes

STORAGE
Leftovers will keep in the fridge for up to 1 day.

2 tbsp plain (all-purpose) flour
½ tsp paprika
4 sardines, cleaned and descaled
2 tbsp olive oil
½ tsp harissa (optional)
juice and grated zest of 2 oranges
2 tbsp raisins
1 orange, peeled and sliced
25g/1oz/¼ cup pine nuts, toasted
2 tbsp chopped coriander (cilantro) leaves

① Mix the flour and paprika on a plate, then turn the sardines in the mixture to coat them all over.

② Mix half the oil with the harissa, if using, orange juice and zest, raisins and orange slices.

③ Heat the remaining oil in a frying pan (skillet) and fry the sardines for 2–3 minutes on each side until browned and crisp. Add the orange slices and their sauce and boil for 1 minute until slightly thickened.

④ Scatter the pine nuts and coriander (cilantro) over the fish and serve immediately.

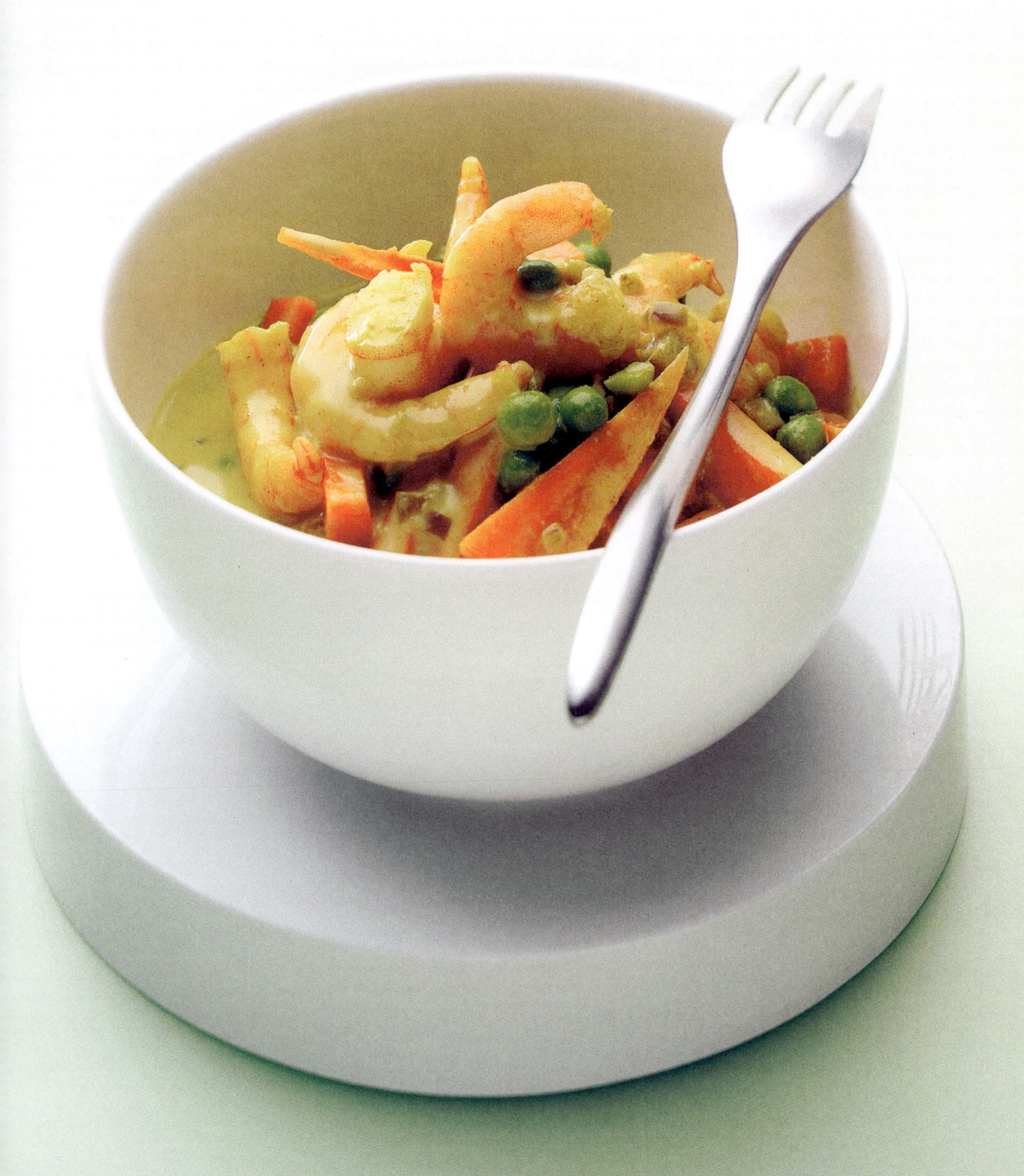

346 CREAMY FISH PIE

SERVES 4–6
PREPARATION 20 minutes
COOKING 55 minutes

STORAGE
Assemble and chill the pie up to 1 day in advance of cooking. If the prawns (shrimp) have not been frozen, the uncooked pie can be frozen for 1 month. Defrost in the fridge before cooking. Cooked leftovers will keep in the fridge for up to 1 day.

- 750g/1lb 10oz sweet potatoes, peeled and cut into chunks
- 1 tbsp olive oil
- 1 clove garlic, crushed
- 150g/5½oz skinless salmon fillet
- 125g/4½oz each skinless smoked haddock fillet and skinless firm white fish fillet
- 2 tbsp lemon juice
- 455ml/16fl oz/scant 2 cups low-fat crème fraîche
- 2 tbsp chopped parsley
- 75g/2½oz Cheddar cheese, grated
- 150g/5½oz peeled, cooked prawns (shrimp) (thawed if frozen)
- 100g/3½oz/¾ cup frozen peas
- 100g/3½oz/¾ cup canned sweetcorn, drained
- 2 hard-boiled eggs, quartered

1. Preheat the oven to 190°C/375°F/gas mark 5. Boil the sweet potatoes for 15 minutes, or until tender, then drain.

2. Meanwhile, heat the oil in a large frying pan (skillet). Fry the garlic and all the fish for 4–5 minutes, then add the lemon juice. Transfer the fish to a baking dish, breaking it into large chunks.

3. Add the crème fraîche, parsley and half the cheese to the frying pan (skillet) and simmer for 2 minutes. Stir in the prawns (shrimp), peas and sweetcorn.

4. Mash the sweet potatoes with 1 tbsp of the sauce. Pour the prawn (shrimp) mixture over the fish and mix gently. Top with the potato and eggs and sprinkle with the remaining cheese. Bake for 30–40 minutes until golden, then serve.

347 PASTA with SMOKED TROUT and BROCCOLI

SERVES 4
PREPARATION
10 minutes
COOKING
12 minutes

STORAGE
Leftovers will keep in the fridge for up to 1 day.

400g/14oz pappardelle or tagliatelle
1 tbsp olive oil
1 clove garlic, crushed
2 shallots, finely chopped
200g/7oz sprouting broccoli or broccoli florets
juice and grated zest of 1 lemon
4 tbsp low-fat crème fraîche
2 tbsp chopped basil leaves
2 tbsp pine nuts
450g/1lb smoked trout, skinned and flaked into large chunks
2 tbsp grated Parmesan cheese

1. Cook the pasta in boiling water according to the package instructions, for about 12 minutes or until al dente.

2. Meanwhile, heat the oil in a frying pan (skillet) and cook the garlic and shallots, stirring, for 2 minutes. Add the broccoli and lemon juice and zest and cook for a further 3–4 minutes.

3. Stir in the crème fraîche, basil and pine nuts and heat through for a few seconds.

4. Drain the pasta well, then add it with the trout to the broccoli mixture. Mix well, sprinkle with the Parmesan and serve.

348 SPAGHETTI with CREOLE SAUCE

SERVES 4
PREPARATION
15 minutes
COOKING
15 minutes

STORAGE
Leftovers will keep in the fridge for up to 1 day.

4 tbsp olive oil
200g/7oz mushrooms, sliced
250g/9oz cod fillet, cut into chunks
4 tbsp parsley, chopped
2 tsp dried thyme
2 tsp turmeric
2 tsp black pepper
350g/12oz pumpkin, diced
400g/14oz spinach, chopped
6 tbsp dried mixed seaweed flakes, soaked in water for 10 minutes
200ml/7fl oz/1 cup coconut milk
400g/14oz spaghetti pasta
sea salt to taste

1. Heat the oil in a frying pan (skillet) and sauté the mushrooms and the cod for 3 minutes. Add the herbs and spices, followed by the pumpkin and spinach, then add the seaweed (with its soaking water). Add the coconut milk, partially cover and simmer for 10 minutes.

2. Cook the pasta in boiling water according to the package instructions, then divide between serving plates, top with the sauce and serve.

349 WINTER TAPAS TARTS

SERVES 4
PREPARATION
20 minutes
COOKING
30 minutes

STORAGE
Leftovers will keep in the fridge for up to 2 days.

1 shallot, chopped
2 tbsp tomato purée (paste)
2 tbsp fresh parsley, chopped
2 tsp paprika
large pinch each of sugar and salt
2 dashes Tabasco sauce
4 cloves garlic, chopped
350g/12oz tuna cut into chunks
oil, for stir-frying
200g/7oz cauliflower florets
1 package ready-made puff pastry, rolled out thinly and cut into quarters
20 brown mushrooms, thinly sliced
sea salt and black pepper to taste
2 tbsp capers
50g/2oz mozzarella cheese, grated
2 tbsp grated Parmesan cheese

① Preheat the oven to 220°C/425°F/gas mark 7.

② Blend the shallot, tomato purée (paste), parsley, paprika, sugar, salt, Tabasco sauce and garlic in a bowl with a little water.

③ Stir-fry the tuna chunks in a frying pan (skillet) with a little oil until golden and set aside. Blanch the cauliflower florets in boiling water for 3 minutes, then drain.

④ Line four 4 x 10cm/$1^{1}/_{2}$ x 4in pie dishes with the pastry. Add the blended tomato mixture, followed by a layer of blanched cauliflower and mushroom slices. Season and sprinkle with the capers and the mozzarella. Sprinkle with Parmesan and bake in the middle of the hot oven for 20–25 minutes, until the tarts begin to brown. Serve hot.

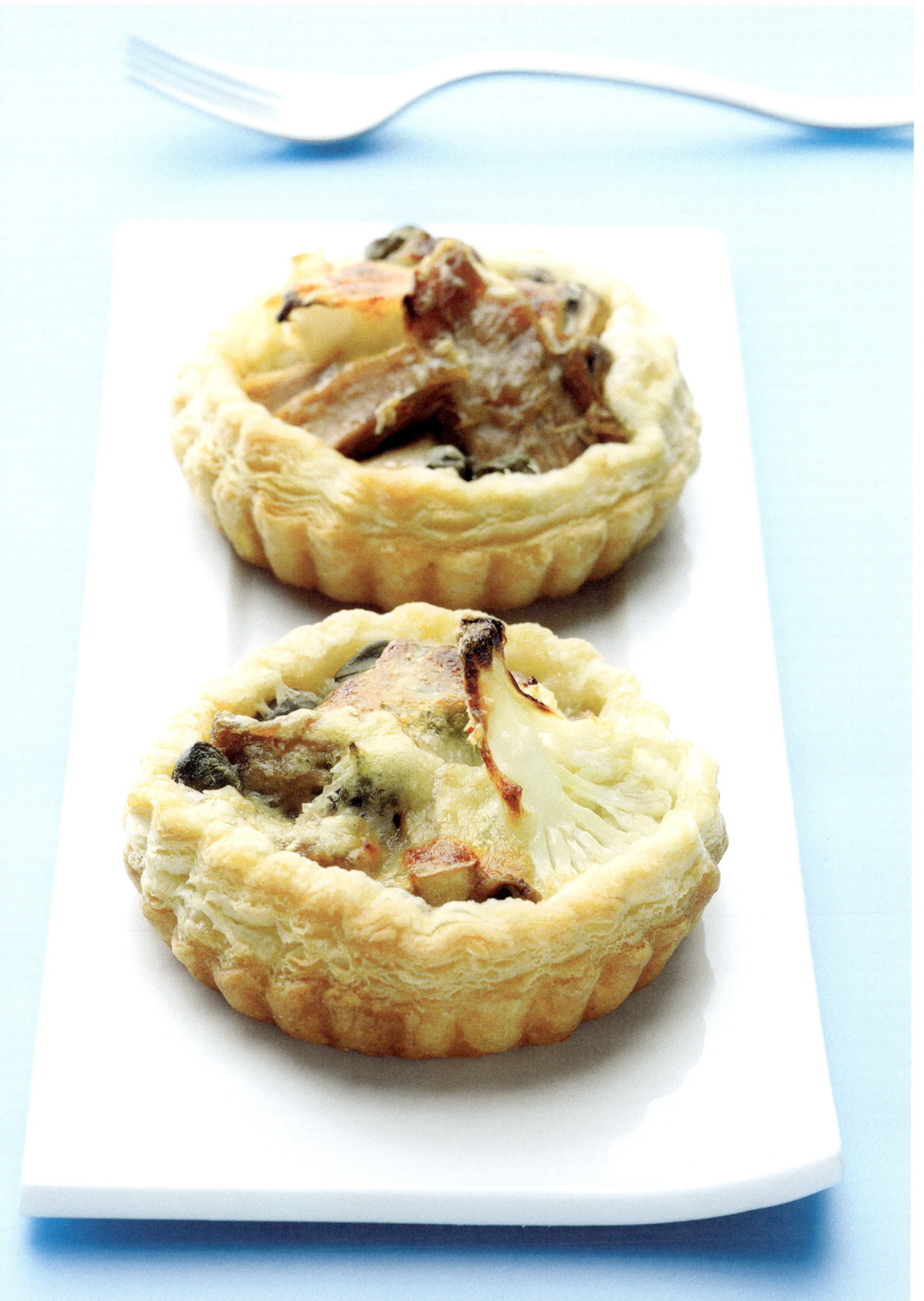

350 GRILLED COD with SALSA

SERVES 4
PREPARATION
10 minutes
COOKING
15 minutes

STORAGE
You can prepare this dish in advance and refrigerate for up to 6 hours before cooking.

2 small yellow (bell) peppers, deseeded and finely diced
6 plum tomatoes, finely diced
1 red onion, peeled and finely diced
½ cucumber, finely diced
3 tbsp olive oil
2 tbsp chopped fresh coriander (cilantro)
4 cod fillets, about 140g/5oz each
1 lemon, sliced

1. Preheat the oven to 200°C/400°F/gas mark 6. Place all the vegetables in a bowl and add the olive oil and coriander (cilantro).

2. Put the cod fillets in a small oven-proof dish and pour the salsa mix over the top.

3. Cover the dish with foil and place in the oven for 15 minutes until the fish is cooked. Serve garnished with the lemon slices.

351 SALMON with MANGO SALSA

SERVES 4
PREPARATION
10 minutes
COOKING
6 minutes

STORAGE
The salsa will keep in the fridge for up to 3 days.

4 salmon fillets, about 140g/5oz each, skinned
1 tbsp olive oil
2 cloves garlic, finely sliced
6 spring onions (scallions), chopped
1 mango, peeled, pitted and diced into small pieces
juice of 2 limes
1 tsp chopped root ginger
1 tsp chilli powder
3 tbsp mango chutney

1. Preheat the grill (broiler) to medium. Place the salmon fillets on a grill pan and grill (broil) for 5-6 minutes on either side.

2. Meanwhile, heat the olive oil in a small saucepan, add the garlic and spring onions (scallions) and sauté for 30 seconds. Add the diced mango, lime juice, ginger and chilli powder and stir over a low heat for 1 minute. Stir in the mango chutney and remove from the heat.

3. Put the salmon onto plates and spoon the salsa equally on top of each fillet.

352 CATALAN TART

SERVES 4
PREPARATION
10 minutes
COOKING
15 minutes

STORAGE
Leftovers will keep in the fridge for up to 2 days.

4 tbsp olive oil
4 shallots, sliced
16 mushrooms, sliced
1 tsp ground cumin
1 tsp ground coriander
large pinch of saffron
1 package ready-made shortcrust pastry, rolled out very thin
4 large tomatoes, sliced
16 anchovy fillets or 12 black olives, pitted and sliced
celery salt and black pepper to taste

1) Preheat the oven to 200°C/400°F/gas mark 6.

2) Heat the oil in a small wok or saucepan and gently stir-fry the shallots and mushrooms. Add the spices and heat through.

3) Place the rolled-out pastry in a 20cm/8in pie dish and add the mushroom mixture. Cover with tomato slices and anchovies or olives. Season, then bake for 10 minutes or until golden, and serve.

353 CUBAN COD

SERVES 4
PREPARATION
10 minutes
COOKING
10 minutes

STORAGE
Leftovers will keep in the fridge for up to 1 day.

600g/1lb 5oz potatoes, finely sliced
corn oil for drizzling and frying
2 onions, chopped
2 cloves garlic, chopped
2 tsp tomato purée (paste)
400ml/14fl oz/1$^{2}/_{3}$ cups fish/vegetable stock
large pinch of saffron
4 dried hot chillies
4 fresh cod fillets, about 200g/7oz each, halved
sea salt and cayenne pepper to taste
lemon wedges, to serve

1) Preheat the oven to 220°C/425°F/gas mark 7.

2) Place the potato slices in a baking dish and drizzle with oil. Bake in a hot oven for 10 minutes.

3) Meanwhile, fry the onion and the garlic in a frying pan (skillet) with a little oil, add the tomato purée (paste), stock, saffron and chillies and bring to the boil. Season to taste and set aside.

4) Place the cod fillets on top of the partially-cooked potato slices. Pour the sauce over and bake for a further 10 minutes (until the fish is tender). Serve with wedges of lemon alongside.

354 EGGLESS SEAWEED OMELETTE

SERVES 4
PREPARATION 10 minutes
COOKING 17 minutes
STORAGE Best eaten immediately.

BATTER
200g/7oz plain (all-purpose) flour
2 tbsp brewer's yeast flakes
2 tsp baking powder
large pinch of saffron
½ tsp sea salt
400ml/14fl oz/1⅔ cups soya or rice milk
2 tsp olive oil, plus some for frying

FILLING
2 sweet potatoes, chopped into thin sticks
200g/7oz fresh shiitake mushrooms, sliced
2 tbsp hiziki seaweed, soaked in hot water
2 tbsp tahini (sesame paste)
sea salt and black pepper to taste
toasted salted sesame seeds (gomasio), to garnish

1. Mix the flour, brewer's yeast flakes, baking powder, saffron and salt in a bowl. Add the milk and the oil and whisk to make a smooth batter. Set aside.

2. To prepare the filling, stir-fry the sweet potato and the shiitake in a frying pan (skillet) with a little hot oil. Add the seaweed with a little of its soaking water and cook for 5 minutes, then add the tahini (sesame paste), season and garnish with toasted sesame seeds. Set aside (keep warm).

3. Heat an oiled frying pan (skillet) over a medium heat. Add a quarter of the batter, swirling to coat the pan, and cook the omelette until the top is dry. Turn and cook the other side, then transfer to a warmed plate. Repeat until you have made 4 omelettes. Top each with the filling, roll and serve.

355 CHINESE FIVE-SPICE NOODLES

SERVES 4
PREPARATION 15 minutes
COOKING 10 minutes

4 tbsp sunflower oil
2 cloves garlic, finely chopped
8 spring onions (scallions), sliced
250g/9oz cooked prawns (shrimp)
250g/9oz fresh spinach, chopped
2 tsp grated root ginger
2 tbsp tamari
2 tsp Chinese five-spice powder
2 tbsp Chinese rice wine or dry sherry
2 tsp raw cane sugar
400g/14oz Chinese rice noodles
2 tbsp salted sesame seeds (gomasio), toasted

STORAGE
Best eaten immediately.

1. Heat the oil in a wok or large pan and stir-fry the garlic, spring onions (scallions) and prawns (shrimp) over a medium heat for 3 minutes. Add the spinach, ginger and tamari and stir-fry for a further minute, then add the five-spice, wine or sherry and sugar. Lower the heat and very gently simmer for 3–4 minutes. Check the seasoning.

2. Cook the noodles as instructed on the package. Serve topped with the sauce and garnished with sesame seeds.

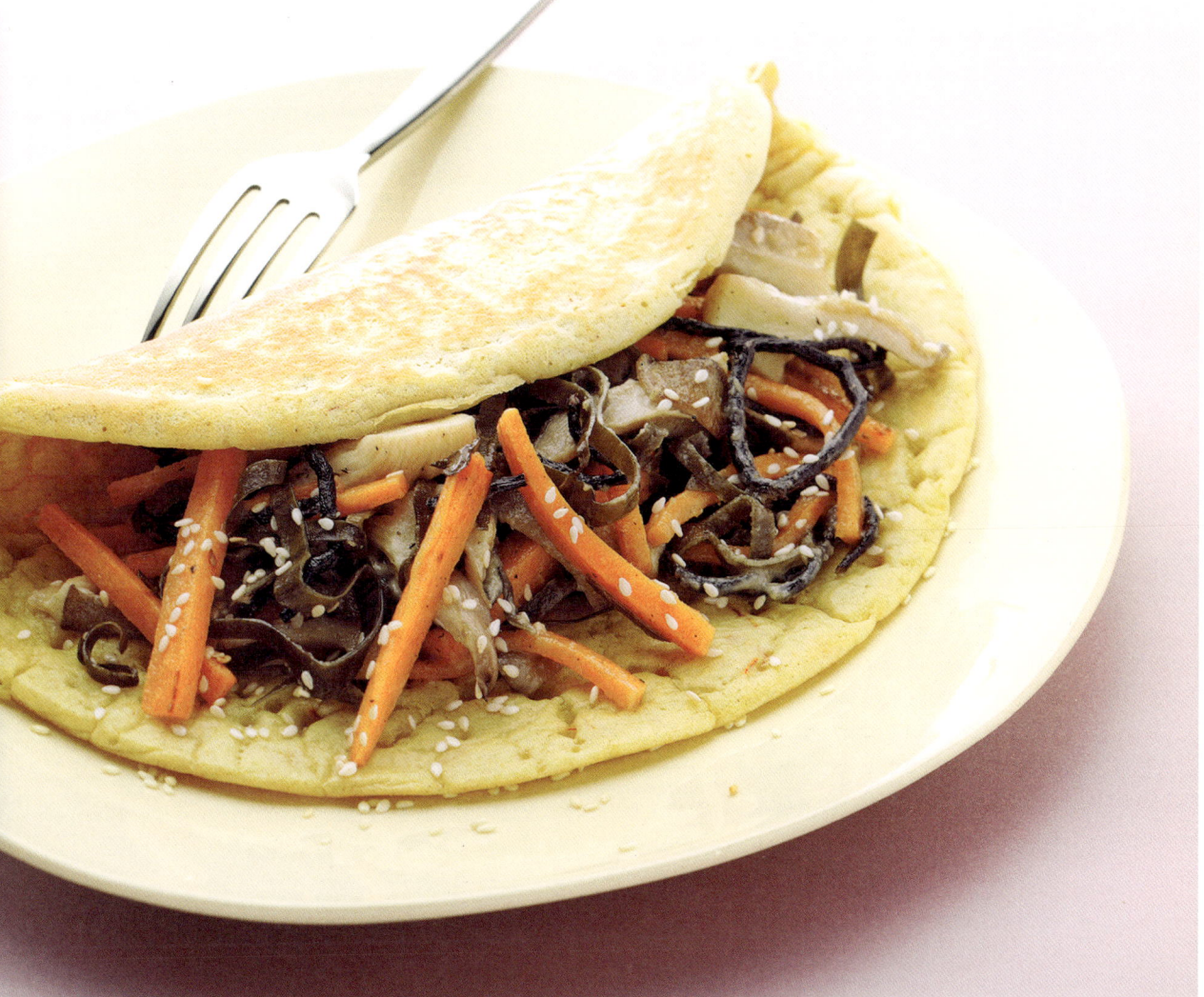

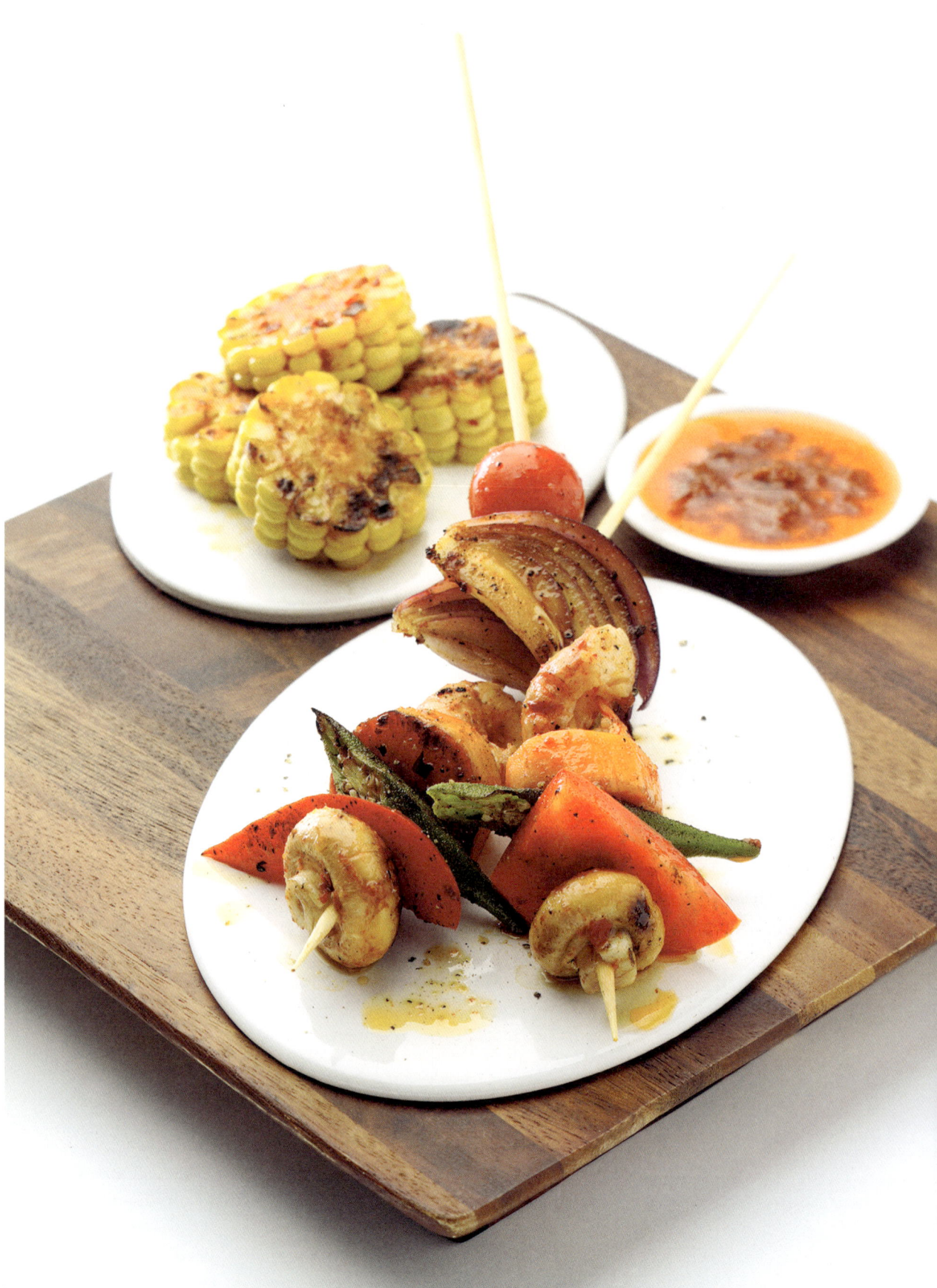

356 BROCHETTES with PILI-PILI SAUCE

SERVES 4
PREPARATION
15 minutes
COOKING
10–15 minutes

STORAGE
Best eaten immediately.

4 red hot chillies, chopped
4 cloves garlic, chopped
juice of 2 lemons
2 tsp paprika
large pinch of salt
100ml/3½fl oz/scant ½ cup olive oil
20 scampi (Dublin Bay prawns), peeled
2 sweet potatoes, cut into chunks
20 button mushrooms, kept whole
2 red onions, quartered
20 okra (lady's fingers), halved
2 red (bell) peppers, cut into chunks
20 cherry tomatoes
4 corn cobs, sliced into chunks

1. In a food processor, blend the chillies, garlic, lemon juice, paprika, salt and oil to a coarse paste and set aside.

2. Alternately spear the scampi (Dublin Bay prawns), sweet potatoes, mushrooms, onions, okra, red (bell) peppers and cherry tomatoes onto four metal barbecue skewers, then place them on a baking sheet with the corn chunks and brush with the pili-pili paste.

3. Place the kebabs under a hot grill (broiler) and cook until golden, brushing with more pili-pili paste as you turn them. Serve hot.

357 FENNEL, MONKFISH and POTATO BAKE

SERVES 4
PREPARATION
15 minutes
COOKING
22 minutes

STORAGE
Leftovers will keep in the fridge for up to 1 day.

2 tbsp olive oil
500g/1lb 2oz trimmed monkfish, cut into chunks and seasoned
500g/1lb 2oz potatoes, quartered and parboiled
2 fennel bulbs, sliced
2 red onions, sliced
8 sun-dried tomatoes, chopped
2 lemons, thinly sliced
200ml/7fl oz/scant 1 cup hot vegetable or fish stock
handful of fresh parsley, chopped
sea salt and black pepper to taste
baguette or cooked rice, to serve

1. Preheat the oven to 220°C/425°F/gas mark 7.

2. Heat the oil in a large frying pan (skillet) over a high heat and fry the monkfish for 2 minutes.

3. Grease an ovenproof dish and arrange the parboiled potatoes on the bottom. Add the slices of fennel, onion, tomato and lemon, in layers, and finish with the monkfish. Add the stock, garnish with parsley and season. Cover and bake for 20 minutes. Serve with rice or baguette.

358 CARIBBEAN CASSEROLE

SERVES 4
PREPARATION
15 minutes
COOKING
22 minutes

STORAGE
Leftovers will keep in the fridge for up to 1 day.

4 tbsp olive oil
2 medium sweet potatoes, peeled and diced
200g/7oz Savoy cabbage, chopped
400g/14oz pumpkin, peeled, deseeded and diced
200g/7oz fresh spinach, chopped
1 strip kombu seaweed, soaked in 100ml/3½fl oz/scant 1 cup water for 10 minutes, then chopped
2 tsp turmeric
400ml/14fl oz/1⅔ cups coconut milk
2 tsp thyme
2 tbsp fresh parsley, chopped
sea salt and black pepper to taste
300g/10½oz cod fillet, diced

1. Heat the oil in a heavy-based casserole dish and stir-fry the sweet potato, Savoy cabbage and pumpkin for 3 minutes until the cabbage begins to soften. Add the spinach, together with the seaweed and its soaking water, followed by the turmeric and coconut milk. Sprinkle with the thyme and parsley, and season. Bring to the boil, cover with a tight-fitting lid and simmer for 10 minutes.

2. Add the cod chunks and sprinkle with a little salt. Cover and simmer for 5 minutes, then remove the lid, turn up the heat a little and reduce for 1 minute. Serve with rice.

359 SEAFOOD PASTA

SERVES 4
PREPARATION
10 minutes
COOKING
12 minutes

STORAGE
Best eaten immediately.

400g/14oz pasta shapes of choice
4 tbsp olive oil
400g/14oz fresh tuna, diced
2 cloves garlic, finely chopped
2 small red (bell) peppers, quartered, deseeded and sliced
4 tbsp dried mixed seaweed, soaked
4 ripe tomatoes, chopped
4 anchovy fillets, chopped or 16 black olives, pitted and chopped
2 tbsp fresh basil, chopped
sea salt and black pepper to taste

1. Cook the pasta according to the package instructions.

2. Heat the oil in a casserole dish, add the tuna and fry until lightly browned. Turn down the heat, add the garlic and red (bell) pepper and cook until soft. Add the seaweed (with its soaking water), tomatoes, anchovies or olives and basil and reduce for 5 minutes, then season.

3. Drain the cooked pasta and divide onto heated plates. Top with the sauce and serve immediately.

360 SEAFOOD RISOTTO

SERVES 4
PREPARATION
15 minutes
COOKING
20 minutes

STORAGE
Leftovers will keep in the fridge for up to 1 day.

- 4 tbsp olive oil
- 2 small red onions, finely chopped
- 2 fennel bulbs, finely chopped
- 4 cloves garlic, crushed
- 1 tsp fennel seeds, crushed
- 1 tsp cayenne pepper
- large pinch of saffron
- 300g/10½oz risotto rice
- 1 cup dried hiziki seaweed, soaked in cold water
- 2 tbsp tomato purée (paste)
- 100ml/3½fl oz/scant 1 cup dry white wine
- 1.5l/52fl oz/6½ cups fish or vegetable stock, heated
- 400g/14oz crab meat
- 4 tbsp lemon juice
- 4 tbsp fresh parsley, finely chopped

1) Heat the oil in a large heavy-based casserole dish and stir-fry the onion and the fennel until soft. Add the garlic, fennel seeds, cayenne pepper, saffron, rice and hiziki and stir-fry for 3 minutes. Add the tomato purée (paste) and stir for 1 minute until the rice is coated. Pour in the wine and stir until it is absorbed, then slowly add the stock. Bring to the boil, cover and gently simmer until the rice is cooked and the liquid is absorbed.

2) Stir in the crab meat and the lemon juice. Heat through. Adjust the seasoning, garnish with parsley and serve.

361 PASTA ALLA PUTTANESCA

SERVES 4
PREPARATION
10 minutes
COOKING
12 minutes

STORAGE
Best eaten immediately.

- 300g/10½oz spaghetti pasta
- 2 tbsp olive oil
- 4 cloves garlic, crushed
- 4–6 anchovy fillets, chopped
- 4 large ripe tomatoes, chopped
- 24 black olives, pitted and chopped
- 2 tbsp capers
- large handful fresh flat-leaf parsley, chopped
- 2 pinches of cayenne pepper
- sea salt and black pepper to taste

1) Cook the pasta in according to the package instructions.

2) Heat the oil in a frying pan (skillet) and add the garlic, then the anchovies. Stir-fry for 1 minute, add the tomatoes and cook for 5 minutes. Add the olives, capers, parsley and cayenne pepper. Season and simmer for 3 minutes.

3) Drain the cooked spaghetti, place in a large serving dish and top with the sauce. Serve immediately.

362 TUNA KEBABS with PINEAPPLE

SERVES 4
PREPARATION
15 minutes +
marinating
COOKING
6 minutes

STORAGE
The sambal will keep in the fridge for up to 2 days. The tuna kebabs are best cooked and eaten on the day they are prepared.

300g/10½oz fresh tuna steak, cut into chunks
1 red (bell) pepper, deseeded and cut into chunks

MARINADE
juice of 2 oranges
2 tbsp honey or agave nectar
2 tbsp tamari
1 tbsp olive oil

PINEAPPLE SAMBAL
2 oranges, peeled, segmented and chopped
½ fresh pineapple, diced
1 spring onion (scallion), finely chopped
3 tbsp chopped coriander (cilantro) leaves

1 Put the tuna in a shallow bowl. Stir the marinade ingredients together in a small bowl and pour this over the tuna. Cover with clingfilm (plastic wrap) and chill for 30 minutes. Meanwhile, soak 8 wooden skewers in cold water.

2 To make the sambal, mix the oranges, pineapple, spring onion

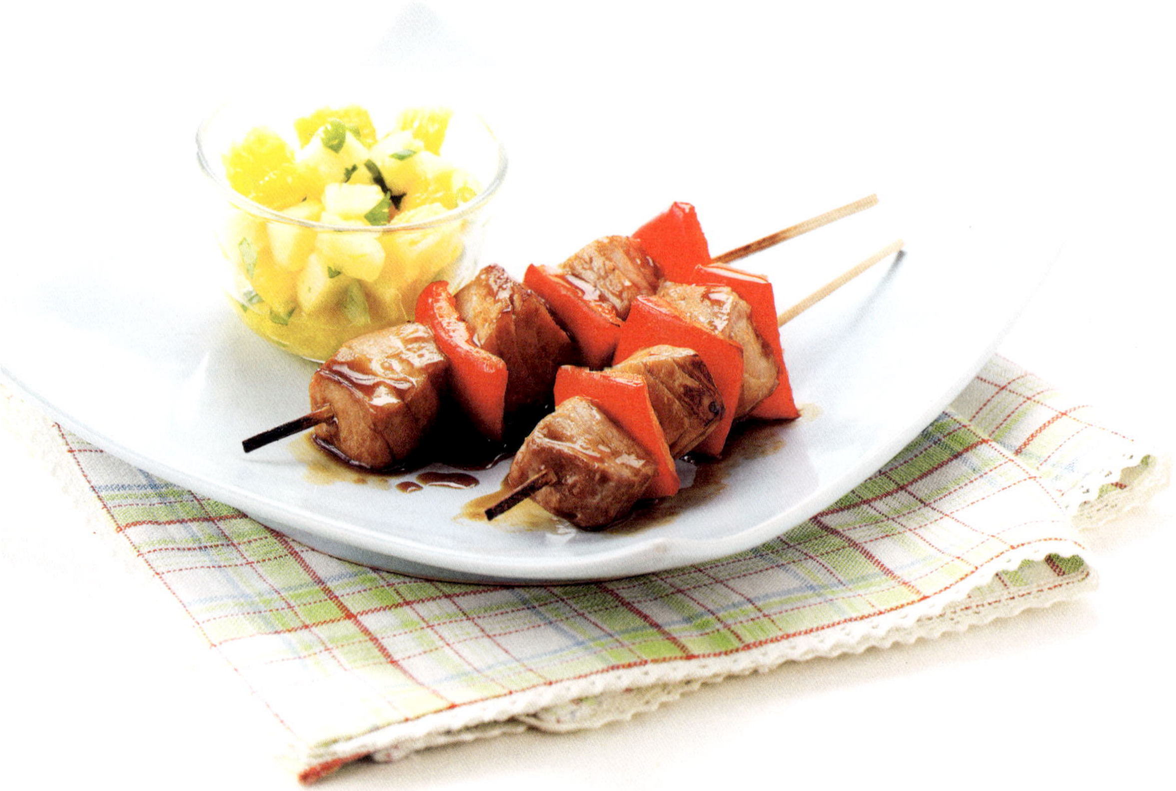

(scallion) and coriander (cilantro) in a bowl, cover with clingfilm (plastic wrap) and chill.

③ Thread the tuna and (bell) pepper chunks onto the skewers. Pour the marinade from the tuna into a small pan and bring to the boil for 1–2 minutes. Remove from the heat.

④ Preheat the grill (broiler) to high. Grill (broil) the kebabs for 2–3 minutes on each side until browned and just cooked. Put 2 kebabs on each plate and drizzle over some of the marinade. Serve with a portion of sambal on the side.

363 TUNA STEAK KEBABS AND SUGAR SNAPS

SERVES 4

PREPARATION
10 minutes

COOKING
10 minutes

STORAGE
Keep the kebabs uncooked in the fridge for no more than 12 hours.

4 tuna steaks, cut into 2cm (³⁄₄in) cubes
32 cherry tomatoes
2 tbsp green pesto
2 tbsp sesame oil
400g/14oz/3 cups sugar snap peas
2 tbsp sesame seeds

① Preheat the grill (broiler) to high. Load four metal skewers with the tuna cubes and cherry tomatoes. Baste the kebabs with the green pesto and place under the grill (broiler) for 10 minutes, turning occasionally.

② Heat the sesame oil in a wok, add the sugar snap peas and stir-fry for about 4 minutes. Add the sesame seeds, stir and remove from the heat.

③ Divide the sugar snap peas between four plates. Remove the kebabs from the heat and place on top of the peas.

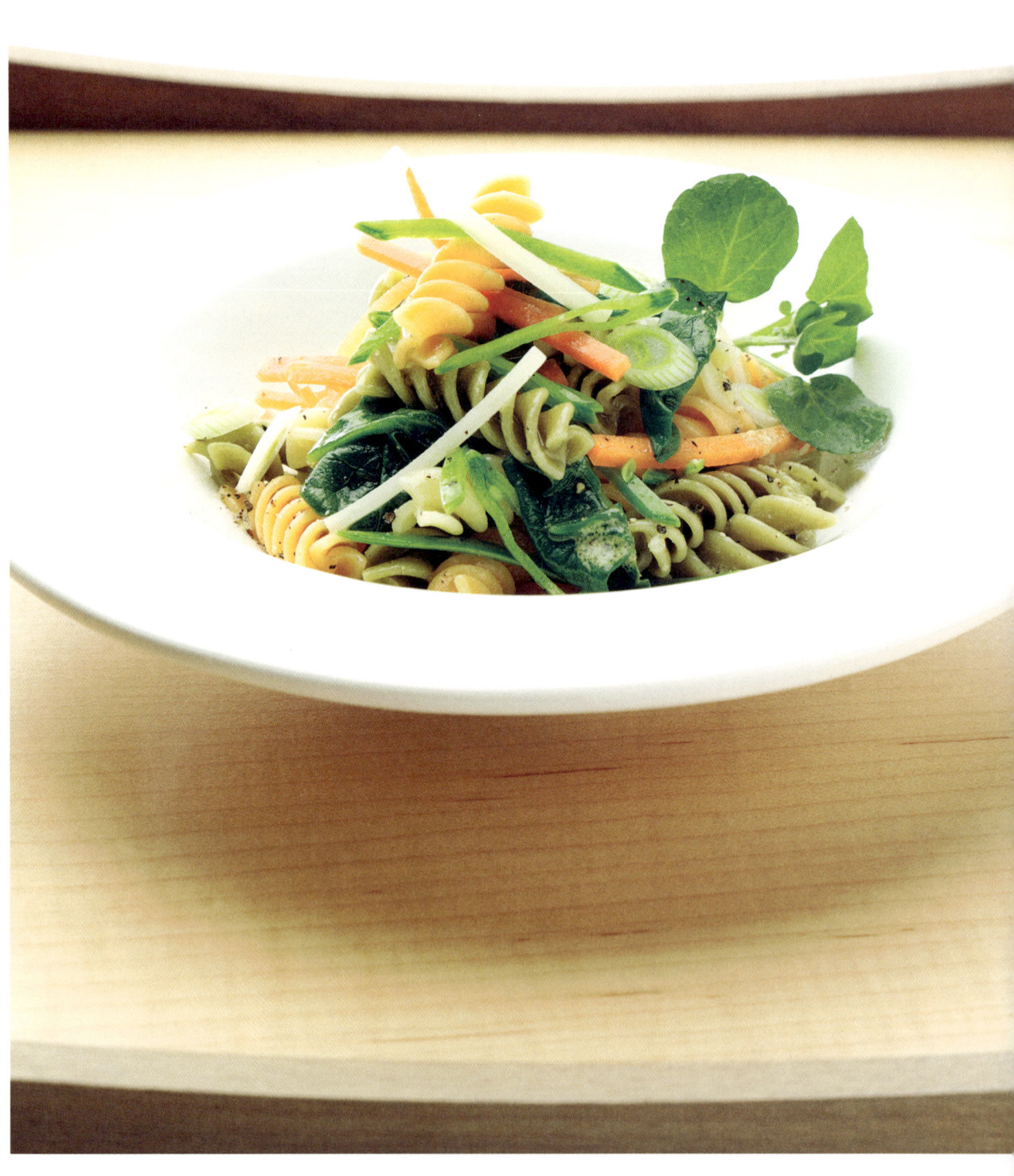

364 PASTA PRIMAVERA

SERVES 4
PREPARATION
10 minutes
COOKING
12 minutes

STORAGE
Best eaten immediately.

400g/14oz tricolor fusilli pasta
4 tbsp olive oil
4 spring onions (scallions), chopped
200g/7oz carrots, cut into thin sticks
200g/7oz celeriac (celery root), cut into thin sticks
200g/7oz mangetout (snow peas)
200g/7oz baby spinach leaves, chopped
200ml/7fl oz/scant 1 cup vegetable stock or water
2 tbsp lemon juice
2 tsp Dijon mustard
sea salt and black pepper to taste
large handful watercress, chopped

1. Cook the pasta according to the package instructions.

2. Meanwhile, heat 2 tablespoons of the oil in a casserole dish and gently stir-fry the spring onions (scallions) for 30 seconds, then add the carrots, celeriac (celery root), mangetout (snow peas) and spinach. Stir-fry for 2 minutes then add the stock or water. Bring to the boil and simmer for 5 minutes. Add the lemon juice, mustard and remaining oil, and season.

3. Drain the cooked pasta and mix with the vegetables. Garnish with watercress and serve hot.

365 PESTO, SPINACH AND MUSHROOM PASTA

SERVES 4
PREPARATION
5 minutes
COOKING
20 minutes

STORAGE
Keep the sauce refrigerated for 2–3 days, but use fresh pasta.

300g/10½oz fresh spinach tagliatelle
5 tbsp olive oil
2 onions, peeled and diced
2 cloves garlic, peeled and finely sliced
110g/4oz/⅔ cup pine nuts
200g/7oz/1 cup spinach, chopped
200g/7oz/2 cups mushrooms, sliced
6 tbsp pesto
200g/7oz/1⅓ cups grated Parmesan

1. Cook the fresh pasta with 1 tablespoon of the oil according to package instructions.

2. Heat the remaining olive oil in a pan. Add the onion, garlic and pine nuts and sauté for 1 minute. Add the spinach and mushrooms and simmer for 5 minutes. Add the pesto, stir, then set aside.

3. Drain the pasta and divide onto individual plates. Serve the sauce over the pasta and garnish with the grated Parmesan.

366 BROCCOLI AND GINGER STIR-FRY

SERVES 4
PREPARATION
5 minutes
COOKING
12 minutes

STORAGE
This meal can be delicious cold and will retain its freshness for up to 2 days if refrigerated.

6 tbsp sesame oil
500g/1lb 2oz broccoli, chopped
300g/10½oz curly kale, shredded
2 cloves garlic, peeled and chopped
4 tsp chopped root ginger
12 spring onions (scallions), sliced
6 tbsp tamari
300g/10½oz udon noodles (check that they are gluten-free)
4 tbsp sesame seeds
2 tbsp chopped coriander (cilantro)

1 Heat the sesame oil in a wok, then add the broccoli and curly kale and stir-fry for 3–5 minutes. Add the garlic, ginger, spring onions (scallions) and tamari. Continue to stir.

2 Add the udon noodles, sesame seeds and, if required, a little more tamari. Keep stirring over the heat for another 3–5 minutes until the vegetables are lightly cooked and still crunchy.

3 Remove from the heat and serve on individual plates, garnished with the coriander (cilantro).

367 ROAST PEPPERS

SERVES 4
PREPARATION
10 minutes
COOKING
30 minutes

STORAGE
Keep the in the fridge for up to 2 days.

12 yellow (bell) peppers
250ml/9fl oz/1 cup water
110g/4oz/½ cup couscous
2 tbsp olive oil, plus extra for drizzling
2 red onions, peeled and diced
4 cloves garlic, peeled and sliced
450g/1lb asparagus, chopped
230g/8oz/2 cups spinach
50g/2oz/⅔ cup pine nuts
110g/4oz/⅔ cup feta cheese
2 tsp dried oregano
50g/2oz/⅔ cup chopped parsley

1 Preheat the oven to 200°C/400°F/gas mark 6. Cut the tops off the (bell) peppers, core them, and remove the seeds. Pour the water into a saucepan, bring to the boil and add the couscous. Let simmer until the water has been absorbed (about 10 minutes). Remove from the heat.

2 In a wok, heat the olive oil and stir-fry the onion, garlic, asparagus, spinach and pine nuts for 1–2 minutes or until the asparagus is soft. Remove from the heat, add the feta cheese, oregano and couscous, mixing well. Spoon into the (bell) peppers and place in a shallow, ovenproof dish.

③ Drizzle with olive oil and bake for 10–15 minutes until lightly browned. Serve garnished with the chopped parsley.

368 CORN PANCAKES with SPICY PEAS

SERVES 4
PREPARATION 10 minutes
COOKING 30 minutes

STORAGE
Best eaten immediately.

PANCAKES
250g/9oz/2½ cups cornflour (cornstarch)
250g/9oz/scant 2 cups plain (all-purpose) flour
2 tbsp baking powder
1 tsp sea salt
4 tbsp corn oil, plus some for frying
600ml/21fl oz/2½ cups water

FILLING
2 spring onions (scallions), sliced
2 tsp ground cumin
2 cloves garlic, crushed
500g/1lb 2oz/3¾ cups chickpeas (garbanzo beans), canned
200g/7oz/1⅓ cups green peas
200ml/7fl oz/1 cup vegetable stock
2 dashes Tabasco sauce
sea salt and black pepper to taste

① Mix the two flours with the baking powder, salt, corn oil and water, and whisk to a smooth consistency. Set aside.

② Stir-fry the spring onions (scallions) in a casserole dish with 2 tbsp oil, then add the cumin and the garlic. Heat through, add the chickpeas (garbanzo beans) and stir for 1 minute. Add the green peas, stock and Tabasco sauce, and season. Leave the peas to simmer while you make the pancakes.

③ Heat a little more oil in a frying pan (skillet) and fry approximately twelve pancakes. Divide the filling between the pancakes and serve.

369 PROVENÇAL PANCAKES

SERVES 4
PREPARATION 15 minutes
COOKING 22 minutes

STORAGE
Best eaten immediately.

PANCAKES
200g/7oz/1½ cups spelt flour
70g/2½oz/½ cup soya flour
300ml/10½fl oz/1½ cups milk
4 tbsp olive oil
grapeseed oil for frying

FILLING
2 leeks, chopped
2 green (bell) peppers, sliced
4 large ripe tomatoes, chopped
24 black olives, pitted and chopped
2 tbsp fresh basil, chopped
sea salt and black pepper to taste

1. Whisk the two flours with the milk, olive oil and a pinch of salt to make a batter. Set aside.

2. Sweat the leek in a pan with a little olive oil for 2 minutes. Add the green (bell) pepper, tomatoes, olives and fresh basil. Cover and simmer for 5 minutes, then season.

3. Heat a little grapeseed oil in a frying pan (skillet) and fry eight pancakes. Place 2 tbsp filling on each pancake, fold and serve.

370 SPINACH PANCAKES with HUMMUS and WILD MUSHROOMS

SERVES 4
PREPARATION 10 minutes
COOKING 15 minutes

STORAGE
Best eaten immediately.

PANCAKES
250g/9oz plain (all-purpose) flour
2 eggs, beaten
250ml/9fl oz/1 cup milk or soya milk
250ml/9fl oz/1 cup water
2 tbsp grapeseed oil or butter
large pinch of sea salt
400g/14oz fresh spinach, chopped, cooked and drained
olive oil for frying

FILLING
600g/1lb 5oz wild mushrooms, chopped
4 cloves garlic, crushed
200g/7oz/¾ cup hummus
sea salt and black pepper to taste

1. Mix the flour, eggs, milk, water, oil or butter and salt, then add the spinach and mix well.

2. Heat a little oil in a frying pan (skillet) and cook the pancakes over a medium-low heat.

3. Add more oil to a separate pan and stir-fry the mushrooms with the garlic, and season. Spread a spoonful of hummus over each pancake, add the seasoned mushrooms, fold and serve hot.

371 CHEESY POTATO AND ROCKET PANCAKES

SERVES 4
PREPARATION 10 minutes
COOKING 30 minutes
STORAGE Best eaten immediately.

PANCAKES
250g/9oz plain (all-purpose) flour
2 eggs, beaten
250ml/9fl oz/1 cup milk or soya milk
250ml/9fl oz/1 cup water
2 tbsp grapeseed oil or butter
large pinch of sea salt
olive oil for frying

FILLING
1kg/2lb 3oz potatoes, chopped
4 cloves garlic, crushed
2 small fresh or dried red chillies, chopped or crumbled
400g/14oz) fresh rocket (arugula), chopped
100g/3½oz Gruyère cheese, grated
sea salt to taste

1. Boil the potatoes in salted water until soft. Meanwhile, mix all the batter ingredients and set aside.

2. Heat 2 tablespoons of oil in a large heavy pan and fry the garlic and chilli for 30 seconds. Add half the rocket (arugula) and stir. Remove from the heat. Stir in the cooked potatoes, the Gruyère cheese and the remaining rocket (arugula). Mash, mix and season.

3. Heat a little more oil in a frying pan (skillet) and fry the pancakes for 2 minutes on each side. Top with 2 tablespoons of the filling. Roll the pancakes and serve as you go.

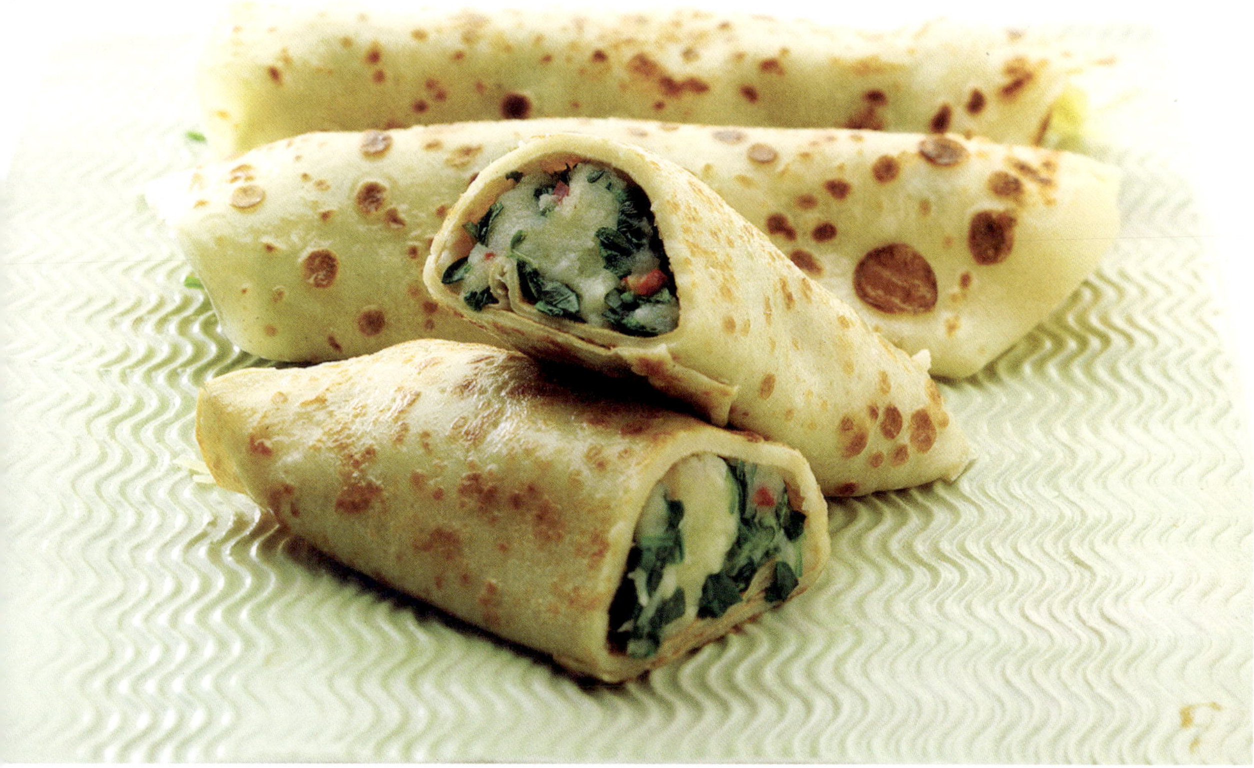

372 BUCKWHEAT NOODLES WITH SPICY COURGETTE SAUCE

SERVES 4
PREPARATION 10 minutes
COOKING 16 minutes
STORAGE Best eaten immediately.

2 tbsp olive oil
2 small white onions, finely chopped
2 cloves garlic, crushed
2 medium courgettes (zucchini), thinly sliced
100g/3½oz sun-dried tomatoes, chopped
2 small red chillies, deseeded and finely sliced
200ml/7fl oz/scant 1 cup crème fraîche
2 tbsp fresh oregano, finely chopped
sea salt and black pepper to taste
400g/14oz Japanese buckwheat noodles
a little grated cheese (optional)

1) Heat the oil in a casserole dish and sweat the onion and garlic for 5 minutes until soft (don't let them brown). Add the courgettes (zucchini) and cook for 2–3 minutes. Then add the sun-dried tomatoes and the chilli, cover and simmer for 5 minutes, stirring from time to time. Add the crème fraîche and fresh oregano, and season. Heat through and very gently simmer for 2–3 minutes.

2) Cook the noodles as instructed on the package. Drain and toss with the sauce. Sprinkle with cheese (if using) and serve immediately.

373 SPICY CHICKPEAS WITH AUBERGINE

SERVES 4
PREPARATION 10 minutes
COOKING 25 minutes
STORAGE Leftovers will keep in the fridge for up to 3 days.

4 tbsp olive oil
2 leeks, sliced
800g/1lb 12oz/6 cups chickpeas (garbanzo beans), cooked or canned
2 aubergines (eggplant), diced
2 cloves garlic, crushed
1 tsp ground cumin
1 tsp ground coriander
1kg/2lb 3oz tomatoes, chopped
sea salt and black pepper to taste

1) Heat the oil in a casserole dish and gently sweat the leeks for 5 minutes. Turn up the heat a little and add the chickpeas (garbanzo beans), aubergines (eggplant), garlic, cumin and coriander. Stir-fry for 5 minutes. Add the tomatoes and bring to the boil. Cover and simmer for 15 minutes (adding a little water if necessary). Season and serve with rice.

374 TOFU NOODLES

SERVES 4
PREPARATION
10 minutes + marinating
COOKING
12 minutes

STORAGE
Leftovers will keep in the fridge for up to 2 days

- 2 tsp honey or agave nectar
- 5 tbsp tamari
- 2 cloves garlic, crushed
- 1 tsp grated root ginger
- 250g/9oz firm tofu
- 150g/5½oz rice noodles
- 3 tbsp smooth peanut butter (without added sugar)
- 2 tbsp olive oil
- 350g/12oz mixed stir-fry vegetables, such as broccoli, mushrooms, (bell) peppers, beansprouts, mangetout (snow peas).

1. Mix the honey or agave nectarz, tamari, garlic and ginger and pour half into a shallow dish, then add the tofu. Turn the tofu in the sauce to coat; cover and marinate for at least 30 minutes.

2. Put the noodles in a bowl, cover with boiling water and soak for 2 minutes. Drain and rinse under cold water. The noodles should still be crisp.

3. Mix the peanut butter into the remaining tamari mixture with 125ml/4fl oz/½ cup boiling water.

4. Drain the tofu and reserve the marinade. Heat a wok, add the oil and cook the tofu in batches for 2–3 minutes until well browned. Transfer to a plate.

5. Stir-fry the vegetables for 2 minutes. Add the noodles, tofu, peanut sauce and reserved marinade. Stir-fry for 2–3 minutes until the vegetables are tender but crisp and the liquid has reduced slightly. Serve immediately.

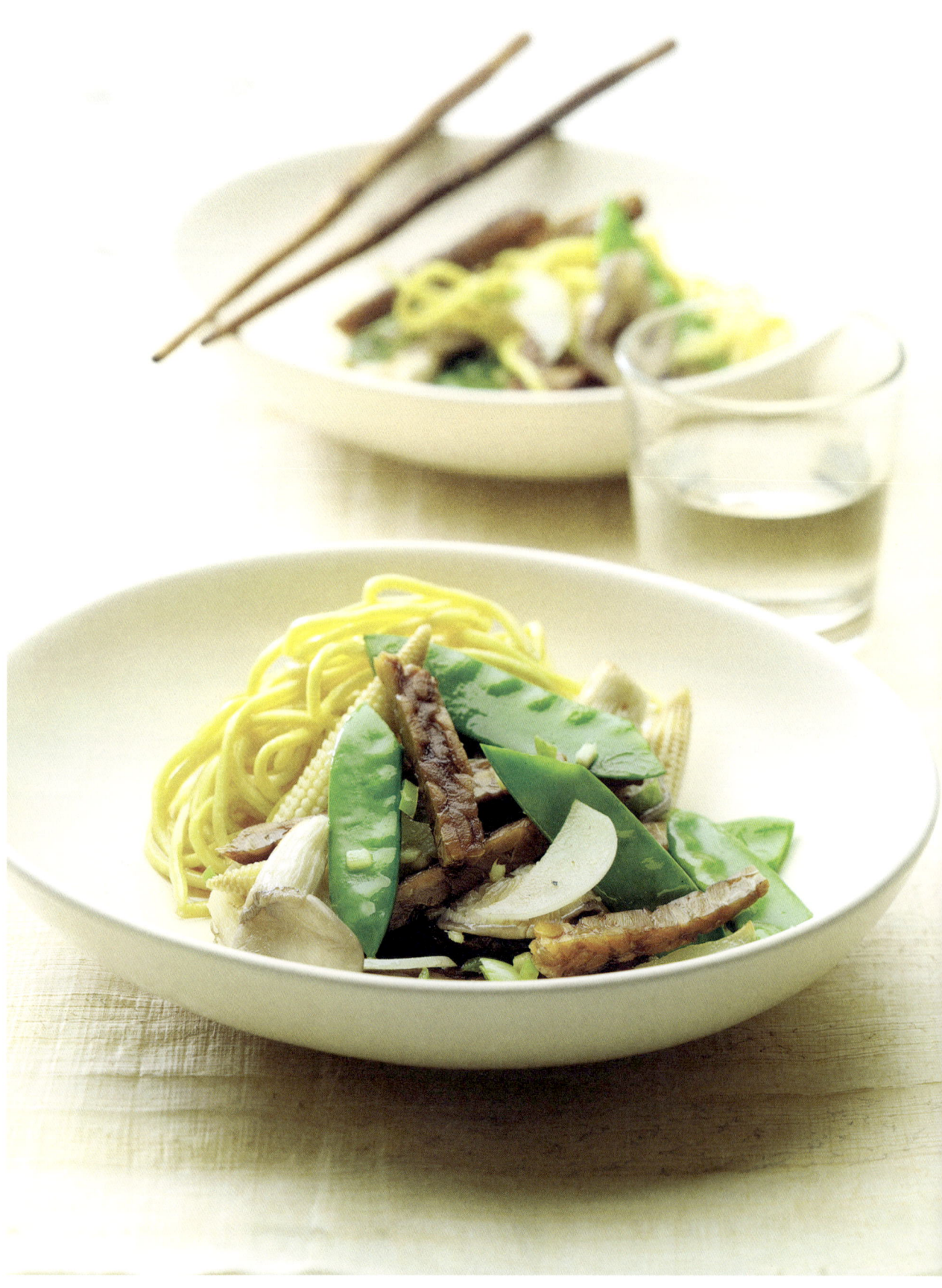

375 INDONESIAN TEMPEH AND VEGETABLES

SERVES 4
PREPARATION 10 minutes
COOKING 10 minutes
STORAGE Best eaten immediately.

- 8 tempeh strips, cut into sticks
- 4 tbsp tamari
- 4 tbsp olive oil
- 2 cloves garlic, sliced
- 2 tbsp chopped fresh root ginger
- 2 green chillies, deseeded and sliced
- 200g/7oz baby corn, kept whole
- 200g/7oz mangetout (snow peas)
- 200g/7oz oyster mushrooms
- 4 spring onions (scallions), sliced
- 2 tbsp toasted sesame oil
- sea salt and black pepper to taste

1. Marinate the tempeh in the tamari while you prepare the other ingredients.

2. Stir-fry the marinated tempeh with the olive oil in a large pan or wok, add the remaining ingredients (except for the sesame oil), one by one, and stir-fry for a few more minutes. Add the sesame oil, season and serve with noodles.

376 MOROCCAN APRICOT PARCELS

SERVES 4
PREPARATION 5 minutes
COOKING 30 minutes
STORAGE Refrigerate raw and use within a week, or freeze for up to 3 weeks.

- 1 tbsp olive oil
- 85g/3oz/½ cup pine nuts
- ½ red (bell) pepper, chopped
- 2 cloves garlic, peeled and sliced
- 115g/4oz/½ cup dried apricots, chopped
- 4 spring onions (scallions), chopped
- 400-g/14-oz can chickpeas (garbanzo beans), drained
- 115g/4oz/½ cup feta cheese
- 25g/1oz/¼ cup chopped basil
- ½ tsp freshly ground black pepper
- 175g/6oz/¾ cup crème fraîche
- 280g/10oz filo (phyllo) pastry

1. Heat the oven to 190°C/375°F/gas mark 5. Heat the olive oil in a pan. Add the pine nuts, red (bell) pepper and garlic and sauté for 2 minutes. Add the apricots, spring onions (scallions) and chickpeas (garbanzo beans) and cook, stirring, over a low heat for 2 minutes. Set aside.

2. Crumble the feta into a bowl and mix in the ingredients from the pan along with the basil, black pepper and crème fraîche.

3. Roll out the filo (phyllo) pastry, large enough to cut four 7.5 x 7.5cm (3 x 3in) squares. Spoon the feta mixture into the middle of each square, fold over to make a triangle and press the edges together. Cook on a baking sheet for 15–20 minutes.

377 POLENTA and PEPPER CAKES with PESTO

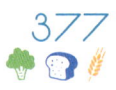

SERVES 4
PREPARATION
10 minutes
COOKING
20 minutes

STORAGE
You can refrigerate the uncooked mixture for up to 2 days or freeze it for up to a month.

- 4 tbsp olive oil
- 2 red (bell) peppers, diced
- 230g/8oz baby courgettes (zucchini), sliced
- 2 red onions, peeled and diced
- 230g/8oz broccoli, chopped
- 230g/8oz/2 cups mushrooms, sliced
- 4 cloves garlic, finely sliced
- 3l/105fl oz/12 cups water
- 540g/1lb 4oz/3⅔ cups polenta (cornmeal)
- 170g/6oz/1 cup grated Cheddar cheese
- 4 tsp green pesto

1. Preheat the oven to 150°C/300°F/gas mark 2 and heat the oil in a frying pan (skillet). Add the vegetables and garlic and sauté for 5–6 minutes until lightly brown.

2. Meanwhile, in a pan, bring the water to the boil, add the polenta and simmer, stirring, for 15–20 minutes, until it leaves the sides of the pan and thickens. Remove from the heat and mix in the cheese and sautéed vegetables.

3. Mould the mixture into cakes, place on a non-stick baking sheet and put in the oven for 20 minutes or until browned lightly. Serve on individual plates with a teaspoon of pesto drizzled over each cake.

378 CELERIAC SCHNITZEL

SERVES 2–4
PREPARATION
10 minutes
COOKING
20 minutes

STORAGE
Best eaten immediately.

- 1 large celeriac (celery root), peeled and cut into thick slices
- 2 tbsp grapeseed oil
- 1 egg, beaten
- 2 tbsp seasoned breadcrumbs
- 1 lemon, thinly sliced
- 2 tbsp grated horseradish
- 1 handful fresh parsley, chopped
- 1 tbsp capers

1. Blanch the celeriac (celery root) in a saucepan of boiling salted water for 3 minutes.

2. Heat the oil in a large frying pan (skillet). Dip the celeriac (celery root) slices into the egg, then the breadcrumbs, and fry until golden. Place a slice of lemon, a little grated horseradish and a few capers on each schnitzel to garnish. Serve with boiled potatoes and chopped parsley.

379 LENTIL MOUSSAKA

SERVES 2–4
PREPARATION
20 minutes
COOKING
1 hour 10 minutes

STORAGE
Assemble and freeze, uncooked, for up to 1 month. Defrost in the fridge before cooking. Leftovers will keep in the fridge for up to 2 days.

3 tbsp olive oil
1 large aubergine (eggplant), thickly sliced
1 red onion, chopped
1 clove garlic, chopped
180g/6¼oz red lentils, rinsed
2 carrots, chopped
400g/14oz canned chopped tomatoes
4 tbsp sun-dried tomato purée (paste)
600ml/21fl oz/scant 2½ cups vegetable stock
200g/7oz/1 cup Greek yogurt
2 eggs
4 tbsp grated Parmesan cheese

1. Preheat the grill (broiler) to high and line a grill pan with foil. Use 2 tablespoons of the oil to brush the aubergine (eggplant) slices on both sides. Grill (broil) for 3–4 minutes on each side until golden. Set aside.

2. Preheat the oven to 190°C/375°F/gas mark 5. Heat the remaining oil in a saucepan. Cook the onion and garlic for 2 minutes. Stir in the lentils, carrots, chopped tomatoes, tomato purée (paste) and stock and bring to the boil. Reduce the heat, cover and simmer for 20 minutes, or until the lentils are soft.

3. Spread half the lentils in a baking dish. Top with half the aubergines (egplant), then the remaining lentils and finish with a layer of aubergines (eggplant). Mix the yogurt, eggs and half the cheese and spoon over the aubergines (eggplant). Sprinkle with the remaining cheese.

4. Bake for 30–35 minutes, or until golden, then serve.

380 CHICKPEA VEGGIE PATTIES

SERVES 4
PREPARATION 15 minutes + chilling
COOKING 20 minutes

STORAGE Leftovers will keep in the fridge for up to 3 days or in the freezer, uncooked, for 1 month. Defrost in the fridge before cooking.

1 tbsp olive oil, plus extra for greasing
400g/14oz canned chickpeas (garbanzo beans), drained
½ red onion, grated
1 carrot, grated
1 clove garlic, crushed
2 tbsp chopped parsley
1 tsp ground cumin
1 tsp ground coriander
1 egg
75g/2½oz/generous ½ cup wholemeal breadcrumbs
4 wholemeal rolls or pitta breads
handful of mixed salad leaves

1. Grease a baking sheet with oil. Pulse the chickpeas (garbanzo beans), onion, carrot, garlic, parsley, cumin and coriander in a food processor to form a coarse paste. Transfer to a bowl, and stir in the egg and breadcrumbs.

2. Wet your hands to prevent the mixture from sticking and shape it into 8 patties. Put on the baking sheet and chill for 30 minutes.

3. Preheat the oven to 200°C/400°F/gas mark 6. Brush the patties with the oil and bake for 20 minutes until golden brown.

4. Meanwhile, split the rolls or pittas in half and toast or warm them in the oven. Fill the breads with salad and a couple of patties and serve.

381 SCANDINAVIAN BEETROOT BURGERS

SERVES 4
PREPARATION 15 minutes
COOKING 30 minutes

400g/14oz/3 cups well-cooked rice
200g/7oz tofu, grated
2 medium beetroot (beets), grated
100g/3½oz/1¾ cups breadcrumbs
2 tbsp red wine vinegar
2 tbsp olive oil, plus some for frying
2 tsp dried basil
sea salt and black pepper to taste
plain (all-purpose) flour for dipping

1. Mix together the cooked rice, grated tofu, beetroot (beets), breadcrumbs, red wine vinegar, olive oil and basil in a bowl. Season and shape into twelve 70-g/2½-oz flat patties. Dip the patties in the flour to coat.

2. Heat a little oil in a frying pan (skillet) over a high heat and fry the

STORAGE
You can refrigerate the uncooked mixture for up to 2 days or freeze it for up to a month.

patties in batches for another 2 minutes on each side. Turn down the heat and continue to fry for about 5 minutes on each side.

③ Serve each burger in a bun with some mustard, tomato ketchup, red onion, lettuce, tomato and pickled cucumber.

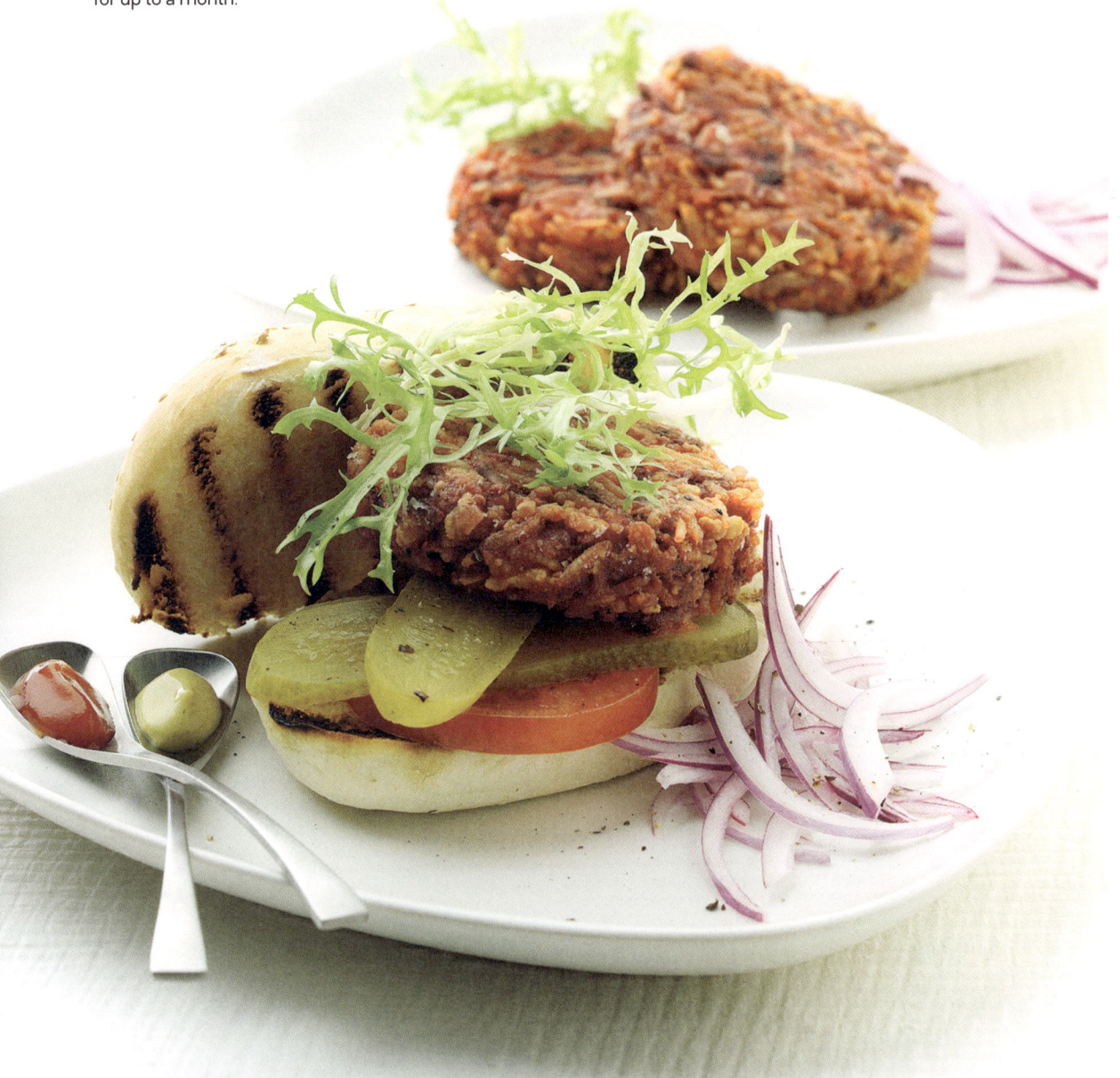

382 MUSHROOM AND SPINACH QUICHE

SERVES 4
PREPARATION
30 minutes
COOKING
20 minutes

STORAGE
You can keep the cooked quiche refrigerated for up to 3 days.

200g/7oz/1 2/3 cups rye flour
3 tbsp ground almonds
125g/4 1/2 oz butter
3 tbsp water
115g/4oz/1 cup spinach
1 onion, peeled and chopped
115g/4oz/1 cup mushrooms, sliced
2 whole eggs
2 egg yolks
250ml/9fl oz/1 cup single (light) cream
1 pinch of celery salt
115g/4oz/2/3 cup goat's cheese

1. Preheat the oven to 200°C/400°F/gas mark 6.

2. Put the flour, ground almonds and 115g/4oz of the butter into a bowl. Mix in the butter with your fingers until the mixture resembles breadcrumbs. Add the water and knead together to form a dough. Roll out on a work surface into a large circle and place in a greased 20cm/8in quiche tin (pan).

3. Heat the remaining butter in a wok and add the spinach, onion and mushrooms. Stir-fry for 5 minutes until browned.

4. Whisk together the eggs and yolks, cream and celery salt. Pour the vegetables into the pastry case. Crumble the goat's cheese on top and pour over the egg mixture. Bake for 20 minutes.

383 STUFFED MUSHROOMS

SERVES 4
PREPARATION 5 minutes
COOKING 25 minutes

STORAGE Leftovers will keep in the fridge for up to 1 day.

12 large flat mushrooms, stalks removed and chopped
4 tbsp almonds, chopped
olive oil, for frying and brushing
4 tbsp breadcrumbs
200g/7oz/scant 1 cup soft cheese
2 tbsp lemon juice
4 tbsp fresh parsley, chopped
2 tbsp paprika

1. Preheat the oven to 200°C/400°F/gas mark 6.

2. Fry the mushroom stalks and the almonds in a frying pan (skillet) with a little oil, then mix them with the breadcrumbs and the cheese. Season and set aside.

3. Place the mushroom caps upside down on a baking sheet and brush with the lemon juice and olive oil. Add the filling and bake in a hot oven for 20 minutes. Garnish with fresh parsley and paprika, and serve with toast and salad.

384 WILD MUSHROOM PIE

SERVES 4
PREPARATION 10 minutes
COOKING 45–50 minutes

STORAGE Leftovers will keep in the fridge for up to 2 days.

400g/14oz puff pastry, rolled out
6 small shallots, halved and sliced
4 tbsp olive oil
500g/1lb 2oz wild mushrooms
2 tsp thyme
200ml/7fl oz/scant 1 cup milk or soya milk
4 eggs
large pinch of nutmeg

1. Preheat the oven to 220°C/425°F/gas mark 7. Place the rolled-out pastry on greaseproof paper in a 23cm/9in round baking tin (pan). Scatter with baking beans and bake blind for 10–15 minutes. Allow to cool and remove the beans.

2. Gently sweat the shallots in a heavy-based frying pan (skillet) with the oil for 5 minutes. Add the mushrooms and the thyme and stir-fry for 10 minutes. Blend the milk, eggs and nutmeg to a smooth consistency, and season. Place the mushrooms on the pastry, pour the blended egg mixture over, return to the oven and bake for 15–20 minutes until the pastry is crisp and golden and the filling is set, and serve.

385 ROASTED TOMATO AND BASIL PASTA

SERVES 4
PREPARATION 5 minutes
COOKING 20 minutes

STORAGE
You can refrigerate the sauce for up to 2 days or freeze it for up to a month.

- 450g/1lb fresh spinach tagliatelle (ensure egg-free if necessary)
- 4 tbsp olive oil
- 2 onions, peeled and diced
- 2 cloves garlic, finely sliced
- 2 x 400-g/14-oz cans chopped tomatoes
- 200g/7oz cherry tomatoes
- 2 tsp dried oregano
- 200g/7oz spinach
- 50g/2oz/$^2/_3$ cup chopped basil
- large handful pine nuts

1. Cook the tagliatelle according to the package instructions.

2. Meanwhile, heat the olive oil in another saucepan. Add the onion and garlic and gently sauté.

3. Add the tomatoes, oregano and spinach and stir over a medium heat. Cover and let simmer for 10 minutes.

4. When the pasta is cooked, drain and arrange on individual plates. Divide the sauce over the pasta and serve garnished with basil leaves and pine nuts.

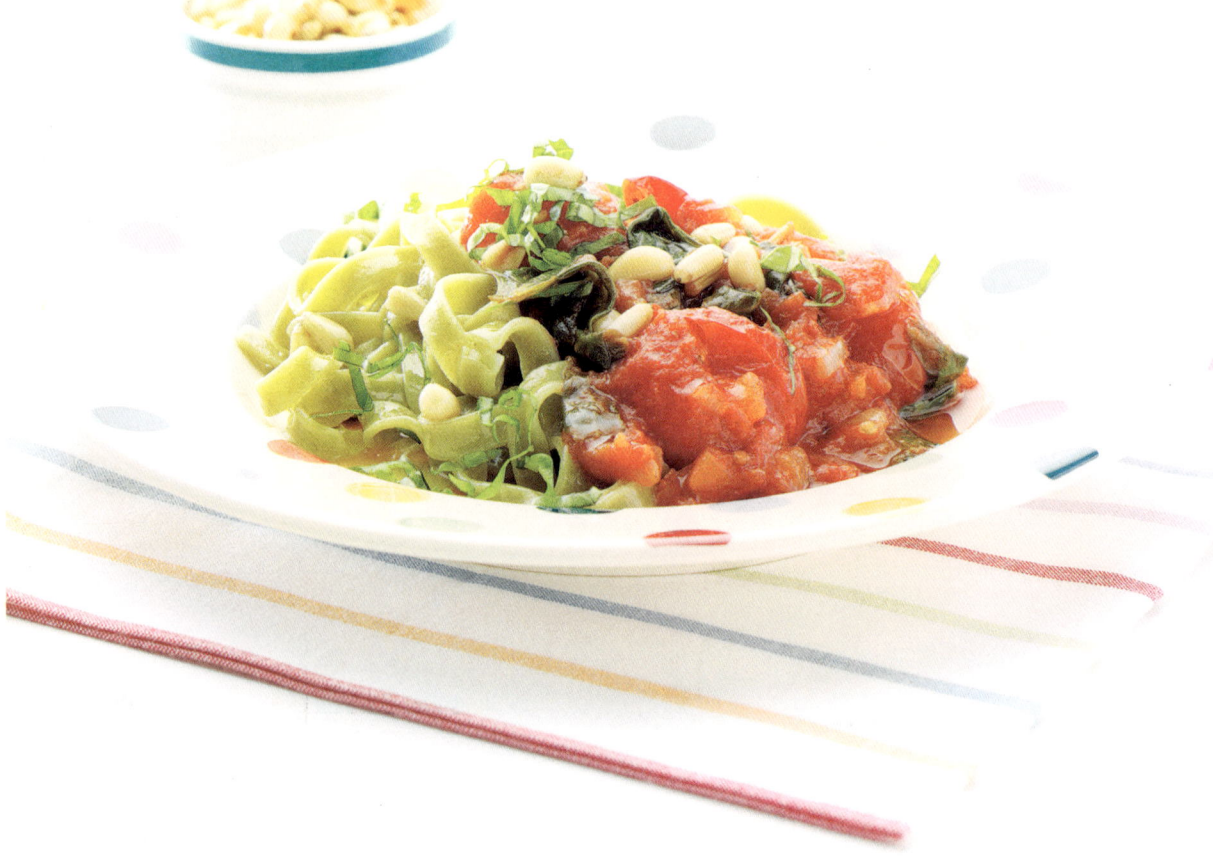

386 SPAGHETTINI with COOL HERBS and HOT TOMATOES

SERVES 4
PREPARATION
10 minutes
COOKING
10 minutes

STORAGE
Keep the sauce refrigerated for 2–3 days, but use freshly cooked pasta.

- 400g/14oz spaghettini pasta
- 4 cloves garlic
- large handful fresh mint
- large handful fresh basil
- large handful fresh oregano
- 4 large ripe beef tomatoes, quartered
- 2 tbsp capers
- 2 tsp Tabasco sauce
- 2 tsp maple syrup
- 4 tbsp olive oil
- sea salt and black pepper to taste
- 4 tbsp chopped walnuts

1. Cook the pasta in boiling water according to the package instructions, for about 12 minutes or until al dente.

2. Coarsely chop the garlic and the herbs, then blend them in a food processor with the tomatoes, capers, Tabasco sauce, maple syrup and oil. Season and set aside.

3. Drain the cooked pasta and divide between four large plates. Top with the blended tomato sauce and garnish with chopped walnuts. Serve immediately.

387 SPAGHETTI with ARTICHOKES, BEANS and SPINACH

SERVES 4
PREPARATION 10 minutes
COOKING 13 minutes
STORAGE Keep the sauce refrigerated for 2–3 days, but use freshly cooked pasta.

300g/10½oz spaghetti pasta
4 tbsp olive oil
2 spring onions (scallions), sliced
2 cloves garlic, chopped
2 red (bell) peppers, halved and sliced
200g/7oz/1¾ cups broad (fava) beans, fresh or frozen
250g/9oz fresh spinach, chopped
8 artichoke hearts, sliced
4 tbsp tomato purée
1 tsp raw cane sugar
2 tbsp fresh marjoram
sea salt and black pepper to taste

1) Cook the pasta in boiling water according to the package instructions, for about 12 minutes or until al dente.

2) Meanwhile, gently heat the oil in a large saucepan. Add the spring onions (scallions), garlic and red (bell) pepper and gently fry for 2 minutes. Stir in the beans, spinach and artichoke hearts. Add the tomato purée (paste), sugar and marjoram, and a little water if necessary. Cover and very gently simmer for 10 minutes. Season and serve with the cooked spaghetti.

388 PASTA with VEGETABLES and CREAMY MUSTARD SAUCE

SERVES 4
PREPARATION 15 minutes
COOKING 15 minutes
STORAGE Best eaten immediately.

400g/14oz pasta shapes of choice
2 small leeks, finely sliced
1 small hokkaido pumpkin, deseeded, peeled and diced
2 small heads broccoli, cut into small florets
large handful fresh parsley, finely chopped, plus extra to garnish
2 tbsp fresh tarragon (or 2 tsp dried), finely chopped
4 tbsp Dijon mustard
2 cloves garlic, crushed
6 tbsp olive oil
sea salt and black pepper to taste

1) Cook the pasta according to the package instructions. After 4 minutes, add the vegetables and continue to boil until the pasta is just cooked. Drain the cooked pasta and vegetables in a colander.

2) Mix the parsley and tarragon with the mustard, garlic, oil, salt and pepper in a bowl.

3) Gently heat the mustard sauce in the pasta pan. Return the pasta and vegetables to the pan and gently mix. Check the seasoning and serve garnished with parsley.

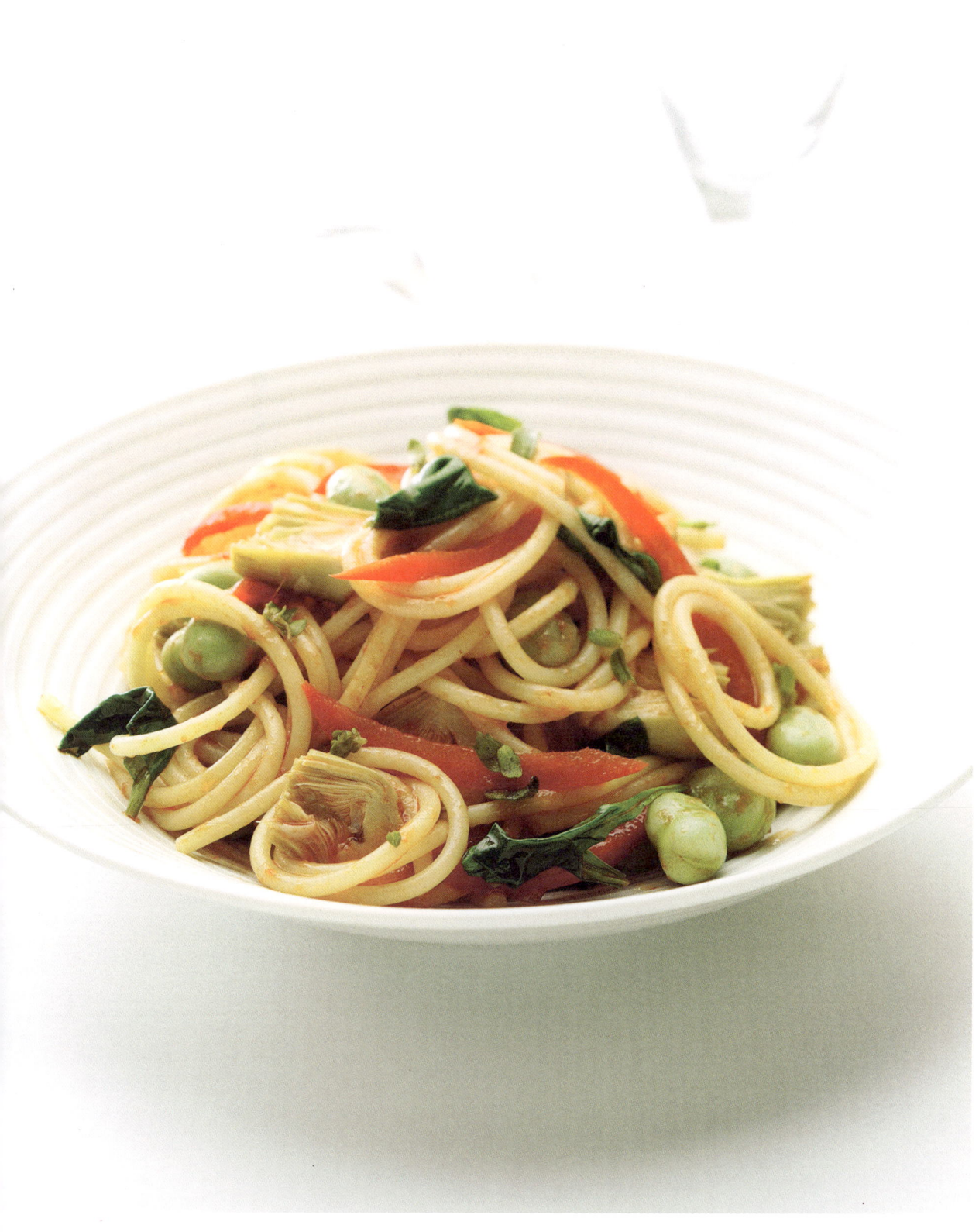

389 PENNE with ASPARAGUS and MUSHROOM SAUCE

SERVES 4
PREPARATION
10 minutes
COOKING
12 minutes

STORAGE
Best eaten immediately.

400g/14oz penne pasta
2 bunches green asparagus
4 tbsp olive oil
2 shallot, finely chopped
200g/7oz mushrooms, sliced
200ml/7fl oz/scant 1 cup vegetable stock
2 tsp cornflour (cornstarch) dissolved in a little cold water
2 tbsp tamari
sea salt and black pepper to taste

1. Cook the pasta in boiling water according to the package instructions.

2. Cut the asparagus into penne-sized lengths, then stir-fry them in the olive oil together with the shallot and the mushrooms for 5 minutes. Add the stock, bring to the boil and simmer for 2–3 minutes, or until the asparagus is tender. Pour in the dissolved cornflour (cornstarch) and the tamari and cook until the sauce thickens. Season with salt (if necessary) and plenty of black pepper.

3. Drain the cooked pasta and add to the asparagus and mushroom sauce. Serve hot.

390 RIGATONI with HERB PANGRATTATO

SERVES 4
PREPARATION
10 minutes
COOKING
12 minutes

STORAGE
Best eaten immediately.

400g/14oz mascarpone cheese
6–7 tbsp olive oil
6 cloves garlic, crushed
4 tbsp Parmesan
sea salt and black pepper to taste
400g/14oz rigatoni pasta
4 thick slices ciabatta bread, coarsely crumbled
2 tsp thyme
2 tsp oregano

1. Mix the mascarpone with 2 tablespoons of the oil in a bowl. Add 2 cloves of garlic and the Parmesan, and season. Set aside.

2. Cook the pasta in boiling water according to the package instructions.

3. To make the pangrattato, heat 4–5 tablespoons of oil in a small saucepan, add the remaining 4 cloves of garlic and the breadcrumbs and stir-fry until golden. Add the herbs at the last minute and remove from the heat.

4. Drain the cooked pasta and mix with the cheese sauce. Garnish with the herb pangrattato and serve immediately.

391 FETTUCCINE with WALNUT PESTO

SERVES 4
PREPARATION 10 minutes
COOKING 12 minutes
STORAGE Keep the sauce refrigerated for 2–3 days, but use fresh pasta.

- 400g/14oz fettuccine pasta
- 100g/3½oz/¾ cup walnuts (shelled weight)
- 2 cloves garlic, crushed
- 2 tbsp fresh flat-leaf parsley, chopped
- 2 thick slices bread, crumbled and soaked in milk or soya milk
- 2 tbsp olive oil
- 4 tbsp fresh basil, chopped
- sea salt and black pepper to taste

1 Cook the pasta in boiling water according to the package instructions, for about 12 minutes or until al dente.

2 Meanwhile, pound the walnuts in a mortar (reserving a few to garnish) together with the garlic, parsley and a little salt, until you have a rough paste. Squeeze the milk from the crumbled bread, add the bread to the mortar and mix well. Then add the oil and the basil (and a little of the soaking milk if necessary), and mix until you have a thick green sauce.

3 Drain the cooked pasta and mix with the pesto sauce. Season, garnish with the reserved walnut halves and serve with Parmesan.

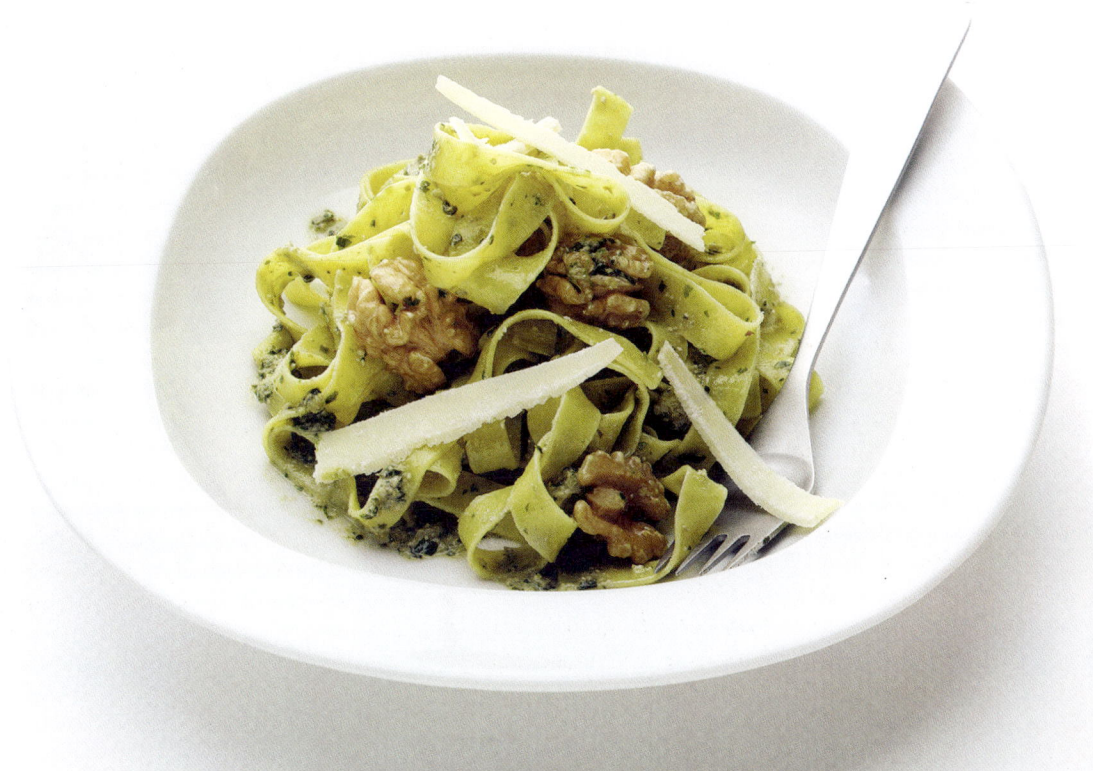

392 LEMON RISOTTO with FRESH BASIL

SERVES 4
PREPARATION
10 minutes
COOKING
20 minutes

STORAGE
Leftovers will keep in the fridge for up to 2 days.

- 4 tbsp olive oil
- 2 leeks, sliced
- 4 celery stalks (with leaves), sliced
- 2 cloves garlic, crushed
- 300g/10½oz/1½ cups risotto rice
- 150ml/5fl oz/⅔ cup dry vermouth
- 1l/35fl oz/4¼ cups hot vegetable stock
- 1 lemon, quartered and sliced
- 6 tbsp fresh basil, chopped
- 4 tbsp Parmesan

1) Heat the oil in a large, heavy saucepan and gently stir-fry the leek and the celery until soft. Add the garlic and the rice, stir for 1 minute, then add the vermouth. Stir for a further minute, then add the stock. Bring to the boil, cover and very gently simmer until the rice is cooked. Add the lemon pieces and most of the basil, gently stir and heat through. Sprinkle with the Parmesan and the remaining basil, and serve immediately.

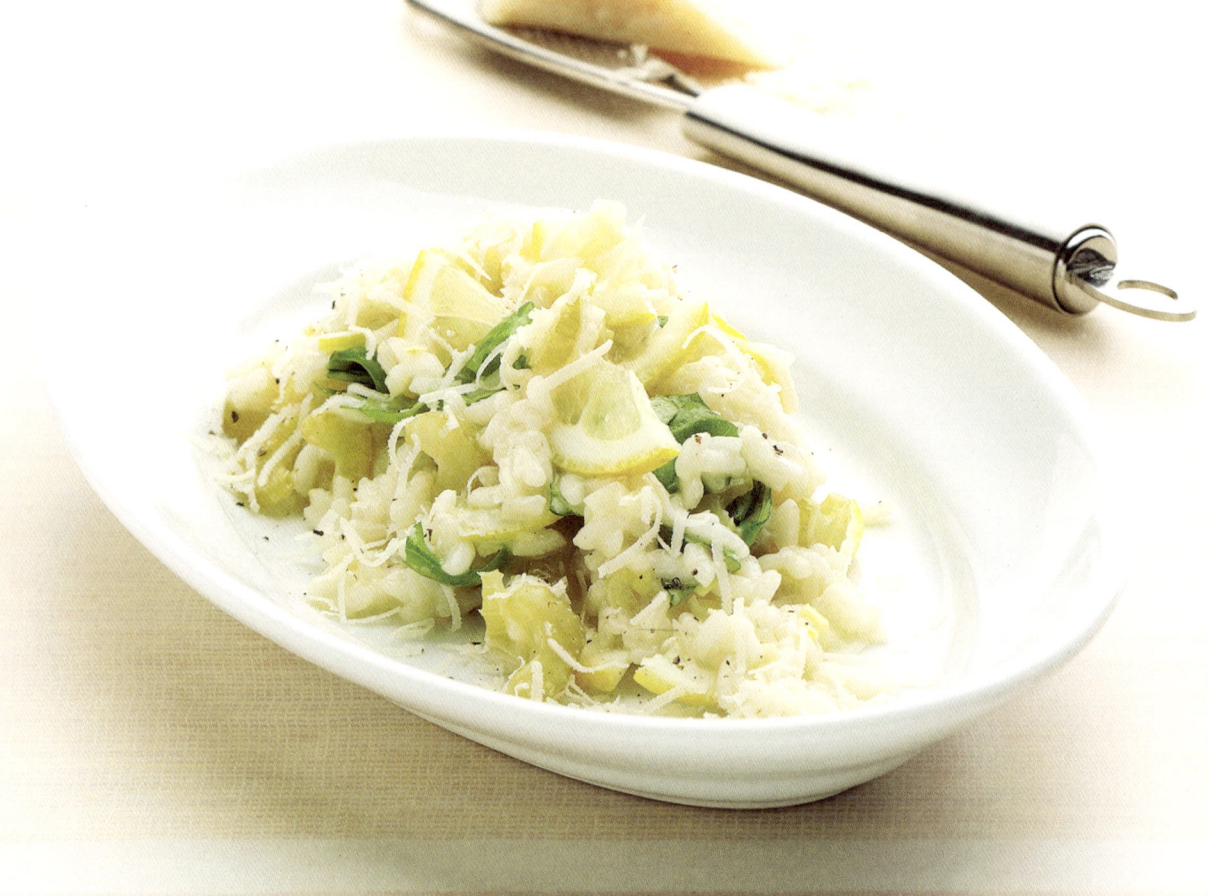

393 GREEK RAGOUT

SERVES 4
PREPARATION 10 minutes
COOKING 22 minutes

STORAGE
Leftovers will keep in the fridge for up to 2 days.

4 tbsp olive oil
2 leeks, sliced
1kg/2lb 3oz new potatoes, chopped
400g/14oz fresh green beans, trimmed
800ml/28fl oz/scant 3½ cups hot vegetable stock
2 tbsp tomato purée (paste)
2 tsp honey
2 tsp fresh or dried oregano, plus extra to garnish
sea salt and black pepper to taste
2 tbsp lemon juice

1. Heat the oil in a medium casserole dish and sauté the leek for 3 minutes. Add the potatoes and the trimmed beans and sauté for a further 2 minutes, then add the hot stock, tomato purée (paste), honey and oregano, and season. Bring to the boil and cook until the potatoes are tender (about 15 minutes). Add the lemon juice and serve.

394 BARLEY RISOTTO

SERVES 4
PREPARATION
15 minutes
COOKING
1 hour 5 minutes

STORAGE
Leftovers will keep in the fridge for up to 2 days.

100g/3½oz/½ cup pearl barley
15g/½oz dried mushrooms
2 tbsp olive oil
1 onion chopped
2 cloves garlic, crushed
125g/4½oz/¾ cup brown basmati rice
700ml/24fl oz/3 cups hot vegetable stock
1 tbsp tahini (sesame paste)
175g/6oz mushrooms, sliced
2 tbsp chopped parsley
4 tbsp grated Parmesan cheese
freshly ground black pepper

1. Cover the pearl barley with water, bring to the boil and simmer for 35 minutes, or until just tender, then drain. Soak the dried mushrooms for 15 minutes in enough boiling water to cover. Drain, reserving the liquid.

2. Heat half the oil in a large pan. Fry the onion and garlic until soft. Add the cooked barley and rice. Mix the stock, mushroom soaking liquid and tahini (sesame paste) and slowly pour into the rice, stirring continuously.

3. Add the drained mushrooms, bring to the boil and reduce the heat. Simmer, uncovered, for 20–25 minutes, or until the rice is tender and most of the stock has been absorbed.

4. Meanwhile, heat the remaining oil in a frying pan (skillet). Fry the fresh mushrooms, stirring, for 3–4 minutes until browned. Add to the risotto with the parsley, Parmesan and black pepper to taste, then serve immediately.

395 PEA and PARMESAN QUINOA RISOTTO

SERVES 4
PREPARATION
5 minutes
COOKING
15 minutes

STORAGE
This meal is delicious cold and will retain its freshness for up to 3 days if refrigerated.

250ml/9fl oz/1 cup water
1 tsp olive oil
140g/5oz/heaped ¾ cup quinoa
2 tbsp sesame oil
2 courgettes (zucchini), sliced
140g/5oz asparagus, chopped
1 onion, peeled and sliced
100g/3½oz/ heaped ¾ cup frozen peas
3 cloves garlic, peeled and sliced
2 heaped tsp green peppercorns
100g/3½oz Parmesan cheese, grated

1. Heat the water in a saucepan, add the olive oil and quinoa and simmer for 15 minutes, until the quinoa becomes thick and all the water is absorbed.

2. Meanwhile, heat the sesame oil in a wok, add the courgettes (zucchini), asparagus and onion and stir-fry over a high heat for 5-6 minutes until the vegetables are softened.

3. Add the frozen peas, garlic and peppercorns. Reduce the heat and stir-fry for another 2 minutes. Drain the quinoa and add to the wok. Stir in the Parmesan cheese until melted and serve in individual bowls.

396 SPRING GREEN RISOTTO

SERVES 4
PREPARATION
5 minutes
COOKING
20 minutes

STORAGE
Leftovers will keep in the fridge for up to 2 days.

4 tbsp olive oil
2 small leeks, sliced
400g/14oz risotto rice
250g/9oz fresh curly kale leaves
1l/35fl oz/4¼ cups hot vegetable stock
4 tbsp white wine
sea salt and black pepper to taste

1. Heat the oil in a large pan or wok and gently soften the leek for 2-3 minutes. Add the rice and stir-fry for 2 minutes, then add the curly kale leaves and let them wilt for 1 minute. Add the stock and the wine, season, cover and very gently simmer until the rice is cooked. Check from time to time (and add a little water if necessary). Serve with walnut bread.

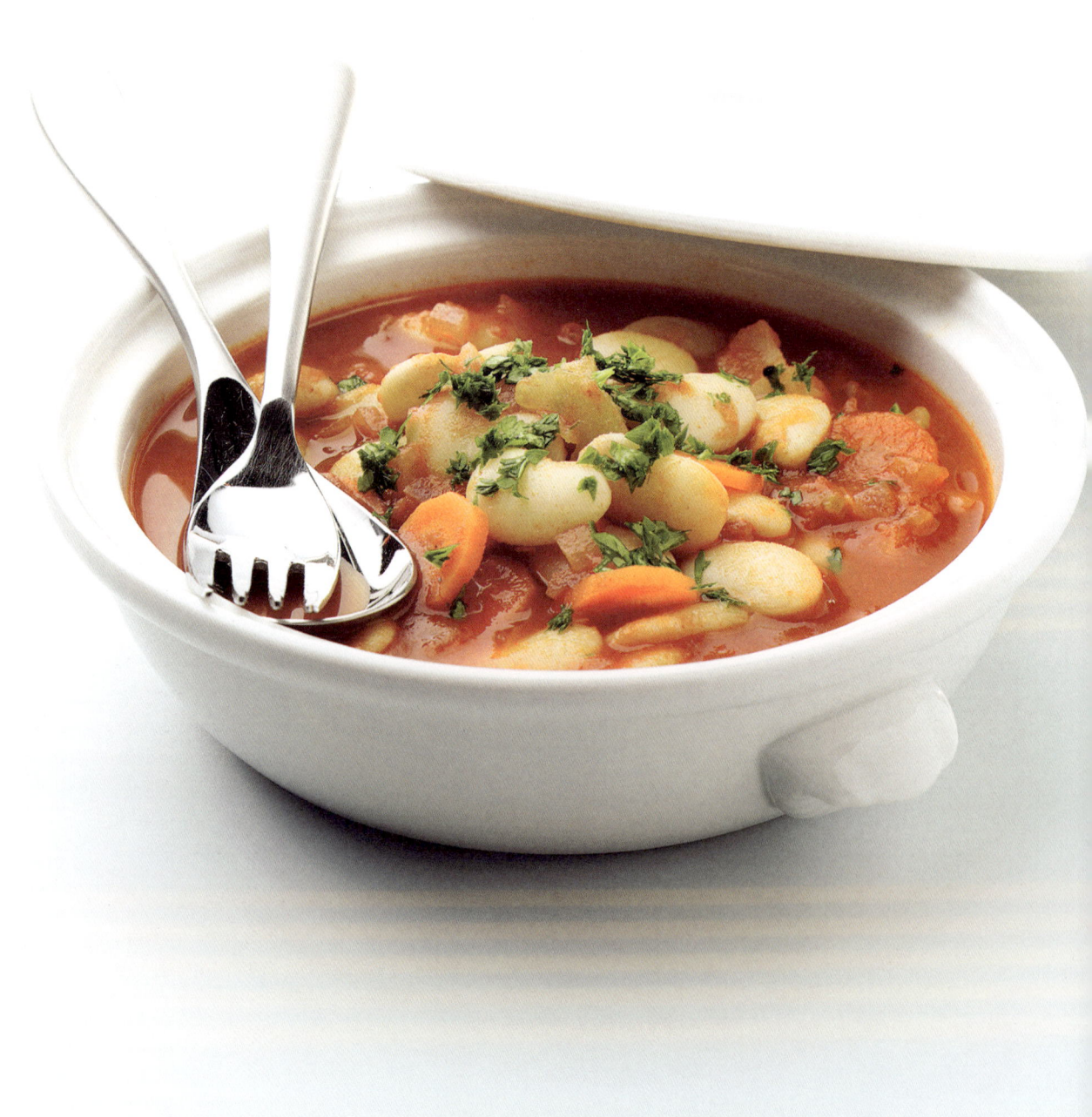

397 SPICED BEAN AND JUNIPER CASSEROLE

SERVES 4
PREPARATION
15 minutes
COOKING
20 minutes

STORAGE
Leftovers will keep in the fridge for up to 2 days.

4 tbsp olive oil
2 red onions, chopped
2 cloves garlic, crushed
2 potatoes, cut into chunks
2 carrots, sliced
2 celery stalks, sliced
2 tsp ground cumin and coriander
sea salt and cayenne pepper to taste
800g/1lb 12oz butterbeans (lima beans), cooked or canned and drained
500g/1lb 2oz tomatoes, chopped
2 sprigs each of fresh thyme and rosemary
600ml/21fl oz/2½ cups hot vegetable stock
8 juniper berries, lightly crushed
2 tbsp fresh parsley, finely chopped

1. Heat the olive oil in a casserole dish and gently sauté the red onion, garlic, potato, carrot and celery for 5 minutes. Add the cumin and coriander, and season. Sauté for a couple more minutes, then add the beans, followed by the tomatoes, thyme and rosemary. Sauté for a further 2 minutes, then add the stock and the juniper berries.

2. Bring to the boil, cover and gently simmer until the vegetables are cooked. Garnish with parsley and serve with rice or thick slices of wholemeal bread.

398 SPINACH BOUILLABAISSE

SERVES 4
PREPARATION
10 minutes
COOKING
25 minutes

STORAGE
Leftovers will keep in the fridge for up to 2 days.

2 leeks, sliced
4 potatoes, chopped
2 tbsp olive oil
4 cloves garlic, chopped
500g/1lb 2oz spinach, chopped
375ml/13fl oz/1½ cups hot vegetable stock
1 tsp ground coriander
1 tsp turmeric
sea salt and cayenne pepper to taste
handful fresh parsley, chopped
4 eggs

1. Gently stir-fry the leek and potatoes in a large pan or casserole dish with the olive oil for 5 minutes. Add the garlic and the spinach and stir-fry for 5 minutes, then add the stock and the spices, and season. Bring to the boil, add the parsley and simmer for 5 minutes.

2. Crack the eggs on top and continue to simmer for 10 minutes. Serve immediately with bread and cheese.

399 VEGETABLE LASAGNE

SERVES 4
PREPARATION
5 minutes
COOKING
40 minutes

STORAGE
Once cooked, refrigerate for up to 3 days, then reheat.

2 tbsp olive oil
1 onion, peeled and diced
2 cloves garlic, peeled and sliced
1 red (bell) pepper, deseeded and sliced
115g/4oz/1 cup mushrooms, sliced
150g/5½oz/⅔ cup cabbage greens, chopped
1 handful sunflower seeds
1 handful pumpkin seeds
1 tsp celery salt
1 tsp ground cinnamon
100g/3½oz/½ cup tomato purée (paste)
1 tbsp sweet chilli sauce
400-g/14-oz can chickpeas (garbanzo beans), drained and rinsed
2 x 400-g/14-oz cans chopped tomatoes
25g/1oz/⅓ cup chopped basil
200g/7oz feta cheese
10 sheets lasagne pasta
15g/1/2oz butter
1 tbsp plain (all-purpose) flour
425ml/15 fl oz/1¾ cups milk
115g/4oz/⅔ cup grated Cheddar cheese

1) Preheat the oven to 190°C/375°F/gas mark 5. In a wok, heat the oil and fry the vegetables over a low heat until they are soft but still bright in colour. Remove from the heat.

2) In a mixing bowl, stir in the next nine ingredients, then add the wok mixture. Spread half in an ovenproof dish, crumble over half the feta. Cover with half the lasagne, then the rest of the feta. Layer with the tomato mix and the lasagne.

3) Heat the butter in a pan. Add the flour and mix, then the milk, always stirring. Add the cheese, stir until the sauce thickens and pour it over the lasagne. Cook for 30 minutes.

400 SWEET POTATO AND SPINACH CURRY

SERVES 4
PREPARATION
5 minutes
COOKING
20 minutes

STORAGE
You can refrigerate the curry for up to 3 days, or freeze it for up to a month.

280g/10oz/2²⁄₃ cups brown basmati rice
1 tbsp olive oil
1 onion, peeled and diced
2 cloves garlic, peeled and sliced
2 large sweet potatoes, peeled and chopped
½ cinnamon stick
2 tsp coriander seeds
1 tsp curry powder
2 tsp vegetable bouillon powder
375ml/13fl oz/1½ cups water
225g/8oz/2 cups spinach
55g/2oz/½ cup pumpkin seeds
55g/2oz/½ cup raisins
400-g/14-oz can coconut milk
25g/1oz/⅓ cup chopped parsley

1) Half fill a large saucepan with water, bring to the boil and add the rice. Cover and let simmer for 15 minutes.

2) Meanwhile, heat the oil in a separate saucepan, add the onion and garlic and sauté. Add the sweet potato, cinnamon, coriander seeds, curry powder, bouillon powder and water and simmer for 10 minutes.

3) Add the spinach, seeds, raisins and coconut milk to the curry and simmer for another 5–10 minutes. Remove both pans from the heat, drain the rice and serve garnished with the chopped parsley.

401 BEAN CASSOULET

SERVES 4
PREPARATION
10 minutes + overnight soak
COOKING
50 minutes

STORAGE
You can refrigerate for up to 3 days, or freeze and then reheat within a month.

115g/4oz/½ cup haricot (navy) beans
115g/4oz/½ cup mung beans
115g/4oz/½ cup broad (fava) beans
1l/35fl oz/4¼ cups vegetable stock
175g/6oz mushrooms, sliced
400g/14oz can chopped tomatoes
3 cloves garlic, peeled and sliced
2 celery stalks, sliced
4 tbsp tomato purée (paste)
8 shallots
5 tbsp olive oil
1 tsp oregano
4 sprigs basil

1) Soak all the beans in water overnight. Preheat the oven to 190°C/375°F/gas mark 5.

2) Drain the beans and pour into a large casserole dish with a lid. Add the remaining ingredients, except the basil, and stir well.

3) Cover with the lid and place in the oven for 40–50 minutes, stirring every 20 minutes. Remove and serve on plates, garnished with the basil.

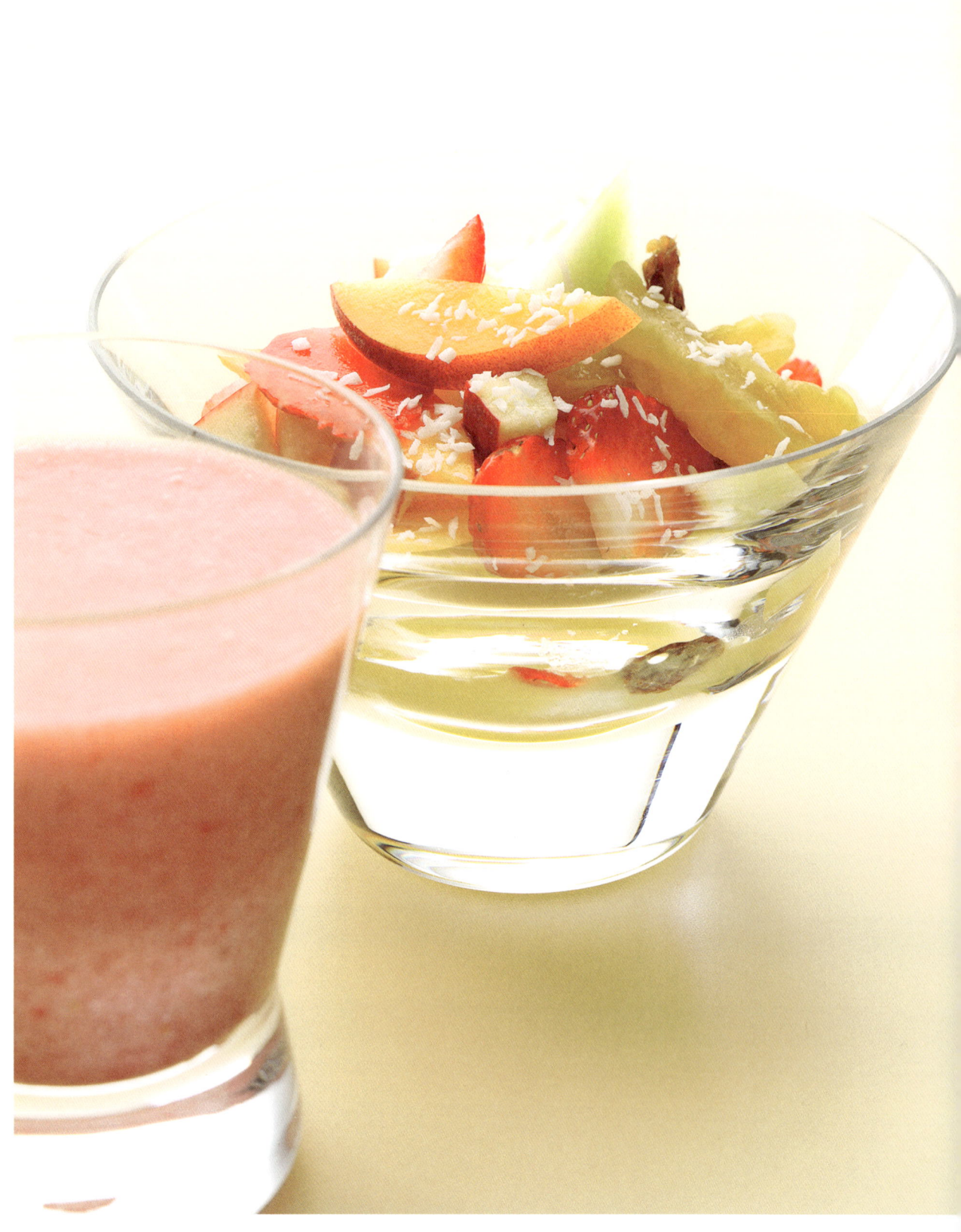

Desserts

Desserts are often loaded with refined sugar, saturated fats and other ingredients that have no – or even negative – nutritional value. The great news for parents is that it doesn't have to be that way. The recipes in this chapter contain a few treats, but they are mainly packed full with healthy ingredients, such as a variety of different fruits that provide natural, rather than artificial, sweetness.

Whether choosing to serve a delicious Fruit Parfait (see page 304) or a Banana and Coconut Ice Cream (see page 316), you can rest assured that these indulgences are both nutritious and delicious and that there are plenty of ideas here to satisfy even the sweetest tooth.

402 HONEY FRUIT SALAD

SERVES 4
PREPARATION
20 minutes

200g/7oz ready-to-eat dried apricots, raisins and peaches
400ml/14fl oz/1²⁄₃ cups orange juice
2 tsp honey
2 bananas, peeled and sliced
16 strawberries, thinly sliced
1 honeydew melon, peeled, deseeded and cubed
4 ripe peaches, halved and thinly sliced
2 apples, cored and diced
4 tbsp coconut, freshly grated or desiccated (dried shredded)

1. Place the dried fruit in a small bowl, cover with the orange juice and honey and leave to marinate for 10 minutes.

2. Make a sauce by blending the bananas and strawberries with a little water.

3. Mix the remaining fresh fruit in a large bowl, add the marinated fruit and sprinkle with the coconut. Serve with the sauce.

403 FRUIT PARFAIT

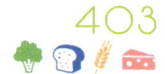

SERVES 4
PREPARATION
15 minutes

STORAGE
Best eaten immediately.

1 cantaloupe melon, deseeded
200g/7oz/1¼ cups raspberries
16 cherries, pitted
2 peaches, quartered and diced
200g/7oz/1¼ cups blackberries
4 passionfruit, halved and flesh scooped out
2 tbsp lemon juice
4 cloves, crushed in a mortar
½ tsp each of cinnamon and ground coriander
2 tbsp almond butter
2 bananas, peeled
50g/2oz plain chocolate, grated (optional)
4 tbsp pistachio nuts, chopped

1. Scoop out the melon flesh with a melon baller.

2. Layer the fruit (except for the banana) and berries in tall parfait glasses.

3. Blend the lemon juice and spices with the almond butter, bananas and enough water to make a thick cream. Spoon the cream over the fruit and berries and allow it to run down through the layers. Garnish with chocolate (if using) and nuts, and serve immediately with a scoop of ice cream, if wished.

404 RUBY-RED SALAD

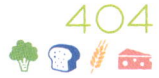

SERVES 4
PREPARATION
10 minutes

STORAGE
Best eaten immediately.

2 ruby-red grapefruit, peeled and chopped
2 papayas, peeled, deseeded and cubed
1 large bunch fresh mint, chopped
2 tsp ground cinnamon
2 tsp maple syrup (optional)

1 Divide the grapefruit and papaya between serving plates, garnish with fresh mint, sprinkle with cinnamon and the maple syrup (if using), and serve.

405 SILKY FRUIT SALAD

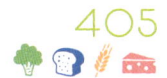

SERVES 4
PREPARATION
10 minutes

STORAGE
Best eaten immediately.

4 tbsp dried apricots, sliced
200ml/7fl oz/scant 1 cup grape juice
2 bananas, peeled and sliced
2 sharon fruit, halved and sliced
2 large ripe pears, cored and sliced
4 plums, pitted and sliced
1 pomegranate, peeled and chopped
4 tbsp pine kernels, chopped

1 Soak the dried apricots in the grape juice while you prepare the other fruit.

2 Place all the fresh fruit in a serving bowl, add the soaked apricots together with the grape juice and gently toss. Garnish with chopped pine kernels and serve.

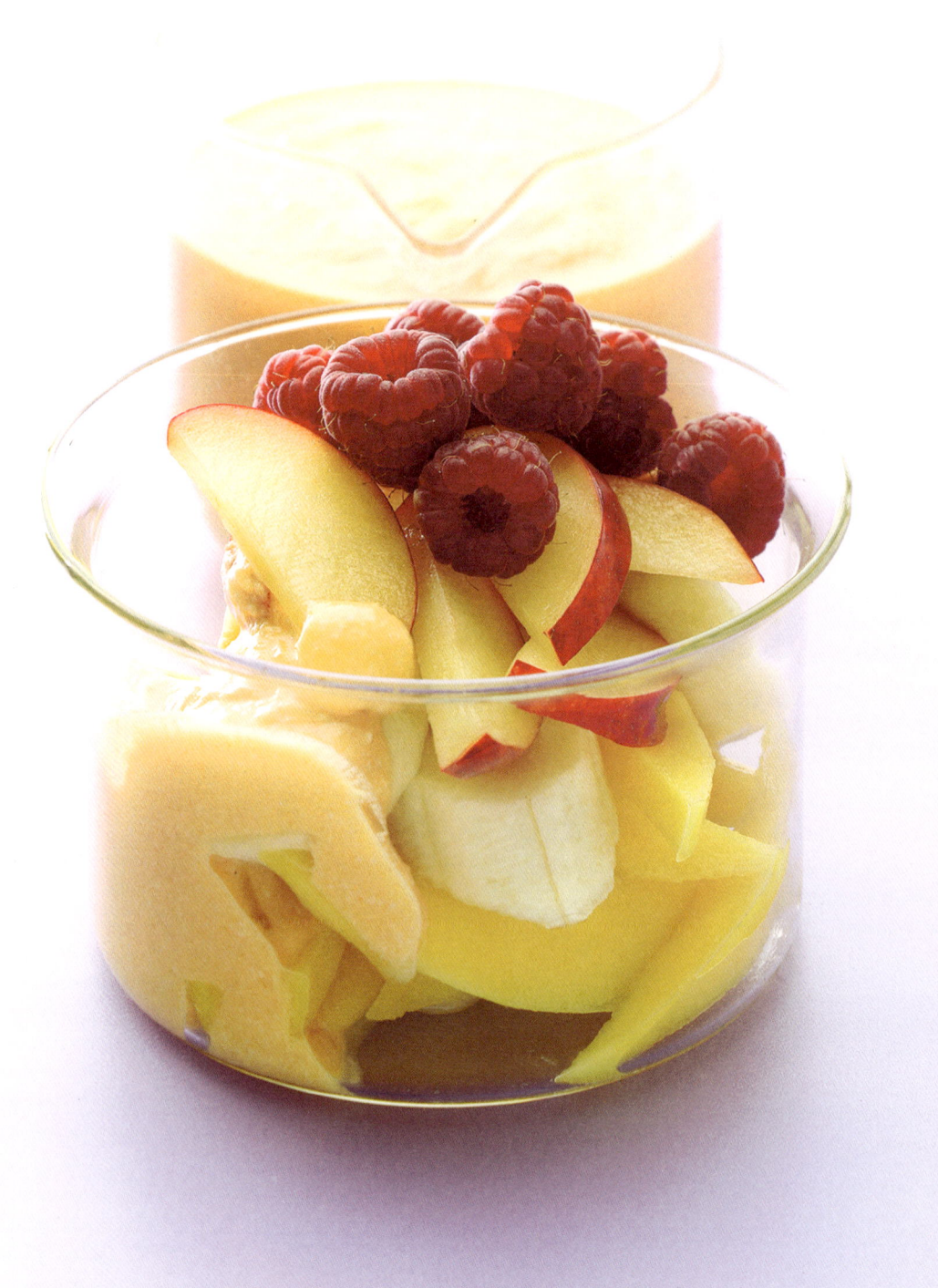

406 LAYERED FRUIT SALAD

SERVES 4
PREPARATION
15 minutes

STORAGE
Best eaten immediately.

2 mangoes, peeled and sliced
2 bananas, peeled and sliced lengthways
8 plums, pitted and sliced
200g/7oz/1¼ cups raspberries
2 papayas, peeled, deseeded and diced
4 tbsp cashew nuts
2 tbsp maple syrup
200ml/7fl oz/scant 1 cup plain or soya yogurt

1. Arrange the mangoes, bananas, plums and raspberries in layers in a dish.

2. Blend the papayas with the cashew nuts, maple syrup and yogurt. Pour the sauce over the fruit layers and serve.

407 FRUIT FLOWERS

SERVES 4
PREPARATION
15 minutes

STORAGE
Best eaten immediately.

4 oranges, peeled and sliced horizontally
2 bananas, peeled and sliced diagonally
4 kiwis, peeled and sliced horizontally
2 papayas, peeled, deseeded and sliced lengthways
4 tsp maple syrup (optional)

1. Arrange the fruit in layers on four flat plates, beginning from the middle and making flower–petal and leaf shapes with the fruit slices.

2. Drizzle with the maple syrup (if using) and serve.

408 APRICOT AND APPLE PURÉE

SERVES 4
PREPARATION
5 minutes + chilling
COOKING
10 minutes

STORAGE
You can keep the purée in the fridge for up to 4 days.

250ml/9fl oz/1 cup water
2 apples, peeled, cored and cut into chunks
115g/4oz/½ cup dried apricots
225g/8oz/1 cup plain yogurt

1. Pour the water into a small saucepan and add the apples and apricots.

2. Bring the water to the boil and then let simmer for 10 minutes until the fruit is soft. Remove from the heat, leave to cool for 10 minutes and then pour into a blender and process until smooth. Refrigerate for 30–40 minutes until chilled.

3. Pour the yogurt into individual bowls and spoon equal amounts of the purée on top.

409 PINEAPPLE BOATS

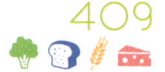

SERVES 4
PREPARATION
20 minutes

STORAGE
Best eaten immediately.

2 small pineapples, halved lengthways
1 large bunch red grapes, halved
2 kiwi fruits, peeled and diced
2 bananas, peeled and sliced
zest and juice of 1 lime
2 tbsp maple syrup
juice of 2 oranges
2 tsp fresh ginger, finely chopped

1. Scoop out the pineapple flesh to make 4 "boats" and set the boats aside while you prepare the filling.

2. Cut the pineapple flesh into chunks and place them in a bowl with the remaining ingredients. Gently toss, then spoon into the pineapple boats and serve with plain or soya yogurt or custard, if wished.

410 BLUEBERRY SALAD

SERVES 4
PREPARATION
15 minutes

STORAGE
Best eaten
immediately.

200g/7oz/1½ cups fresh
   blueberries
400g/14oz red grapes, halved
2 bananas, peeled and sliced
2 sharon fruit, halved and sliced
2 papayas, peeled and deseeded
8 fresh figs, chopped

1) Mix the blueberries, grapes, bananas and sharon fruit in a glass bowl.

2) Chop the papayas and blend with the figs and a little water to make a thick sauce. Pour the sauce over the berries and fruit and serve.

411 SHARON FRUIT with JUICY PEARS

SERVES 4
PREPARATION
10 minutes

STORAGE
Best eaten
immediately.

2 sharon fruit, sliced
2 large ripe pears, halved, cored
   and sliced
1 large bunch red grapes, halved
8 fresh dates, pitted and chopped
200ml/7fl oz/scant 1 cup apple
   juice
large pinch of ground cinnamon
juice of 2 mandarins

1) Place the sharon fruit, pear and grapes in a bowl.

2) In a food processor or blender, blend the dates with the apple juice, cinnamon and mandarin juice. △310

Pour the mixture over the fruit salad and serve.

412 BERRY JUICY YOGURT

SERVES 4
PREPARATION 10 minutes
STORAGE You can refrigerate for up to 24 hours.

400g/14oz/2 cups plain yogurt
juice of 1 lime
115g/4oz/½ cup granola, or similar crunchy cereal
550g/12oz/2 cups summer fruits, such as blueberries, strawberries and raspberries
4 sprigs mint

1. Pour the yogurt into a large mixing bowl. Stir in the lime juice, add the granola and mix thoroughly with a wooden spoon.

2. Spoon 2 tablespoons of the yogurt into each of 4 glasses, then spoon in 2 tablespoons of the summer fruits. Repeat these layers until each glass is full, finishing with a layer of yogurt with a small dollop of summer fruits on top.

3. Garnish each glass with a sprig of mint.

413 SWEET CHERRY SOUP

SERVES 4
PREPARATION 15 minutes
STORAGE Keep in the fridge for up to 2 days.

500g/18oz fresh ripe cherries, pitted
juice of 4 oranges
2 tbsp maple syrup
400ml/14fl oz/1⅔ cups hot water
8 Brazil nuts, chopped
4 slices lime
4 tbsp fresh mint, chopped

1. Blend the cherries with the orange juice, maple syrup and hot water. Refrigerate until cool, and garnish with Brazil nuts, slices of lime and fresh mint just before serving.

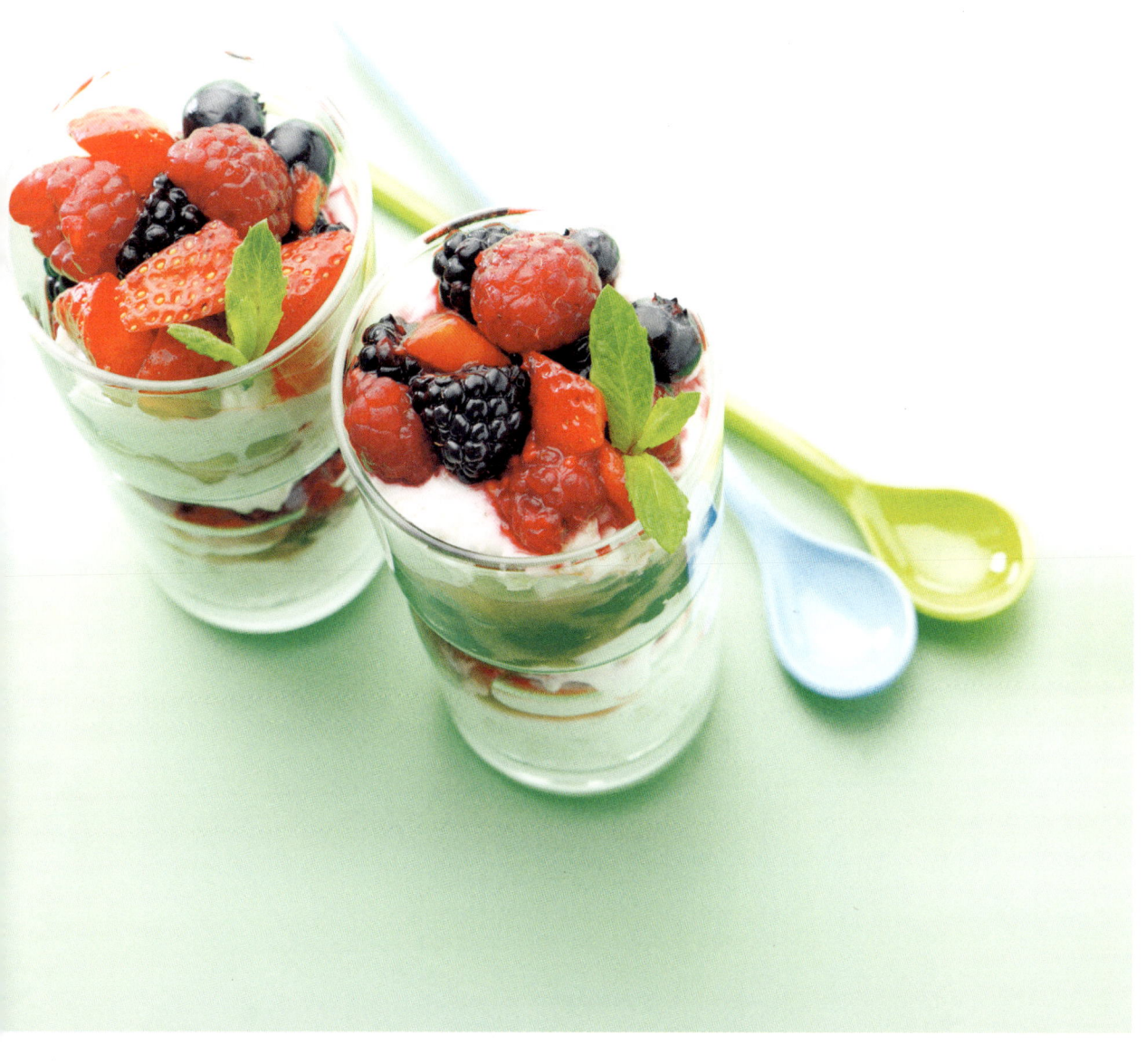

414 CREAMY ORANGE SALAD

SERVES 4
PREPARATION 15 minutes
STORAGE Best eaten immediately.

4 oranges, peeled and diced
8 lychees, peeled, halved and pitted
4 dates, pitted and sliced
4 mandarins, peeled and sliced
2 bananas, peeled and chopped
2 tbsp cashew nuts
4 tsp maple syrup
about 4 tbsp almond milk

1. Divide the oranges, lychees, dates and mandarins between four serving bowls.

2. In a food processor or blender, blend the bananas with the cashews, maple syrup and enough almond milk to make a smooth cream. Pour the cream over the salad and serve.

415 WINTER SUNSHINE SALAD

SERVES 4
PREPARATION 15 minutes
STORAGE Best eaten immediately.

1 pineapple, peeled, cored and cut into chunks
4 mandarins, peeled and divided into segments
2 sharon fruit, sliced
1 papaya, peeled, deseeded and sliced
200ml/7fl oz/scant 1 cup orange juice
seeds from 1 pomegranate
maple syrup, to taste

1. Divide the pineapple chunks, mandarins, sharon fruit and papaya between serving bowls. Sprinkle with the orange juice and pomegranate seeds, then drizzle over maple syrup to taste.

416 APPLE SALAD WITH CASHEW CREAM

SERVES 4
PREPARATION
15 minutes

STORAGE
Best eaten immediately.

4 dessert apples, cored and grated
4 mandarins, peeled and chopped
8 dates, pitted and chopped
100g/3½oz/scant 1 cup cashew nuts
4–5 tbsp apple juice

1. Mix the apples, mandarins and dates in a bowl.

2. Blend the cashews with the apple juice to make a thick cream. Divide the apple salad between glasses, top with the cashew cream and serve immediately.

417 WATERMELON ZEST

SERVES 4
PREPARATION
10 minutes

STORAGE
You can refrigerate for up to 24 hours.

1 watermelon
3 passionfruit
3 limes

1. Cut the watermelon lengthways, then cut into triangular slices or cubes, removing the skin. Place the watermelon pieces onto a large plate.

2. Cut the passionfruit in half. Scoop out the flesh with a spoon into a small bowl and remove the seeds. Squeeze the juice from two of the limes and add to the passionfruit. Mix together, then pour the mixture evenly over the melon.

3. Cut the remaining lime in half, then into wedges and decorate the edge of the plate with these.

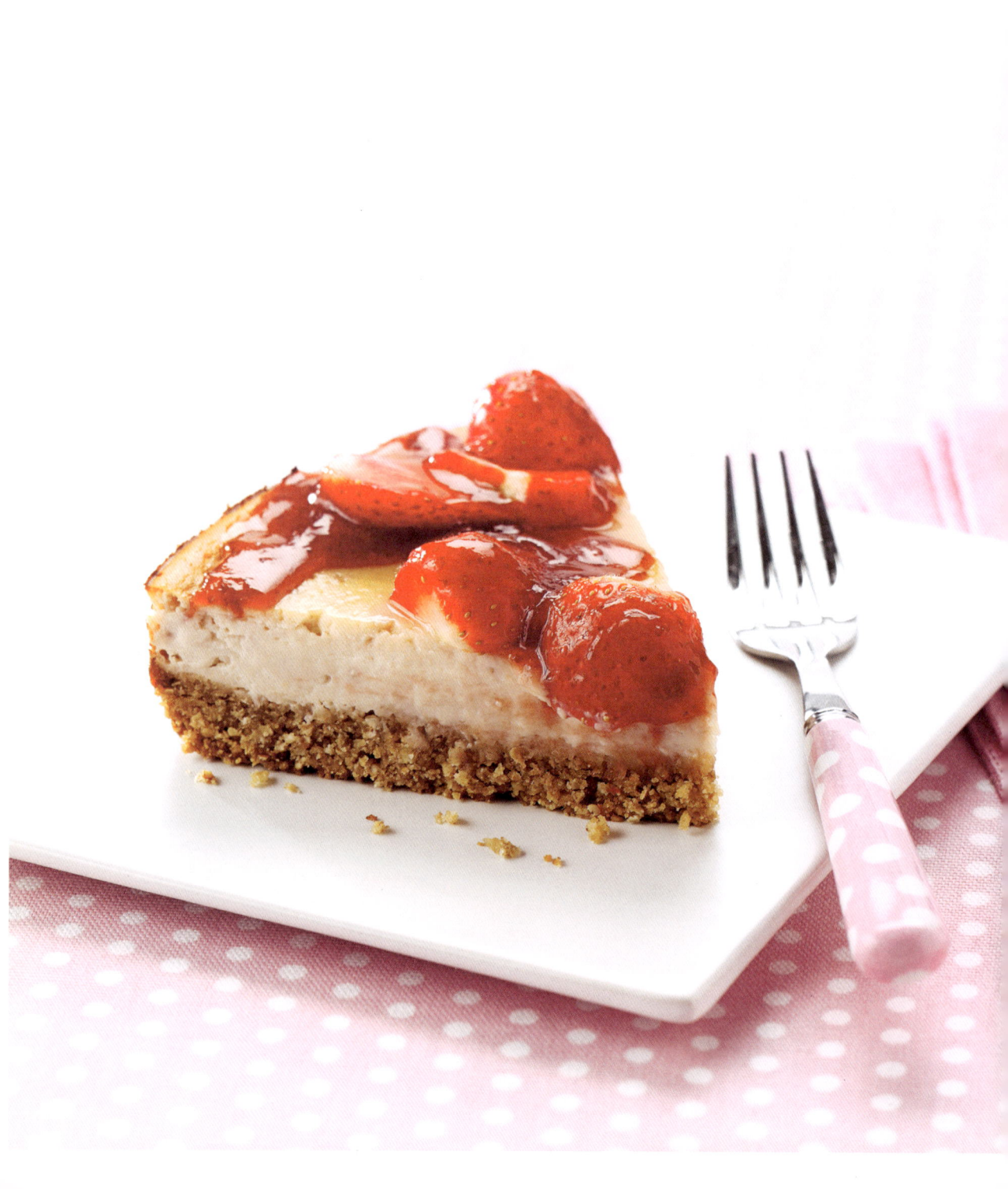

418 STRAWBERRY CHEESECAKE

SERVES 6
PREPARATION 20 minutes + chilling
COOKING 55 minutes

STORAGE Leftovers will keep in the fridge for up to 3 days.

175g/6oz oat cakes
50g/2oz/¼ cup ground almonds
90g/3¼oz butter, melted
5 tbsp honey
3 eggs, beaten
450g/1lb low-fat ricotta cheese
2 tbsp cornflour (cornstarch)
150g/5½oz/1½ cups strawberries

TOPPING
125g/4½oz/½ cup strawberry jam (jelly) or pure fruit spread
150g/5½oz/1½ cups strawberries, sliced

1. Preheat the oven to 200°C/400°F/gas mark 6. Process the oat cakes to fine crumbs in a food processor. In a bowl, mix the crumbs with the almonds. Add the melted butter and 2 tablespoons of the honey and mix thoroughly. Press evenly into a 20cm/8in round springform tin (pan) and bake for 10 minutes.

2. Put the eggs, cheese, cornflour (cornstarch), whole strawberries and remaining honey in a food processor and process until smooth. Pour onto the base and bake for 10 minutes. Reduce the heat to 150°C/300°F/gas mark 3 and bake for a further 30 minutes. Leave to cool in the tin (pan), and then chill for 3 hours. Remove from the tin (pan), before topping.

3. For the topping, heat the jam (jelly) or fruit spread in a pan until runny. Mix in the sliced strawberries and arrange on top of the cheesecake. Chill for a further 30 minutes before serving.

419 CHOCO-NUT ICE CREAM

SERVES 4
PREPARATION
15 minutes + 4 hours freezing

STORAGE
Freeze for up to 3 months. Place in the fridge for 30 minutes before serving.

200g/7oz silken tofu
3 bananas
150ml/5fl oz/scant ⅔ cup soya milk
75g/2½oz/¾ cup hazelnuts, toasted
2 tbsp honey or agave nectar
125g/4½oz plain chocolate (75% cocoa solids), melted

1. Cut the tofu and bananas into small pieces and freeze for 3–4 hours.

2. Put the soya milk and toasted hazelnuts in a food processor or blender and process until smooth and creamy.

3. Add the honey and melted chocolate and process until combined, then add the frozen bananas and tofu and process to form a thick, soft 'ice cream'.

4. Serve immediately or pour into a freezerproof container and freeze until required.

420 BANANA AND COCONUT ICE CREAM

SERVES 4
PREPARATION
15 minutes + cooling + freezing
COOKING
5 minutes

STORAGE
You can keep ice cream in the freezer for up to 2 months.

60ml/2fl oz/¼ cup boiling water
2 tsp gelatine
4 tbsp honey
500ml/17fl oz/2 cups vanilla soy milk
2 bananas, mashed
1 tsp vanilla extract
55g/2oz/¼ cup fresh coconut, grated
400-g/14-oz can coconut milk

1. Pour the boiling water into a large mixing bowl. Add the gelatine and allow it to dissolve for 10 minutes, stirring.

2. Meanwhile, in a saucepan, whisk together the honey and soya milk. Do not let it boil, but stir over a low heat for 2 minutes until hot.

3. Add the gelatine mixture, stir well and then stir in the remaining ingredients. Pour into a bowl and leave to cool for 10 minutes before refrigerating for at least 3 hours.

4. Spoon the chilled mixture into the canister of an ice-cream maker, or pour into a freezer-proof container and leave to freeze overnight.

421 JELLY ISLANDS

SERVES 4
PREPARATION 20 minutes + chilling
COOKING 10 minutes

STORAGE Refrigerate the jellies for up to 4 days. You can refrigerate the sauce for up to a month.

85-g/3-oz pack tropical-flavour vegetarian jelly crystals
600ml/21fl oz/2½ cups boiling water
1 lime, sliced
175g/6oz/1 cup frozen raspberries
2 tbsp icing (confectioners') sugar
4 basil leaves

1. Put the jelly crystals in a bowl and pour the boiling water over the top. Stir the crystals until dissolved.

2. Place a slice of lime in the bottom of 4 ramekin dishes and fill with jelly. Leave to refrigerate for at least an hour until the jelly is set.

3. Blend together the raspberries and icing (confectioners') sugar, then push through a sieve to remove any pips.

4. Turn out the jellies onto side plates and pour the raspberry sauce around the bottom. Decorate with a basil leaf.

422 HAWAIIAN HULAS

SERVES 4
PREPARATION 20 minutes + chilling

STORAGE Keep for no longer than 24 hours in the fridge.

400-g/14-oz can coconut milk
2 vanilla pods
4 small pineapples
1 coconut, cut into 5 chunks and flesh of 1 chunk grated
4 sprigs mint

1. Put the coconut milk into a bowl, add the vanilla pods and refrigerate for 2 hours.

2. Cut off the tops from the pineapples and set aside. Cut out the flesh, leaving the skin intact, and remove the hard core of the pineapple from the flesh and discard. Chop the flesh into chunks, put 4 chunks to one side and place the rest in a blender. Add the infused coconut milk and process until smooth. Pour into the hollowed-out pineapple shells.

3. Sprinkle the grated coconut flesh into the pineapples. Spear 4 cocktail sticks (toothpicks) with the remaining pineapple and a chunk of coconut. Stick into the side of the pineapple, decorate with mint and replace the pineapple tops.

423 FRUIT JELLY

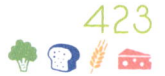

SERVES 4
PREPARATION
15 minutes +
chilling

STORAGE
Store in the fridge
for up to 4 days.

- 2 bananas, peeled and chopped
- 2 sweet apples, cored and chopped
- 50g/2oz dates, pitted
- 200ml/7fl oz/scant 1 cup apple juice
- 2 tsp agar-agar

1. In a food processor or blender, blend the bananas, apples, dates and apple juice, and pour into a saucepan. Whisk in the agar-agar until it is dissolved. Bring to the boil, then pour the mixture into serving bowls and refrigerate until set. Serve with crème fraîche or soya cream.

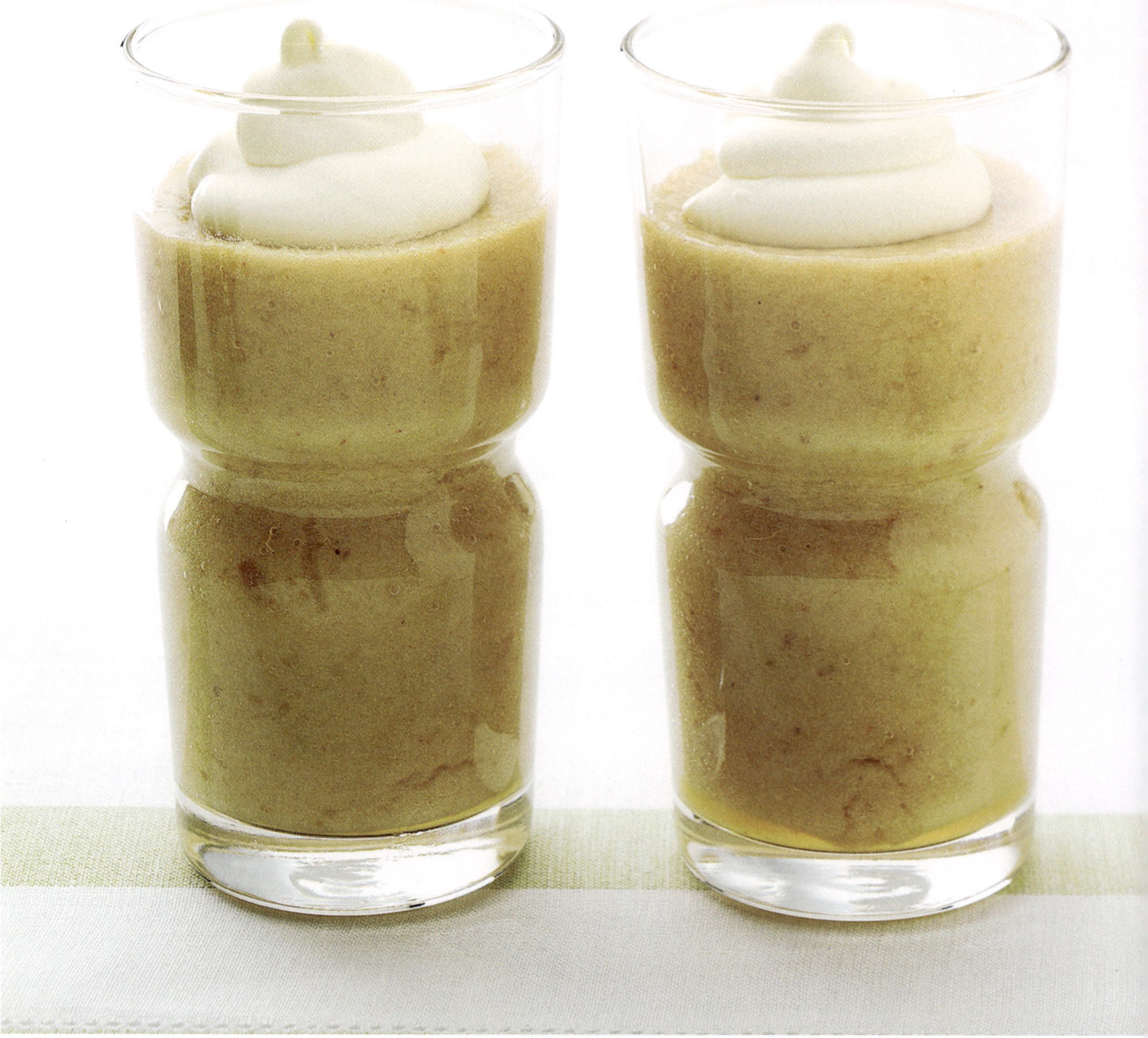

424 ORANGE ESKIMO BOWLS

MAKES 10
PREPARATION 30 minutes + freezing
STORAGE Use within a month from the date of freezing.

10 oranges
grated zest and juice of 1 lemon
grated zest and juice of 1 lime
grated zest and juice of 1 orange
600ml/21fl oz/2½ cups boiling water
200g/7oz/scant 1 cup brown sugar
1 egg white

1. Cut the tops off the oranges and set aside. Scoop out the flesh and juice from 10 of the oranges, discarding this for 8 of them (don't waste it – set aside for use in another recipe). Place the flesh and the juice of the remaining 2 oranges in a blender and add the juice and grated zest of the lime, lemon and other orange.

2. In a separate bowl, pour the boiling water onto the sugar and stir until dissolved. Leave to cool before adding to the blender with the egg white, then process until smooth.

3. Pour the mixture into the hollow oranges, place the tops back on, wrap the oranges in clingfilm (plastic wrap), and freeze.

425 MANGO AND ORANGE FOOL

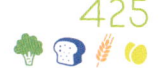

SERVES 4
PREPARATION 10 minutes + chilling
STORAGE Best eaten immediately.

1 large mango, peeled, pitted and chopped
juice and grated zest of 1 orange
150g/5½oz/¾ cup plain yogurt
100g/3½oz/½ cup Greek yogurt
1 tsp flaxseed oil
grated zest of 1 orange, to decorate

1. Purée the mango, orange juice and zest in a food processor or blender until smooth.

2. Add the yogurts and oil and blend until smooth and creamy.

3. Divide the fool among four glasses and chill until required. Decorate with orange zest and serve.

426 MINTY STRAWBERRIES

SERVES 4

PREPARATION
10 minutes

STORAGE
Best eaten immediately.

500g/18oz strawberries, halved
2 pears, cored and diced
2 tsp lemon juice
2 tbsp fresh mint, finely chopped
2 tbsp maple syrup
grated plain (bittersweet) chocolate (optional)

1. Place the strawberries and the pear in a serving bowl. Sprinkle with the lemon juice, fresh mint, maple syrup and a little grated chocolate (if using). Serve with crème fraîche or soya cream.

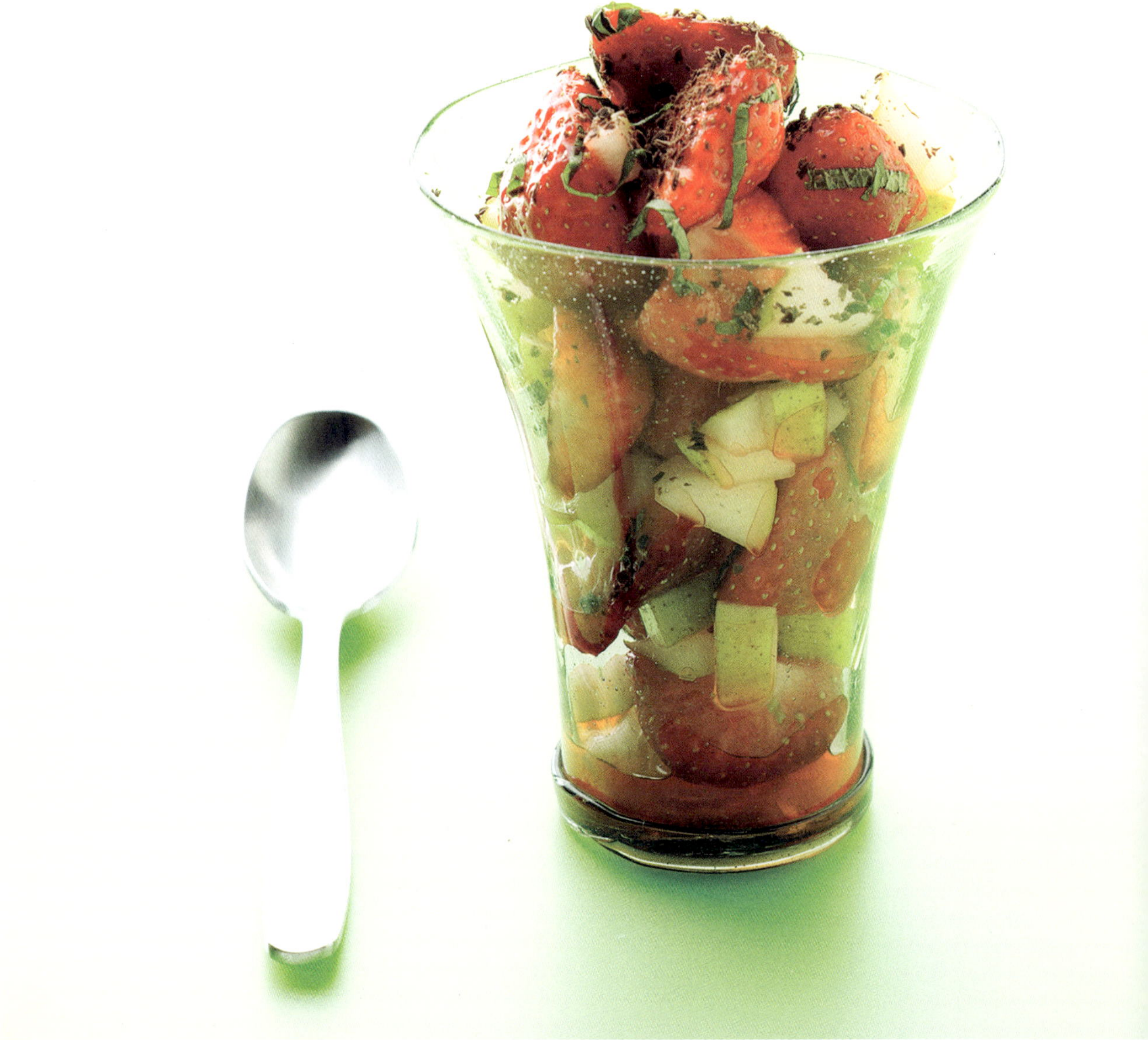

427 SUMMER FRUIT SALAD

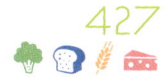

SERVES 4
PREPARATION
10 minutes

STORAGE
Best eaten immediately or make the day before and keep overnight in the fridge.

16 strawberries, hulled and halved or quartered, if large
2 nectarines, pitted and cut into bite-sized chunks
2 kiwi fruit, peeled, quartered and cut into bite-sized chunks
2 apples, cored and cut into bite-sized chunks
16 seedless grapes, halved
8 tbsp orange juice

1. Divide the fruit between four serving bowls. Pour 2 tablespoons of the orange juice over each fruit salad and serve.

428 PINEAPPLE COCKTAIL

SERVES 4
PREPARATION
15 minutes

STORAGE
Best eaten immediately or make the day before and keep overnight in the fridge.

1 pineapple, peeled, cored and cut into chunks
juice of 2 oranges
juice of 2 pomelos
2 pears, cored and cut into chunks
2 tsp finely chopped fresh ginger
4 slices of lemon
4 tsp fresh mint, finely chopped

1. Blend the pineapple chunks with the orange juice, pomelo juice, pear chunks and chopped fresh ginger. Pour the mix into tall glasses, garnish with slices of lemon and chopped fresh mint, and serve.

429 SUMMER BERRY PUDDINGS

SERVES 4
PREPARATION
20 minutes+
chilling
COOKING
5 minutes

STORAGE
Make up to 1 day in advance and chill in the fridge for up to 2 days.

3 tbsp apple juice
400g/14oz mixed berries, such as blackberries, raspberries and blueberries, plus extra to serve
10–12 slices wholemeal bread, crusts removed

1. Put the apple juice and berries into a pan. Bring to a gentle simmer and cook for 2–3 minutes, or until the juices begin to run from the fruit.

2. From 8 slices of bread, cut 8 circles large enough to fit the base and top of individual pudding moulds or ramekins. Cut the remaining bread slices in half. Gently flatten all the pieces of bread with a rolling pin.

3. Line the base and side of each mould with half the circles and the strips of bread. Spoon the berries into each mould and top with the remaining bread circles.

4. Fit a saucer on top of each mould and place a weight on the saucer. Stand the puddings on a tray and chill for 12 hours or overnight.

5. Run a knife around the inside edge of each mould and turn out onto serving plates. Serve with extra berries.

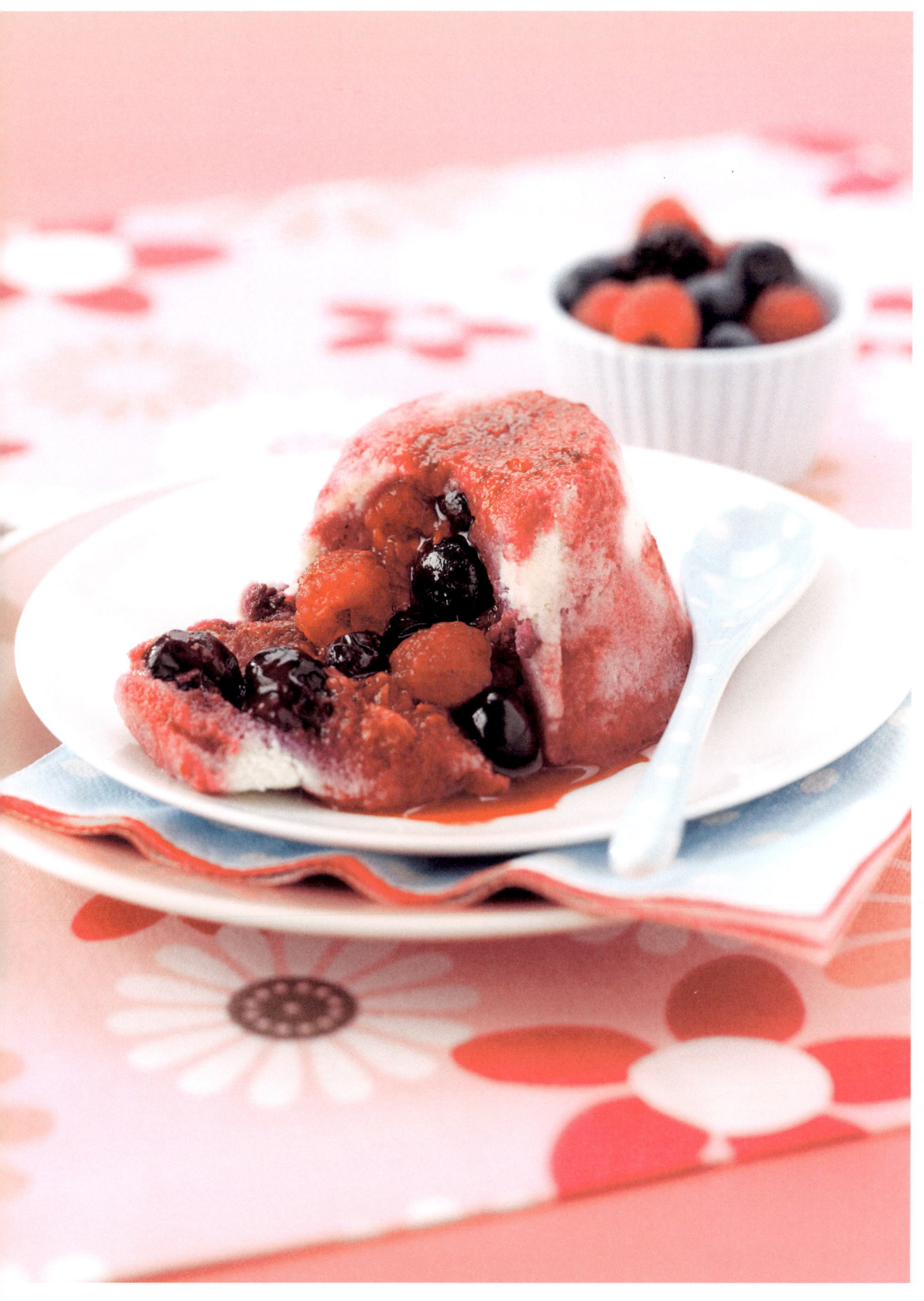

430 ORANGE and CHOCOLATE MOUSSE

SERVES 4
PREPARATION
10 minutes + chilling
COOKING
2 minutes

STORAGE
Make this up to 1 day ahead and chill in the fridge until required. Leftovers will keep in the fridge for up to 2 days.

175g/6oz plain (bittersweet) chocolate (75% cocoa solids), chopped
350g/12oz silken tofu
grated zest and juice of 2 oranges
grated orange zest, to decorate
grated chocolate, to decorate

1. Melt the chocolate in a bowl over a pan of simmering water, stirring occasionally. Leave to cool slightly.

2. Purée the tofu, melted chocolate, orange zest and juice in a food processor or blender until smooth and creamy.

3. Spoon the mixture into four individual dishes and chill for 3 hours, or overnight.

4. Decorate with a little orange zest and grated chocolate, then serve.

431 MANGO FOOL

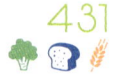

SERVES 4
PREPARATION
10 minutes

STORAGE
Make in advance and keep in the fridge for up to 3 days.

2 mangoes
200ml/7fl oz/scant 1 cup thick plain yogurt
300ml/10½fl oz/1¼ cups low-fat fromage frais
2 tbsp clear honey, or to taste
2 tsp vanilla extract (optional)

1. Peel the mangoes using a vegetable peeler and slice the fruit off the large central stone. Put the mango in a blender with the rest of the ingredients and blend until smooth and creamy.

2. Divide among serving bowls and serve.

432 APRIL FOOL

SERVES 4
PREPARATION
10 minutes + chilling
COOKING
10 minutes

500g/18oz rhubarb, sliced
¼ tsp ground cinnamon
2 tsp honey
4 tsp almond butter
2 frozen bananas, peeled and chopped
6 large dates, pitted and chopped
200ml/7fl oz/scant 1 cup plain or soya yogurt

1. Cook the rhubarb with the cinnamon and a little water in a heavy saucepan until soft, 5–8 minutes. Add the honey and cook for 2 minutes. Transfer the pan to a sink of cold water and let cool.

2. Meanwhile, in a food processor, blend the almond butter with the frozen banana, dates and yogurt. Fold the cooked and cooled rhubarb into the yogurt blend.

3. Spoon into serving bowls and chill before serving.

433 FRUIT LAYER CRISP

SERVES 4
PREPARATION
10 minutes
COOKING
7 minutes
STORAGE
Prepare the oat mixture in advance and store in an airtight container for up to 4 days. Leftovers will keep in the fridge for up to 1 day.

2 tbsp olive oil
75g/2½oz/¾ cup porridge (rolled) oats
50g/2oz/½ cup hazelnuts, chopped
50g/2oz/½ cup flaked almonds
1 tbsp honey
1 tbsp ground flaxseeds
3 tbsp wheat germ
125g/4½oz/1 cup blueberries
125g/4½oz/1 cup raspberries
125g/4½oz/1 cup strawberries, hulled and sliced
300g/10½oz/scant 1¼ cups plain yogurt

1. Heat a non-stick frying pan (skillet) and add the olive oil. Add the oats and stir to coat in the oil, then cook, stirring, for 3–4 minutes until golden brown.

2. Add the hazelnuts and almonds and cook, stirring continuously, for a further 2–3 minutes until the nuts are golden. Pour the mixture into a bowl and stir in the honey, flaxseeds and wheat germ.

3. Mix the blueberries, raspberries and strawberries together in a bowl. Divide half the fruit among four glasses or bowls. Top with half the yogurt, then add a layer of oat mixture. Repeat, finishing with a layer of oat mixture, and serve.

434 TROPICAL FRUIT KEBABS

MAKES 8
PREPARATION 10 minutes
COOKING 15 minutes

STORAGE Keep refrigerated for up to 12 hours.

- 115g/4oz/1 cup raspberries
- 2 tbsp brown sugar
- 1 pineapple
- 2 papaya
- 4 kiwi fruit
- 4 limes, sliced

1. Put the raspberries, sugar and 80ml/2½fl oz/⅓ cup of water in a pan, bring to the boil, then simmer for 10–15 minutes until thickened. Remove from the heat, press through a sieve and chill for 2 hours.

2. Cut the skin off the pineapple and papaya. Remove the seeds from the papaya. Chop the fruit into 2.5cm/1in squares. Peel the kiwi fruit and cut into thick slices.

3. Spear the fruit onto 8 skewers, alternating pineapple, kiwi, papaya and lime until the skewers are full.

4. Place two kebabs on each plate, garnish with a slice of lime and drizzle with raspberry coulis.

435 TROPICAL CRÈME BRÛLÉE

SERVES 4
PREPARATION 15 minutes + chilling
COOKING 35 minutes

STORAGE Make in advance and chill, but do not add the sugar until just before grilling (broiling). This will keep in the fridge for up to 1 day.

- ½ papaya, peeled, deseeded and chopped
- 1 banana, sliced
- 2 tbsp orange juice
- 300g/10½oz/scant 1¼ cups plain yogurt
- 2 tbsp desiccated (dried shredded) coconut
- 4 egg yolks
- 1 tbsp cornflour (cornstarch)
- 4 tsp brown sugar

1. Preheat the oven to 180°C/350°F/gas mark 4. Mix the papaya, banana and orange juice, then divide the mixture among four ramekin dishes.

2. Purée the yogurt, coconut, egg yolks and cornflour (cornstarch) in a food processor until smooth, then spoon the mixture over the fruit.

3. Put the ramekins in a roasting tin (pan) and pour in enough hot water to come halfway up the sides. Bake for 30 minutes until lightly set. Leave to cool, then chill for 4–5 hours or overnight.

4. Sprinkle the sugar over the custards and use a blowtorch to caramelize it. Alternatively, preheat the grill (broiler) to high and caramelize the sugar under the grill (broiler). Cool before serving.

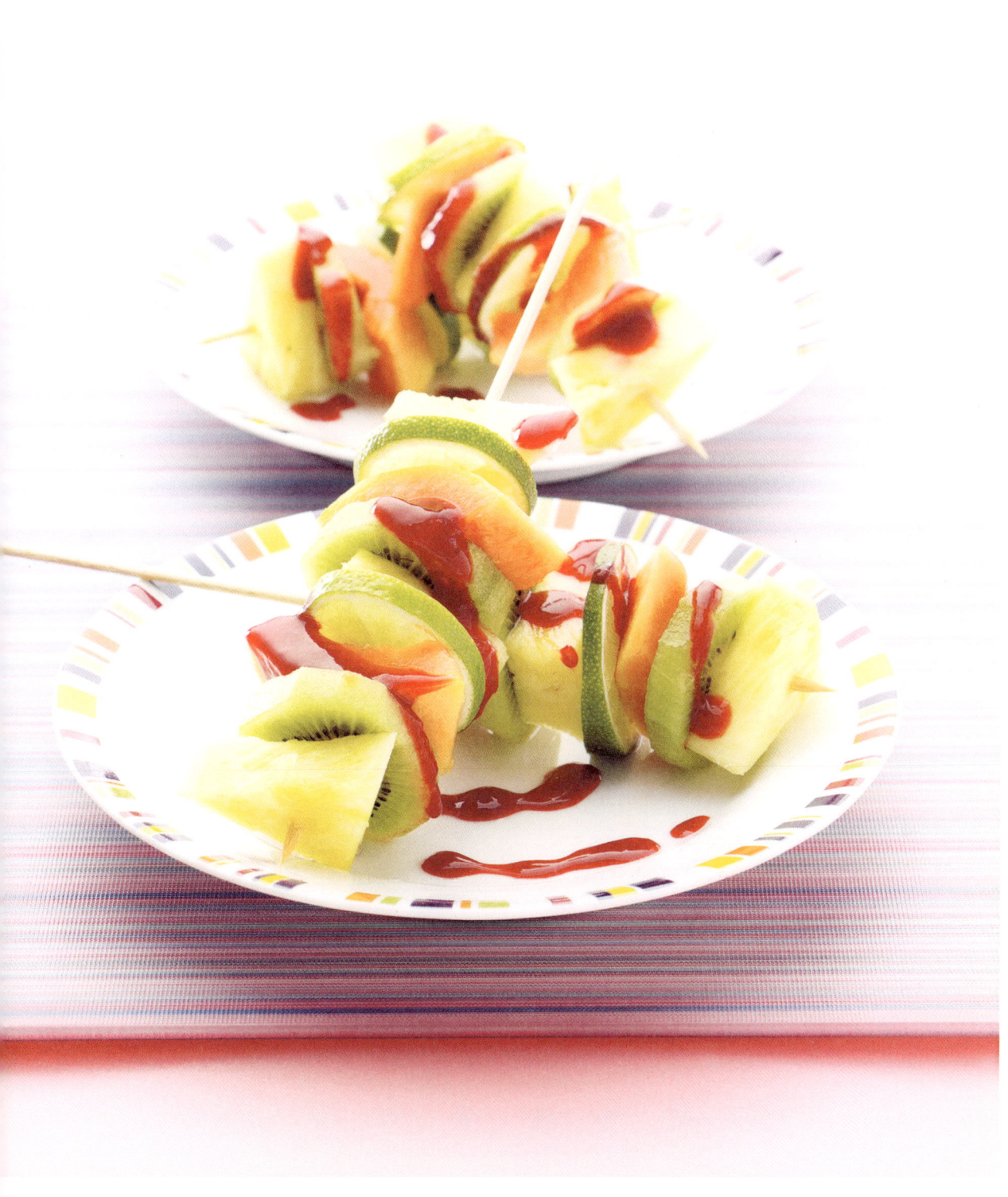

436 FRUIT JELLIES

SERVES 4
PREPARATION
10 minutes + chilling
COOKING
5 minutes

STORAGE
Prepare the jellies up to 1 day in advance and chill. Leftovers will keep in the fridge for up to 2 days.

RED LAYER
250ml/9fl oz/1 cup apple juice
2 tbsp agar-agar flakes
250g/9oz/2 cups fresh or frozen raspberries

ORANGE LAYER
250ml/9fl oz/1 cup orange juice
2 tbsp agar agar flakes
300g/10½ oz/1¼ cups canned mandarin orange segments in natural juice, drained
4 tbsp plain yogurt (optional)

1 Pour the apple juice into a pan and bring to the boil. Add the agar-agar and raspberries and simmer, stirring, for 2 minutes until the agar agar has dissolved.

2 Transfer the mixture to a food processor and process until smooth. Pass through a sieve (strainer), cool slightly, then divide among four tall glasses. Chill for 1-2 hours until set.

3 Pour the orange juice into a pan and bring to the boil. Add the agar-agar and mandarin orange slices and simmer, stirring, for 2 minutes until the agar-agar has dissolved. Transfer the mixture to a food processor and process until smooth. Pass through a sieve (strainer), cool slightly, then pour over the red layer. Chill for a further 1-2 hours, or until set.

4 Top each jelly with some yogurt, if using, and serve.

437 CINNAMON-SPICED APPLE COMPOTE

SERVES 2-4
PREPARATION
10 minutes
COOKING
15 minutes

STORAGE
Keeps in the fridge for up to 5 days or freezes for up to 1 month.

4 apples, cored, peeled and roughly chopped
1 tsp ground cinnamon
1 tsp fresh lemon juice
small knob of butter (optional)

1 Put the apples, cinnamon, lemon juice (this prevents the apples turning brown), butter, if using, and 150ml/5fl oz/⅔cup water in a saucepan. Bring to the boil, then simmer over a medium-low heat for 12-15 minutes, until the apples are tender.

2 Lightly mash the apples with a fork to break them down slightly, then leave to cool.

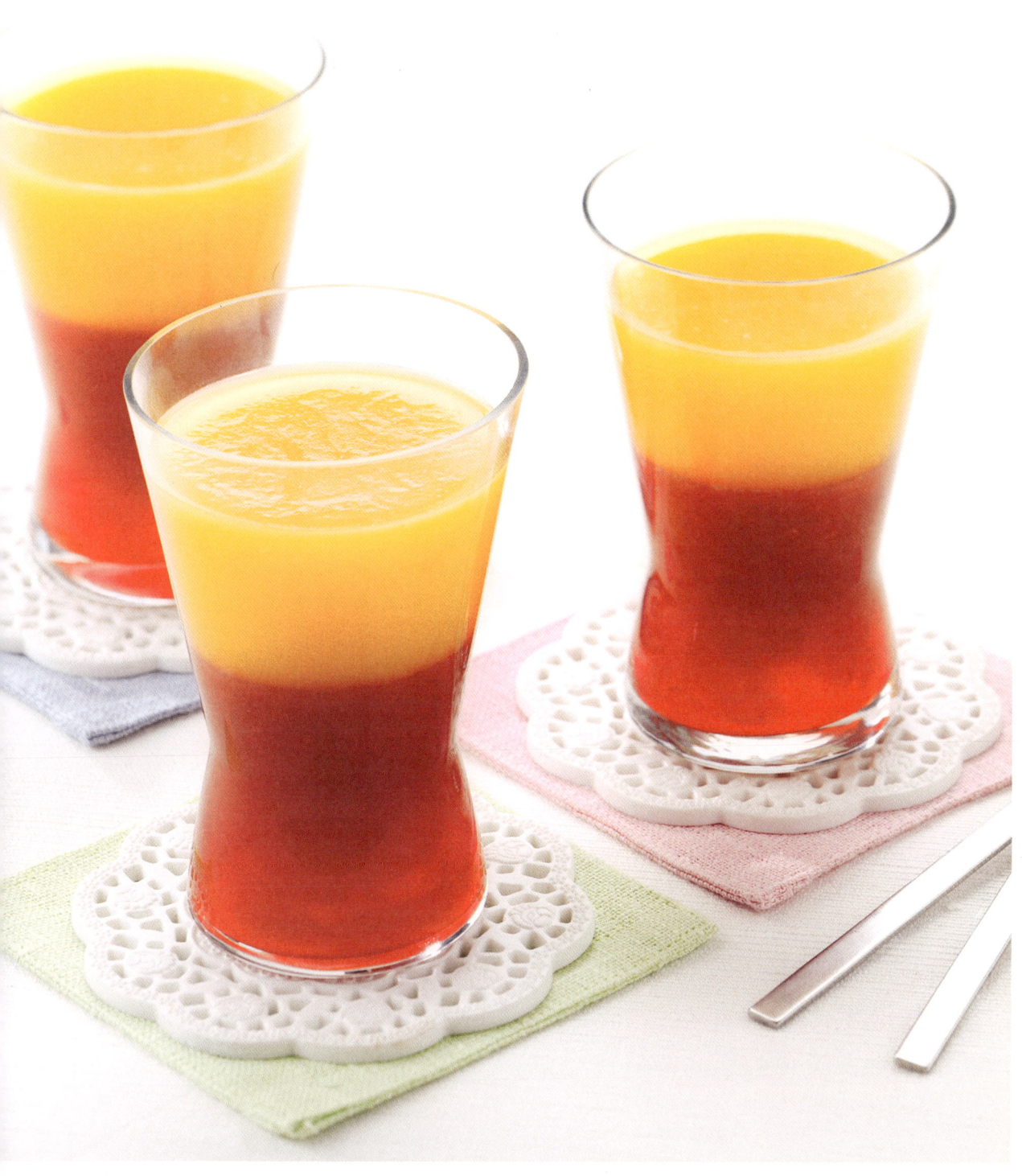

438 STRAWBERRY CRUNCH POTS

SERVES 4
PREPARATION
10 minutes
COOKING
5 minutes

STORAGE
Make the day before and keep in the fridge overnight. The oat and seed mixture will keep in an airtight container for 1 week.

- 100g/3½oz/1 cup porridge (rolled) oats
- 4 tbsp sunflower seeds
- 4 tbsp pumpkin seeds
- 6–8 tbsp clear honey or maple syrup
- 200ml/7 fl oz/scant 1 cup thick plain yogurt
- 1 tsp vanilla extract
- 24 strawberries, hulled and thickly sliced

1. Put the oats in a dry frying pan (skillet) and toast over a medium-low heat for 3 minutes, turning the oats occasionally with a spatula.

2. Next, add the sunflower and pumpkin seeds to the pan and toast for another 2 minutes, tossing the pan frequently until the oats and seeds are light golden.

3. Remove the pan from the heat and stir in the honey or maple syrup. This will sizzle at first, but keep stirring until the oats and seeds are coated. Leave to cool slightly to allow the mixture to crisp up.

4. Mix the yogurt with the vanilla extract in a bowl.

5. Put a layer of the oat mixture in the bottom of 4 tall plastic pots or glasses. Top each with 3 tablespoons of yogurt, then add a layer of strawberries. Repeat with another layer of each, then cover or serve.

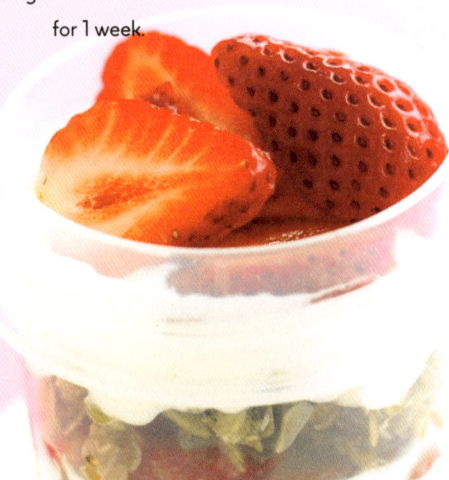

439 RHUBARB AND STRAWBERRY COMPOTE

SERVES 4
PREPARATION
10 minutes
COOKING
15 minutes

STORAGE
Keeps in the fridge for up to 5 days or freezes for up to 1 month.

600g/21oz rhubarb, sliced
2 tsp vanilla sugar
400g/14oz strawberries, hulled and halved
2 tsp finely chopped fresh ginger
maple syrup to taste

1. Put the rhubarb slices in a heavy saucepan, sprinkle with the vanilla sugar and cover with water. Bring to the boil and simmer for 10 minutes. Add the strawberries and the ginger. Heat through and simmer for a further 4–5 minutes.

2. Season with maple syrup and serve warm.

440 HAZELNUT-CHERRY TART

SERVES 6–8
PREPARATION
15 minutes
COOKING
35 minutes

STORAGE
Leftovers will keep in the fridge for up to 3 days.

4 tbsp light olive oil, plus extra for greasing
125g/4½oz/¾ cup hazelnuts
4 tbsp honey
125g/4½oz/¾ cup self-raising wholemeal flour
1 egg, beaten
1 tsp baking powder
150g/5½oz/¾ cup low-fat Greek yogurt
115g/4oz/scant 1 cup cherries, pitted and halved

1. Preheat the oven to 180°C/350°F/gas mark 4 and grease a 20cm/8in springform tin (pan) with oil.

2. Process the nuts in a food processor until finely ground. With the machine running, add the honey, olive oil and flour and process until the mixture resembles breadcrumbs.

3. Put half the mixture into the tin (pan) and press down evenly with the back of a spoon until firm.

4. Add the egg, baking powder and yogurt to the remaining nut mixture in the food processor and process to form a thick batter. Gently mix in the cherries and spoon the mixture over the base.

5. Bake for 30–35 minutes until risen, firm and golden. Leave to cool in the tin (pan), then cut into slices and serve.

441 APPLE, CHERRY AND WALNUT CRÊPES

SERVES 4
PREPARATION
10 minutes
COOKING
20 minutes

STORAGE
Best eaten immediately.

CRÊPE BATTER
250g/9oz/2 cups plain (all-purpose) flour
4 eggs, beaten
250ml/9fl oz/1 cup milk
250ml/9fl oz/1 cup water
2 tbsp vegetable oil or butter
large pinch of sea salt
vegetable oil, for frying

FILLING
2 apples, quartered, cored and thinly sliced
400g/14oz/2½ cups fresh cherries, pitted and halved
4 tbsp chopped walnuts
maple syrup

1. Mix all the batter ingredients and set aside.

2. Combine the apple, cherries and walnuts in a bowl with a little maple syrup.

3. Heat a little oil in a frying pan (skillet), pour in the batter and fry the crêpes for 2 minutes on each side.

4. Top with a couple of tablespoons of filling, roll the crêpes and serve hot.

442 BAKED PEARS WITH HONEY AND BRAZIL NUTS

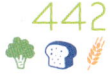

SERVES 4
PREPARATION
5 minutes
COOKING
15 minutes

STORAGE
Leftovers will keep in the fridge for up to 3 days.

1 tbsp grapeseed oil, plus extra for drizzling oiling
4 large, sweet, ripe pears, halved, cored and sliced
2 tbsp runny honey
2 tbsp lemon juice
100g/3½oz/¾ cup Brazil nuts, sliced

1. Preheat the oven to 200°C/400°F/gas mark 6.

2. Grease an ovenproof pie dish with the oil, and cover the bottom with the pear slices. Mix the honey with the lemon juice and pour over the pears. Sprinkle with sliced Brazil nuts and a dash of oil. Bake in a hot oven for approximately 15 minutes until the nuts begin to brown.

3. Serve with plain or soya yogurt.

443 PEACH AND ALMOND RICE PUDDING

SERVES 4
PREPARATION 5 minutes
COOKING 40 minutes

STORAGE Leftovers will keep in the fridge for up to 2 days.

225g/8oz/heaped 1 cup long-grain brown rice
900ml/31fl oz/3¾ cups milk
2 tsp lemon juice
4 tsp ground almonds
2 peaches, peeled, pitted and sliced
handful of flaked almonds, toasted

1. Put the rice, milk and lemon juice in a saucepan. Slowly bring to the boil, then reduce the heat, cover and simmer for 30 minutes, stirring occasionally, until the rice is tender and the milk almost all absorbed.

2. Add the almonds and peaches and cook, stirring, for 5 minutes until the peaches are softened.

3. Spoon into bowls, sprinkle with the flaked almonds and serve.

444 APRICOT AND ORANGE SOUFFLÉS

SERVES 4–6
PREPARATION 15 minutes
COOKING 20 minutes

STORAGE Best eaten immediately. Make the apricot purée in advance and chill for up to 1 day.

olive oil, for greasing
50g/1¾oz/⅓ cup dried apricots
2 tbsp cornflour (cornstarch)
125ml/4fl oz/½ cup orange juice
grated zest of 1 orange
4 eggs, separated
¼ tsp cream of tartar
3 tbsp caster (superfine) sugar

1. Preheat the oven to 190°C/375°F/gas mark 5 and lightly grease four to six ramekins with oil. Put the apricots, cornflour (cornstarch), orange juice and zest in a blender and blend until smooth. Pour into a pan and bring slowly to the boil, stirring continuously for 2–3 minutes until thick. Set aside and leave to cool.

2. Beat the egg yolks into the sauce. In a clean bowl, whisk the egg whites with the cream of tartar until they form soft peaks. Add the sugar and whisk until stiff.

3. Stir a little of the egg white into the sauce, then gently fold in the rest. Divide the mixture among the ramekins, put them on a baking sheet and bake for 12–15 minutes, or until puffed and pale golden. Serve immediately.

445 FRUIT BROCHETTES

SERVES 4
PREPARATION
10 minutes
COOKING
10 minutes

STORAGE
Best eaten immediately.

8 small figs
2 pears, cored and quartered
2 bananas, peeled and cut into chunks
2 thick slices of pineapple, peeled and cut into chunks
8 small apricots, halved and pitted
8 strawberries
4 tbsp maple syrup
4 tbsp lemon juice
4 tbsp toasted sesame oil

1. Thread the fruit onto four metal barbecue skewers. Heat a barbecue or grill (broiler) to medium-hot.

2. Make a marinade of the maple syrup, lemon juice and sesame oil in a bowl.

3. Generously brush the fruit brochettes with the marinade and place on the barbecue (or under the grill/broiler) for 2–3 minutes. Turn, brush again and grill the other side for a further 1–2 minutes. Repeat until the fruit begins to turn golden (don't let it turn soft).

4. Serve hot with plain or soya yogurt.

446 TROPICAL FRUIT FLAMBÉ

SERVES 4
PREPARATION
10 minutes
COOKING
5 minutes

STORAGE
Best eaten immediately.

2 tbsp grapeseed oil
4 thick slices of pineapple, peeled, cored and halved
4 bananas, peeled and halved lengthways
2 papayas, peeled, deseeded and sliced
½ fresh coconut, peeled and thinly sliced
4 tbsp maple syrup
2 tbsp rum

1. Heat the oil in a frying pan (skillet) and fry the fruit pieces for 1 minute. Turn, sprinkle with the maple syrup and fry for a further 1—2 minutes until the fruit is tender (but still firm). Add the rum, heat through and carefully ignite the mixture with a match. Gently shake the pan while allowing the rum to burn for a minute. Serve hot.

447 SUMMER PUDDINGS

SERVES 4
PREPARATION
15 minutes
COOKING
5 minutes

STORAGE
Make in advance and keep in the fridge for up to 3 days or freeze for up to 1 month.

vegetable oil, for greasing
10–12 thin small slices wholemeal bread, crusts removed
2 x 500-g/1lb 2-oz/10-cup bags frozen summer berries
6 tbsp caster (superfine) sugar

1 Lightly oil four 150-ml/5-fl oz dariole moulds or small lidded pots. Cut four circles of bread to fit the base of each mould. Cut each of the remaining bread slices into four triangles. Put a bread round into each mould, then arrange the triangular pieces of bread around the sides, packing them tightly together to avoid any gaps. Allow the bread to overlap the top slightly. Set aside four triangles.

2 Meanwhile, put the fruit in a saucepan with the sugar and 120ml/4fl oz/½ cup water and simmer gently for 4–5 minutes until the berries are defrosted and very juicy.

3 Spoon a little of the berry juice into each mould, then divide the fruit between the moulds, leaving 4 tablespoons of the juice to spoon over the puddings.

4 Fold the bread over the fruit filling, then top with the remaining triangles. Spoon over the juice, then cover each pudding with a plate and a weight and refrigerate overnight.

448 WINTER FRUIT SALAD

SERVES 4
PREPARATION
10 minutes
COOKING
15 minutes

STORAGE
Make in advance and keep in the fridge for up to 1 week.

200g/7oz mixed dried fruit, such as apples, apricots, peaches and prunes, cut into bite-sized pieces
300ml/10fl oz/1¼ cup fresh orange juice
1 cinnamon stick
1 star anise
2 cloves

1 Put the dried fruit, orange juice, cinnamon, star anise and cloves with 6 tablespoons of water in a saucepan. Bring up to boiling point, then reduce the heat, cover and simmer for 10 minutes, until the fruit has softened.

2 Remove from the heat, leave to cool and divide between four small lidded pots or serving bowls.

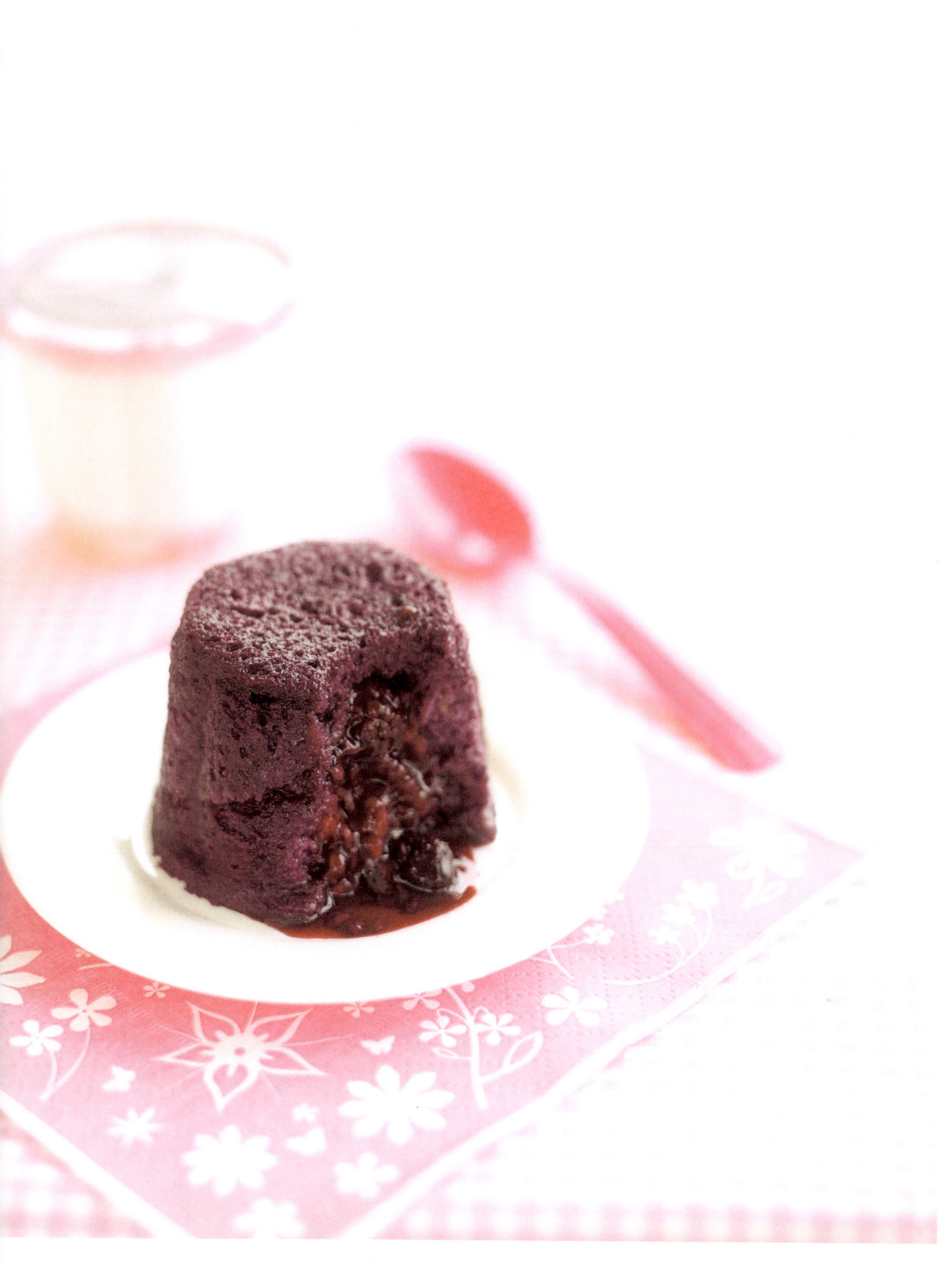

449 FRUITY FILO PARCELS

SERVES 4
PREPARATION 15 minutes
COOKING 12 minutes

STORAGE
Leftovers will keep in the fridge for up to 1 day.

6 tbsp olive oil, plus extra for greasing
2 eating apples, peeled, cored and diced
2 tsp lemon juice
½ tsp ground cinnamon
3 tbsp raisins
4 tbsp chopped mixed nuts (raw, unsalted)
8 sheets of filo (phyllo) pastry, each about 20cm/8in square

1. Preheat the oven to 200°C/400°F/gas mark 6 and grease two baking sheets with oil. Mix the apples, lemon juice, cinnamon, raisins and nuts in a bowl.

2. Put 1 sheet of filo (phyllo) pastry on a board, brush with a little of the oil and cover with another sheet. Put a quarter of the apple mixture lengthways down the middle of the pastry, leaving a small gap at the ends.

3. Fold the two long sides of the pastry over, then roll up from one narrow end to enclose the filling. Place the parcel, seam-side down, on the sheet, then repeat with the remaining filo and filling.

4. Brush the parcels with oil and bake for 10–12 minutes until golden brown. Serve hot or cold.

450 PEAR, BLACKBERRY AND WALNUT CRUMBLE

SERVES 4
PREPARATION
10 minutes
COOKING
35 minutes

STORAGE
Leftovers will keep in the fridge for up to 2 days

- 2 pears, peeled, cored and cut into chunks
- 225g/8oz/scant 2 cups blackberries
- grated zest of 1 lemon
- 1 tbsp lemon juice
- 2 tbsp honey
- 1 tbsp apple juice
- 60g/2¼oz/½ cup walnuts, chopped
- 175g/6oz/2 cups porridge (rolled) oats
- 3 tbsp olive oil
- 3 tbsp apple juice

① Preheat the oven to 180°C/350°F/gas mark 4. Put the pears and blackberries in a shallow baking dish and sprinkle with the lemon zest and juice. Drizzle over the honey and apple juice.

② Mix together the walnuts, oats, oil and apple juice, then spoon the mixture over the fruit and press down gently.

③ Bake for 30 minutes until golden brown, then serve.

451 PUMPKIN AND ORANGE CRUMBLE

SERVES 4
PREPARATION
15 minutes
COOKING
40 minutes

STORAGE
Freeze the raw dish for up to a month.

- 115g/4oz/1 cup self-raising flour
- 175g/6oz/¾ cup brown sugar
- 55g/2oz butter
- 2 eggs
- 1 tsp ground cinnamon
- ¼ tsp ground ginger
- 300-g/10½-oz can evaporated milk
- 400g/14oz pumpkin, chopped
- 3 oranges, peeled and flesh roughly chopped

① Preheat the oven to 200°C/400°F/gas mark 6. Place the flour and 55g/2oz/¼ cup of the sugar in a bowl, add the butter and use your fingers to mix them together until the mixture becomes like breadcrumbs.

② In a mixing bowl, beat the eggs with a fork and add the spices, evaporated milk and remaining sugar.

③ Put the pumpkin and oranges into an ovenproof dish with a high rim. Pour the milk and spice mix on top, then cover with the crumble. Place the dish in the oven and bake for 30–40 minutes or until the top crust has become golden brown. Remove from the oven and serve.

452 APPLE CRUMBLE

SERVES 4
PREPARATION 10 minutes
COOKING 16–20 minutes

STORAGE Freeze the raw dish for up to 1 month.

5 tbsp raisins
4 cooking apples, thinly sliced
2 tbsp grapeseed oil, plus extra for greasing
250g/9oz/2½ cups porridge (rolled) oats
50g/2oz/½ cup chopped walnuts
4 tbsp maple syrup

1. Preheat the oven to 230°C/450°F/gas mark 8. Soak the raisins in a bowl with enough cold water to cover.

2. Place the sliced apples in an oiled, ovenproof dish. Cover with the soaked raisins and their liquid.

3. Heat the oil in a small frying pan (skillet) and stir in the oats and the walnuts. Add the maple syrup and gently heat through for 1 minute, stirring continuously. Evenly spoon the crumble mixture over the apples and bake in a hot oven for about 15 minutes until the topping is golden brown. Serve with ice cream.

453 BAKED CINNAMON APPLES

SERVES 4
PREPARATION 10 minutes
COOKING 20 minutes

STORAGE Best eaten immediately.

4 dessert apples, cored
4 bananas, peeled and mashed
8–12 dates, pitted and chopped
2 tbsp flaked (slivered) almonds
ground cinnamon, to taste
4 tbsp tahini (sesame paste)
2 tbsp lemon juice
6 tbsp maple syrup

1. Preheat the oven to 180°C/350°F/gas mark 4. Cut a horizontal line in the skin of the apples around the middle and set aside.

2. Mix two of the mashed bananas with the dates in a bowl. Stuff the cored apples with the banana and date mixture. Sprinkle the almonds and the cinnamon on top and bake in a hot oven for approximately 20 minutes.

3. Meanwhile, mix the tahini (sesame paste) with the remaining mashed banana, lemon juice and maple syrup in a bowl with enough cold water to make a thick sauce.

4. Place the baked apples on dessert plates, garnish with the sauce and serve.

454 SPICED APPLE VOLCANOS

SERVES 4
PREPARATION
10 minutes
COOKING
15 minutes

STORAGE
Eat immediately. Once cored, you can keep the apples overnight in a bowl of cold water with a squeeze of lemon to prevent them from browning.

4 cooking apples, cored
12 cloves
115g/4oz/1 cup sultanas (golden raisins)
4 tbsp pine nuts
2 tsp ground cinnamon
4 tbsp maple syrup
600ml/21fl oz/2½ cups milk
2 vanilla pods
6 egg yolks
55g/2oz/¼ cup brown sugar

1. Preheat the oven to 220°C/425°F/gas mark 7. Line a baking sheet with foil, keeping enough spare around the sides to cover the apples. Place the apples on the sheet. For each apple, pierce the skin with 3 cloves. Fill with sultanas (golden raisins) and pine nuts. Sprinkle over the cinnamon and drizzle over maple syrup. Wrap in the foil and bake for 15 minutes.

2. Meanwhile, heat the milk in a saucepan but do not boil. Add the vanilla pods and leave to stand off the heat for 10 minutes.

3. Break the egg yolks into a bowl, add the sugar and whisk until thick. Remove the vanilla pods from the milk. Slowly beat the milk into the egg. Pour into a non-stick pan and cook over a low heat, stirring, until thickened. Remove the apples from the oven and serve with the custard.

455 ORCHARD HARVEST WITH CUSTARD

SERVES 4
PREPARATION
15 minutes
COOKING
8 minutes

STORAGE
Best eaten immediately.

4 ripe pears, cored and sliced
2 red apples, cored and sliced
2 sharon fruit, sliced
4 fresh figs, quartered
4 plums, pitted and quartered

CUSTARD
2 tbsp cornflour (cornstarch)
2 tbsp raw cane sugar
2 tsp vanilla extract
large pinch of salt
500ml/17fl oz/2 cups milk

1. Arrange the fruit on plates.

2. To make the custard, put the cornflour (cornstarch) in a bowl with the sugar, vanilla extract, salt and enough milk to make a smooth paste. Heat the remaining milk in a pan (don't let it boil), then slowly add it to the cornflour mixture, stirring continuously. Pour back into the pan, stir and bring to the boil. Serve with the fruit.

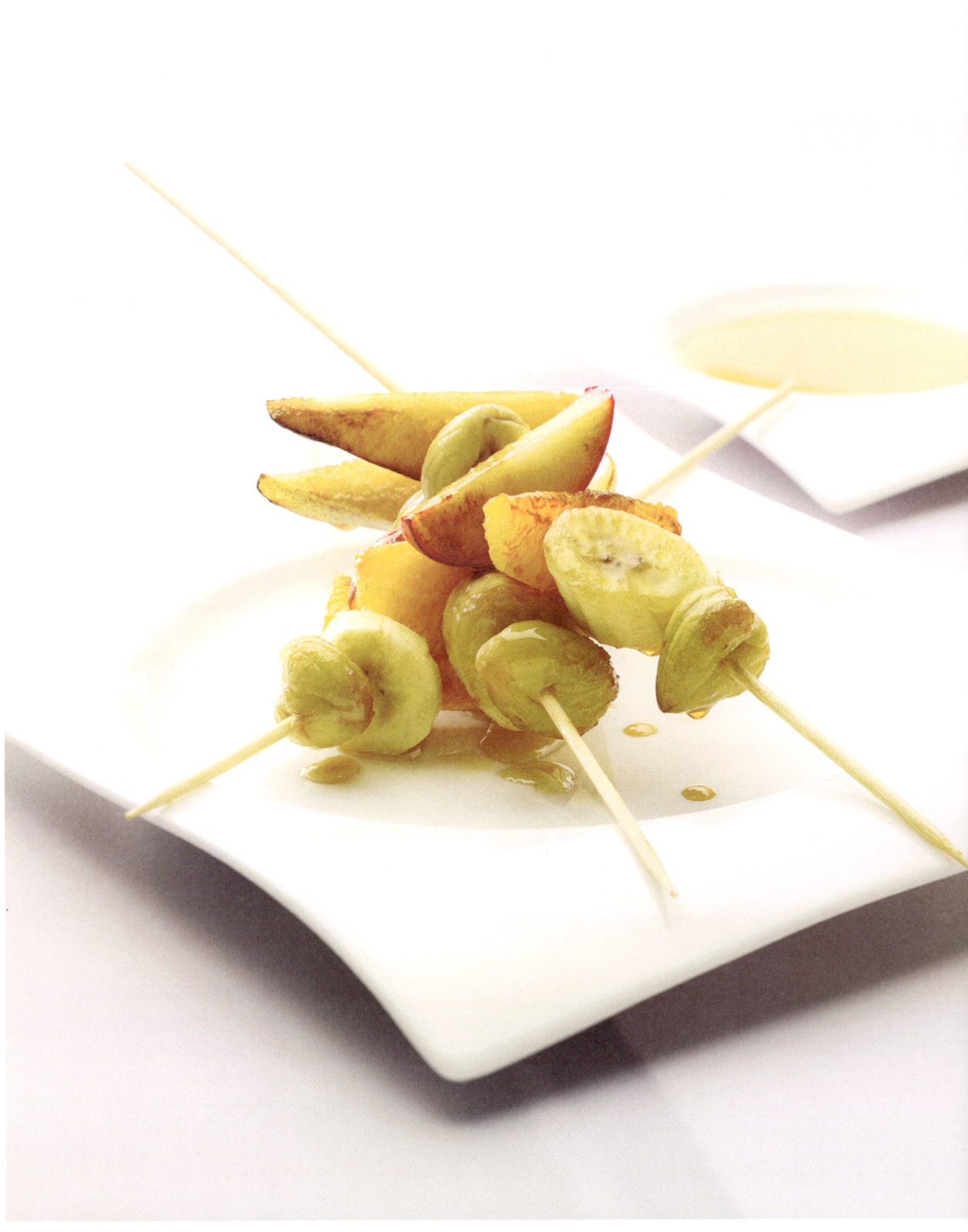

456 BAKED FRUIT KEBABS

SERVES 4
PREPARATION
10 minutes
COOKING
15 minutes

STORAGE
Best eaten immediately.

2 oranges, peeled and cut into chunks
2 pears, cored and cut into chunks
2 apples, cored and cut into chunks
2 bananas, peeled and cut into chunks
16 sweet chestnuts, shelled and peeled
300ml/10½fl oz/1¼ cups grape juice
4 tsp maple syrup
oil, for brushing

1. Preheat the oven to 240°C/475°F/gas mark 9.

2. Thread the fruit and chestnuts onto four barbecue skewers.

3. Mix the grape juice and maple syrup together and brush over the fruit. Place the skewers on greaseproof paper brushed with oil. Roll each skewer in the paper and bake in a hot oven for 15 minutes.

4. Serve with the remaining marinade as a dip.

457 DROP SCONES WITH FRUIT SAUCE

MAKES 10
PREPARATION
10 minutes
COOKING
20 minutes

STORAGE
Make in advance and keep in the fridge for up to 3 days or freeze for up to 1 month.

150g/5½oz/scant 1¼ cups self-raising (self-rising) flour
2 tsp caster (superfine) sugar
200ml/7fl oz/generous ¾ cup milk
1 large free-range egg
vegetable oil, for frying

FRUIT SAUCE
300g/10½oz strawberries
icing (confectioners') sugar, sifted

1. To make the fruit sauce, put the strawberries in a blender and process. Press through a sieve to remove any pips, and sweeten with icing (confectioners') sugar to taste.

2. To make the drop scones, sift the flour into a mixing bowl, then mix with the sugar. Make a well in the middle. Pour the milk into a jug, whisk in the egg, then add to the flour and sugar. Beat to make a smooth batter.

3. Heat a little oil in a non-stick frying pan (skillet) and add three small ladlefuls of batter, one for each drop scone. Cook for about 3 minutes until light golden, then turn and cook for another 2 minutes. Remove and cook the remaining scones.

4. Serve with the fruit sauce.

458 PEAR TART

SERVES 4
PREPARATION 10 minutes
COOKING 30 minutes

STORAGE
Store in an airtight container for up to 1 week.

1 package ready-made shortcrust pastry, rolled out
about 55g/2oz marzipan
2 tbsp flaked (slivered) almonds
2 large sweet, ripe pears, peeled, halved and cored

1 Preheat the oven to 200°C/400°F/gas mark 6.

2 Place the rolled-out pastry in a 20-cm/8-in square, ovenproof pie dish, leaving a generous rim hanging over the edge of the dish. Sprinkle with the almonds. Place a knob of marzipan in the hollow of each pear half, then arrange all four pear halves in the pastry shell, stalk ends meeting in the middle. Fold the pastry into the middle to cover the base of the pears and bake for 30 minutes until golden.

3 Serve with plain or soya yogurt, crème fraîche or soya cream.

459 APPLE TART

SERVES 4
PREPARATION 10 minutes
COOKING 20 minutes

STORAGE
Store in an airtight container for up to 1 week

1 package ready-made shortcrust pastry, rolled out
400g/14oz cooking apples, cored and finely sliced
a little lemon juice
a little grapeseed oil
pinch of raw cane sugar
pinch of ground cinnamon

1 Preheat the oven to 220°C/425°F/gas mark 7.

2 Place the rolled-out pastry in a 20-cm/8-in round baking tin (pan). Sprinkle the apple slices with a little lemon juice to prevent discolouration and add them in concentric circles to cover the whole pastry base. Sprinkle with a little oil, sugar and cinnamon.

3 Bake the tart in the hot oven for 15–20 minutes until the apples begin to golden. Serve with crème fraîche or soya cream.

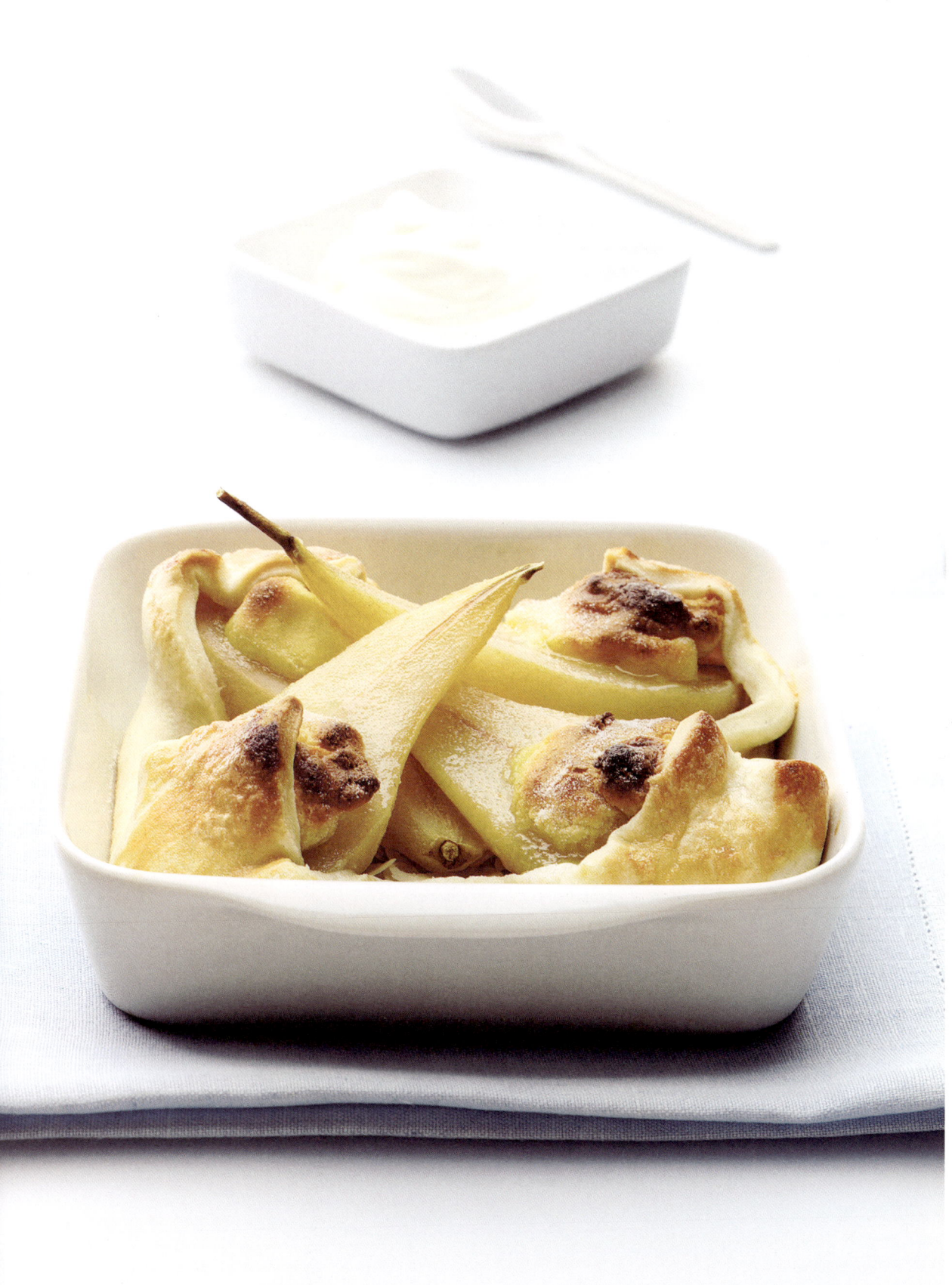

460 PLUM TART

SERVES 4
PREPARATION
10 minutes
COOKING
15 minutes

STORAGE
Store in an airtight container for up to 1 week

1 package ready-made puff pastry, rolled out
300g/10½oz ripe plums, quartered and pitted
1 tbsp runny honey
pinch of ground cinnamon

1. Preheat the oven to 220°C/425°F/gas mark 7.

2. Place the rolled-out pastry in a 20-cm/8-in round baking tin (pan). Line with the plums and brush with the honey. Sprinkle with the cinnamon and bake in a hot oven for 15 minutes.

3. Serve with crème fraîche or soya cream.

461 BREAD, BUTTER AND HONEY PUDDING

SERVES 4
PREPARATION
10 minutes
COOKING
30 minutes

STORAGE
You can freeze this before cooking and keep it for up to a month. After cooking keep it for up to 3 days in the fridge.

400g/14oz wholemeal bread loaf
55g/2oz butter
150g/5½oz clear honey
3 tbsp raisins
2 tbsp pine nuts
2 tbsp pumpkin seeds
300ml/10½fl oz/1¼ cups milk or soya milk
3 eggs
1 tsp ground cinnamon

1. Preheat the oven to 220°C/425°F/gas mark 7. Cut the bread into 11 slices, then spread with butter and honey and remove the crusts. Cut each slice into two triangles.

2. In a bowl, mix the raisins, pine nuts and pumpkin seeds.

3. Line the bottom of an ovenproof dish with the bread slices. Sprinkle over a handful of the nut/raisin mixture. Continue to alternate layers until the dish is full.

4. Pour the milk into a jug (pitcher), add the eggs and cinnamon and whisk together. Pour over the bread dish and leave to stand for 10 minutes. Bake in the oven for 20–30 minutes until golden brown. Serve immediately.

462 PINEAPPLE PIE

SERVES 4
PREPARATION 10 minutes + chilling
COOKING 5 minutes
STORAGE Store in an airtight container for up to 1 week

½ pineapple, peeled, cored and chopped, plus 2 thin slices (halved) to garnish
1 tsp maple syrup
1 tbsp agar-agar
3 tbsp water
1 pre-baked 20cm/8in shortcrust pastry shell
2 tbsp fresh coconut, shredded

1. In a food processor or blender, blend the pineapple and maple syrup until smooth and set aside.

2. Heat the agar-agar with the water in a small saucepan over a low heat, stirring continuously until the mixture bubbles and becomes gelatinous (3–4 minutes). Stir in the blended pineapple and pour into the pre-baked pastry shell. Allow to cool, then garnish with halved pineapple slices and fresh coconut.

3. Chill before serving.

463 FRUITY CHOCOLATE FONDUE

SERVES 4
PREPARATION 25 minutes
STORAGE You can refrigerate the dips for up to 2 days, but eat the fruit immediately.

280g/10oz strawberries
6 bananas, peeled
2 pineapples, peeled
8 peaches
200-g/7-oz can of coconut milk
½ tsp vanilla extract
55g/2oz/¼ cup brown sugar
200g/7oz cream cheese
175g/6oz good-quality milk chocolate
1 tsp cocoa powder
2 sprigs mint

1. Cut the fruit into 2.5cm/1in chunks.

2. Put the coconut milk, vanilla extract, sugar and half the cream cheese into a blender and process until smooth.

3. Melt the chocolate in a saucepan over a very low heat. Stir in the remaining cream cheese and cocoa powder.

4. Pour the two dips into separate bowls and place them in the middle of a large serving platter. Arrange the fruit around the bowls in piles, alternating the colours. Garnish the dips with sprigs of mint and serve with kebab skewers or cocktail sticks.

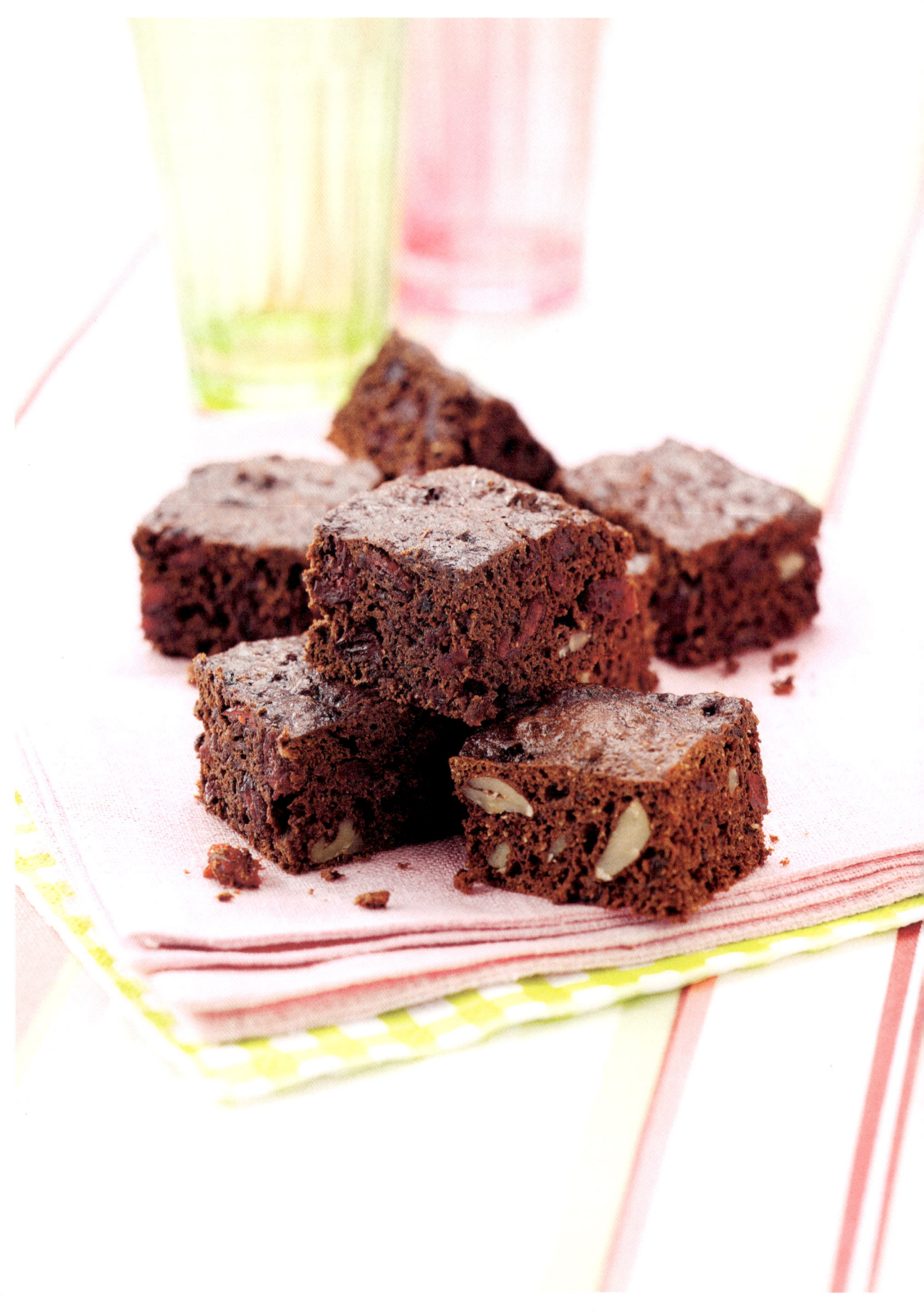

Baked

These treats, cakes and breads have been created with health in mind – with a few concessions to the occasional indulgence. Dried and fresh fruits, nuts and seeds feature heavily. Some of the sweet treats are sufficiently quick and simple to make on the day, while others need a bit more preparation but will keep for a few days.

From muffins and cakes to different takes on the cereal bar, there are plenty of exciting things to try. Chocolate and Cranberry Brownies (see page 350) or Apricot and Cashew Bars (see page 352) are great treats for lunchboxes. The Seeded Dough Balls (see page 367) and Cheese Scones (see page 368) make a good alternative to bread while being just as versatile, and are perfect filled or topped with various sweet or savoury foods. There is even a healthy Party Cake (see page 365) for special occasions.

464 CHOCOLATE and CRANBERRY BROWNIES

MAKES 10–12

PREPARATION
15 minutes

COOKING
30 minutes

STORAGE
Store in the fridge for up to 4 days or in the freezer for up to 3 months, then thaw in the fridge overnight.

- olive oil, for greasing
- 100g/3½oz/½ cup soft prunes
- 50g/2oz/¼ cup caster (superfine) sugar
- 125g/4½oz plain (bittersweet) chocolate, chopped
- 100g/3½oz/heaped ¾ cup dried cranberries
- 25g/1oz/¼ cup pecans, chopped
- 1 tsp vanilla extract
- 50g/2oz/scant ½ cup self-raising wholemeal flour
- 1 tsp baking powder
- 25g/1oz/scant ½ cup wheat germ
- 3 eggs, separated

1. Preheat the oven to 180°C/350°F/gas mark 4 and grease and line the base of a square 15cm/6in cake tin (pan). Blend the prunes, sugar and 3 tablespoons water in a blender.

2. Melt the chocolate in a bowl over a pan of simmering water. Remove from the heat and stir in the prunes, cranberries, pecans, vanilla extract, flour, baking powder, wheat germ and egg yolks.

3. Whisk the egg whites until they form soft peaks and, with a metal spoon, fold them into the chocolate mixture.

4. Spoon the mixture into the tin (pan). Bake for 20–25 minutes until risen and firm to touch. Leave in the tin (pan) to cool. Cut into 10–12 squares and serve.

465 APRICOT MUESLI TRAYBAKE

MAKES 14–16
PREPARATION 15 minutes
COOKING 30 minutes

STORAGE Store in an airtight container in the fridge for up to 4 days.

150ml/5fl oz/scant ⅔ cup light olive oil, plus extra for greasing
375g/13oz/2½ cups dried apricots
150g/5½oz/1¼ cups unsweetened muesli or porridge (rolled) oats
100g/3½oz/1 cup self-raising wholemeal flour
50g/1¾oz/½ cup mixed seeds
1 tsp ground cinnamon
100g/3½oz/1 cup ground almonds
50g/1¾oz/¾ cup desiccated (dried shredded) coconut
2 oranges, peeled, pips removed
5 tbsp honey or agave nectar

1. Preheat the oven to 180°C/350°F/gas mark 4 and lightly grease a shallow 20 x 30cm/8 x 12in tin (pan) with oil.

2. Chop 150g/5½oz/1 cup of the apricots and mix them with the muesli or oats, flour, seeds, cinnamon, almonds and coconut in a bowl.

3. Purée the remaining apricots with the oranges, honey and oil in a food processor. Add the purée to the oat mixture and stir to combine.

4. Spread the mixture evenly in the prepared tin and bake for 25–30 minutes until golden. Cool in the tin (pan), cutting into 14–16 bars while still warm, then serve.

466 MUESLI CRUNCHIES

MAKES 12
PREPARATION 10 minutes
COOKING 20 minutes

STORAGE Store the crunchies for up to a week in an airtight container.

110g/4oz butter
50g/2oz/¼ cup muscovado sugar
1 tbsp molasses
150g/5½oz/1½ cups porridge (rolled) oats
50g/2oz/⅓ cup pecans
50g/2oz/½ cup sunflower seeds
50g/2oz/⅔ cup sultanas (golden raisins)

1. Preheat the oven to 200°C/400°F/gas mark 6. Put the butter, sugar and molasses into a saucepan and heat gently to melt.

2. In a bowl, stir together the remaining ingredients. Add the melted mixture and stir.

3. Press the mixture into a shallow, non-stick baking tin (pan), score into 5cm/2in squares and bake for 20 minutes or until golden brown.

467 APRICOT AND CASHEW BARS

MAKES 8
PREPARATION
10 minutes
COOKING
3 minutes

STORAGE
Make in advance and keep in an airtight container for up to 1 week.

50g/2oz/½ cup whole porridge (rolled) oats
50g/2oz/⅓ cup cashew nuts
150g/5½oz ready-to-eat dried apricots, cut into small pieces
100g/3½oz/¾ cup raisins
4 tbsp fresh orange juice
2 tbsp sunflower seeds
2 tbsp pumpkin seeds

1. Put the oats and cashew nuts in a frying pan (skillet) and toast them over a medium heat for 3 minutes, turning occasionally, until they just golden. Leave to cool.

2. Put the apricots, raisins and orange juice in a food processor and process to a smooth paste. Scrape the fruit purée into a mixing bowl.

3. Put the oats, nuts and seeds in the food processor and process until finely chopped. Tip the mixture into the bowl with the fruit purée. Stir the fruit mixture until all the ingredients are mixed together.

4. Line an 18 x 25cm/7 x 10in tin (pan) with baking paper. Tip the mixture into the tin (pan) and spread evenly. Chill for 1 hour, then cut into 8 bars.

468 OATMEAL COOKIES

MAKES 12
PREPARATION
15 minutes
COOKING
10 minutes

STORAGE
Make in advance and keep in an airtight container for up to 1 week.

vegetable oil, for greasing
50g/1¾oz/½ cup medium oatmeal
85g/3oz/⅔ cup plain (all-purpose) wholemeal flour, plus extra
1 tsp baking powder
pinch of salt
50g/1¾oz butter, diced
1 tbsp caster (superfine) sugar
2 tbsp milk

1. Preheat the oven to 200°C/400°F/gas mark 6. Grease a baking sheet. Sift the oatmeal, flour and baking powder into a bowl. Add the salt and stir to combine.

2. Rub the butter and sugar into the flour mixture until it resembles breadcrumbs. Pour in the milk and mix to make a dough.

3. Turn out onto a lightly floured surface and knead until smooth. Roll out into a 5mm–/¼in-thick rectangle and cut into 12 squares.

4. Place on the baking sheet and prick with a fork. Bake for 10 minutes until golden. Transfer to a wire rack to cool.

469 PEANUT AND OAT COOKIES

MAKES 10–12
PREPARATION
10 minutes
COOKING
15 minutes

STORAGE
Store in an airtight container for up to 4 days.

50g/1¾oz unsalted butter, plus extra for greasing
120g/4¼oz/½ cup crunchy peanut butter
1 tsp ground cinnamon
3 tbsp honey or agave nectar
50g/1¾oz/heaped ½ cup porridge (rolled) oats
1 tbsp ground flaxseeds
50g/1¾oz/¾ cup desiccated (dried shredded) coconut
1 tsp vanilla extract
120g/4¼oz/scant 1 cup plain (all-purpose) wholemeal flour
2 tbsp sesame seeds
2 eggs, beaten

1. Preheat the oven to 180°C/350°F/gas mark 4 and grease and line a baking sheet.

2. Gently heat the butter, peanut butter, cinnamon and honey in a pan until the butter melts. Stir in the oats, flaxseeds, coconut, vanilla extract, flour and sesame seeds. Add the eggs and mix well.

3. Space 10–12 spoonfuls of the mixture well apart on the baking sheet and press down into circles. Bake for 10–12 minutes, or until lightly browned. Leave on the sheet for 5 minutes. Place on a wire rack to cool, then serve.

470 PEANUT BUTTER COOKIES

MAKES 18
PREPARATION
10 minutes
COOKING
15 minutes

STORAGE
You can store the cookies for up to a week in an airtight container; or freeze the uncooked mixture for up to 3 months.

115g/4oz butter
115g/4oz/½ cup brown sugar
3 tbsp wholenut peanut butter
1 banana
150g/5½oz/1⅓ cup rye flour

1. Preheat the oven to 190°C/375°F/gas mark 5. Place the butter, sugar and peanut butter in a small saucepan and heat gently to melt.

2. In a bowl mash the banana with a fork and then add the flour and the melted peanut butter mixture. Stir together until the mixture becomes sticky.

3. Form into walnut-sized balls and press onto a greased baking sheet, leaving a good gap between each cookie. Bake in the oven for 10–15 minutes until golden brown.

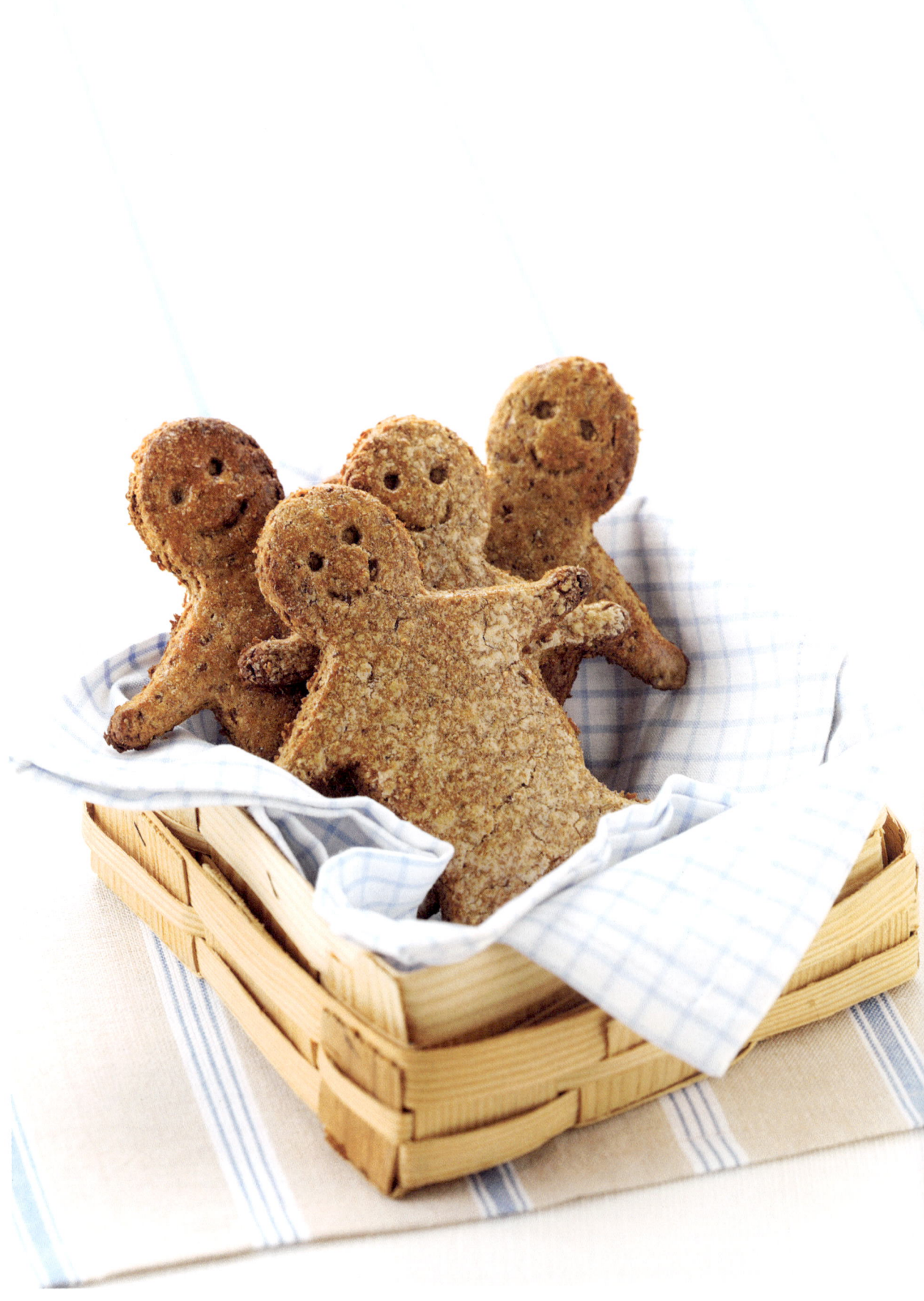

471 FLAXSEED GINGERBREAD MEN

MAKES 12–14
PREPARATION
15 minutes + chilling
COOKING
12 minutes

STORAGE
Store in an airtight container for up to 4 days. Freeze the dough for up to 3 months.

100g/3½oz/scant ½ cup tahini (sesame paste)
60g/2¼oz/heaped ½ cup ground flaxseeds
4 tbsp honey or agave nectar
1 egg, beaten, plus extra for glazing
125g/4½oz/1 cup white or wholemeal plain (all-purpose) flour, plus extra for rolling
1 tsp ground cinnamon
1½ tsp ground ginger
¼ tsp baking soda
olive oil, for greasing

1. In a bowl, mix the tahini (sesame paste), flaxseeds, honey and egg until creamy and smooth.

2. In another bowl, sift together the flour, cinnamon, ginger and baking soda. Add the tahini mixture and mix well to form a stiff dough. Knead lightly, wrap in clingfilm (plastic wrap) and chill for 15 minutes.

3. Preheat the oven to 180°C/350°F/gas mark 4 and lightly grease a baking sheet with oil. Lightly flour a work surface and roll out the dough to 1cm/½in thick. Using a cutter, stamp out 12–14 shapes, place on the baking sheet and brush with beaten egg.

4. Bake for 10–12 minutes, or until a pale golden brown. Leave to cool on the baking sheet for 5 minutes, then transfer to a wire rack to cool.

472 GINGERBREAD STAR COOKIES

MAKES 12–15
PREPARATION
15 minutes
COOKING
20 minutes

STORAGE
Store in an airtight container for up to 2 weeks.

40g/1½oz butter
55g/2oz/¼ cup brown sugar
55g/2oz /⅓ cup golden syrup
115g/4oz/1 cup plain (all-purpose) flour
1 tsp ground ginger
½ tsp allspice
½ tsp baking powder

1. Preheat the oven to 180°C/350°F/gas mark 4. Place the butter, sugar and syrup in a small pan and melt over a low heat. Place the remaining ingredients in a bowl and pour in the melted mixture.

2. Mix until the dough leaves the sides of the bowl. Roll out and cut out 12–15 cookies with a star-shaped cutter. Place the cookies on a non-stick baking sheet and bake for 15–20 minutes, until golden. Remove from the oven and cool.

473 PUMPKIN COOKIES

MAKES 10–12
PREPARATION
10 minutes
COOKING
15 minutes

STORAGE
Store in an airtight container in the fridge for up to 3 days or in the freezer for up to 1 month.

2 tbsp olive oil, plus extra for greasing
125g/4½oz/¾ cup self-raising wholemeal flour
125g/4½oz/¾ cup self-raising white flour, plus extra for rolling
½ tsp baking powder
pinch of cayenne pepper
¼ tsp mustard powder
3 tbsp sesame seeds
150g/5½oz/¾ cup canned unsweetened pumpkin purée
75g/2½oz feta cheese, crumbled
1 egg, beaten
milk, for brushing

① Preheat the oven to 200°C/400°F/gas mark 6 and lightly grease a baking sheet with oil. Sift the flours into a large bowl. Stir in the baking powder, cayenne pepper, mustard powder and 2 tbsp of the sesame seeds. Make a well in the dry ingredients. Add the oil, pumpkin purée and feta and stir in the egg. Mix to form a soft dough, then lightly knead into a smooth ball and roll out on a floured surface to 2.5cm/1in thick.

② Use a 5cm/2in cutter to stamp out 10–12 cookies. Place on the baking sheet, brush with milk and sprinkle with the remaining sesame seeds. Bake for 12–15 minutes, until golden. Cool on a wire rack, then serve.

474 APRICOT COOKIES

MAKES 10
PREPARATION
15 minutes
COOKING
20 minutes

STORAGE
Make in advance and keep in an airtight container for up to 1 week.

70g/2½oz/6 tbsp light brown sugar
125g/4½oz soft unsalted butter
70g/2½oz/½ cup self-raising flour
30g/1oz/¼ cup wholemeal self-raising flour
100g/3½oz/1 cup porridge oats
5 dried apricots, finely chopped

① Preheat the oven to 180°C/350°F/gas mark 4. Line two baking sheets with baking paper.

② Cream the sugar and butter together until light and fluffy. Fold in both flours, the oats and apricots and beat until creamy.

③ Divide the mix into 10 pieces and roll each one into a ball. Arrange on the baking sheets, spaced out to allow for the cookies to spread. Lightly flatten the top of each and bake for 15–20 minutes until golden but still slightly soft.

475 LEMON OATMEAL COOKIES

MAKES 8
PREPARATION
10 minutes
COOKING
20 minutes

STORAGE
Store in an airtight container for up to 3 days.

1 lemon, peeled
grated zest of 2 lemons
100g/3½oz dried dates
25g/1oz butter
25g/1oz/¼ cup porridge oats
100g/3½oz/heaped ¾ cup oatmeal
1 tbsp ground flaxseeds
rice flour, for shaping the biscuits

1. Preheat the oven to 180°C/350°F/gas mark 4 and line a baking sheet with parchment.

2. Cut the lemon into bite-size pieces, discarding the pips. Place in a pan with the zest, dates and butter. Heat gently for 1 minute, or until the butter has melted, then purée in a food processor.

3. Put the oats, oatmeal and flaxseeds in a bowl. Stir in the purée to form a soft dough. Divide the dough into 8 equal pieces and flatten them into rounds.

4. Place on the baking sheet and bake for 15–20 minutes until golden. Cool on a wire rack, then serve.

476 ALMOND SHORTBREAD

MAKES 8
PREPARATION
10 minutes + chilling (optional)
COOKING
20 minutes

STORAGE
Store in an airtight container for up to 3 days. Freeze the dough for up to 1 month.

60g/2¼oz/scant ½ cup unsalted butter, plus extra for greasing
150g/5½oz/scant 1½ cups rice flour, plus extra for rolling
150g/5½oz/1½ cups ground almonds
60g/2¼oz/¼ cup caster (superfine) sugar
60g/2¼oz/¼ cup almond butter
1 egg plus 1 egg yolk, beaten

1. Preheat the oven to 180°C/350°F/gas mark 4 and grease a round 20cm/8in loose-bottomed shallow baking tin (pan) with butter.

2. Put the rice flour and almonds in a bowl. Melt the sugar, butter and almond butter in a pan and pour it into the almond mixture. Add the egg and yolk and mix to a soft dough. Press into the tin (pan).

3. Bake the shortbread for 20 minutes, or until golden brown. Cool completely in the tin (pan), cutting into wedges after about 10 minutes.

477 DATE AND PECAN BROWNIES

MAKES 12
PREPARATION 15 minutes
COOKING 50 minutes
STORAGE Make in advance and keep in an airtight container for up to 1 week.

- 100g/3½oz/1 cup pecans, broken in half
- 150g/5½oz plain (bittersweet) chocolate, broken into chunks
- 150g/5½oz unsalted butter, cut into pieces
- 280g/10oz/1¼ cups caster (superfine) sugar
- 3 free-range eggs, lightly beaten
- 125g/4½oz/1 cup plain (all-purpose) flour
- 1½ tsp baking powder
- 100g/3½oz dried ready-to-eat dates, cut into small pieces

1. Preheat the oven to 180°C/350°F/gas mark 4. Line and grease a 20cm/8in square cake tin (pan). Put the pecans on a baking sheet and roast for about 5 minutes until they are slightly golden and smell toasted.

2. Meanwhile, melt the chocolate and butter in a bowl over a pan of slightly simmering water, stirring very occasionally. Remove from the heat and leave to cool slightly.

3. Whisk together the sugar and eggs in a bowl until pale, and stir into the chocolate mixture. Sift in the flour and baking powder, then add the pecans and dates. Mix with a wooden spoon, then pour the mixture into the cake tin (pan).

4. Cook for 40–45 minutes until the top forms a light crust, but the centre is still slightly gooey. Leave to cool in the tin (pan), then turn out and cut into 12 squares.

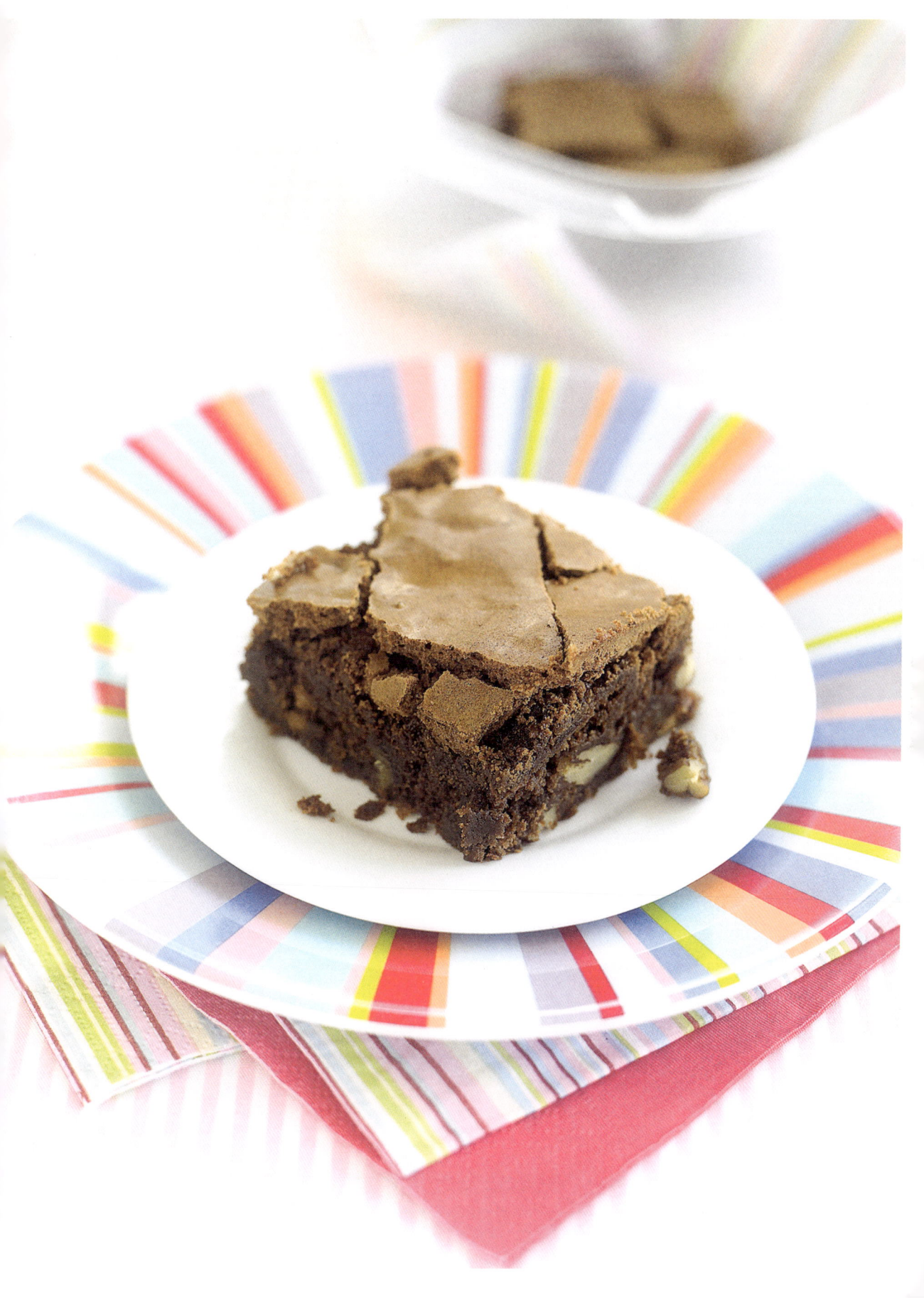

478 CUSTARD TARTLETS

MAKES 8
PREPARATION 10 minutes
COOKING 20 minutes

STORAGE
Make in advance and keep in the fridge for up to 3 days.

3 sheets filo (phyllo) pastry, defrosted if frozen
20g/³/₄oz butter, melted
2 large free-range eggs
3 tbsp caster (superfine) sugar
300ml/10fl oz/1¼ cups milk
1 tsp vanilla extract
freshly grated nutmeg

1. Preheat the oven to 190°C/375°F/gas mark 5. Place the sheets of filo (phyllo) on top of one another and cut into eight 11cm/4½in squares.

2. Brush eight holes of a deep muffin pan with melted butter, then press a three-layered square of filo into each one, leaving the top to overhang the tin. Brush the top of the pastry with more melted butter.

3. Whisk the eggs and sugar in a bowl. Heat the milk, then pour it into the egg mixture with the vanilla and whisk again. Strain the mixture into a jug, then pour into the pastry cases. Grate a little nutmeg over the top.

4. Bake for 20 minutes until the pastry is golden and the filling set. Cool on a wire rack.

479 JAMMY HEART TARTS

MAKES 12–15
PREPARATION 15 minutes
COOKING 20 minutes

STORAGE
Store the tarts in an airtight container for up to 2 weeks.

115g/4oz/1 cup plain (all-purpose) flour
55g/2oz/¼ cup brown sugar
55g/2oz butter
2 tbsp water
115g/4oz/½ cup pure fruit strawberry jam (jelly)

1. Preheat the oven to 200°C/400°F/gas mark 6. Place the flour in a large mixing bowl, add the sugar and butter, and mix together using your fingertips.

2. Add 1 tablespoon of water and mix well. If the mixture is not holding together, add the other tablespoon of water. Press the mixture together with your hands and knead until it holds. Carefully roll out the pastry onto a floured surface.

3. Cut out 12–15 circles using a medium pastry cutter. Grease a non-stick tart pan and lay the circles of pastry into the dents. Put 1 teaspoon of the jam (jelly) into each tart. Bake the tarts for 15–20 minutes, until golden. Cool before serving.

480 BLUEBERRY MUFFINS

MAKES 8–10
PREPARATION
10 minutes
COOKING
20 minutes

STORAGE
Store in an airtight container in the fridge for up to 3 days or in the freezer for up to 1 month.

75ml/2½fl oz/⅓ cup olive oil, plus extra for greasing
225g/8oz/scant 2 cups self-raising wholemeal flour
2 tsp baking powder
2 eggs, beaten
75ml/2½fl oz/⅓ cup milk
2 bananas, mashed
125g/4½oz/1 cup blueberries

1 Preheat the oven to 200°C/400°F/gas mark 6 and grease 8–10 cups of a muffin tin (pan) with oil.

2 Sift the flour and baking powder into a bowl. In another bowl, beat the eggs, oil and milk and stir in the bananas. Pour the wet mixture into the flour and mix well. Gently fold in the blueberries.

3 Spoon the mixture into the muffin cups and bake for 15–20 minutes, or until risen, firm to the touch and golden. Turn out onto a wire rack to cool, then serve.

481 BANANA AND BLUEBERRY MUFFINS

MAKES 10
PREPARATION
15 minutes
COOKING
20 minutes

STORAGE
Make the day before and keep in an airtight container. Muffins are best eaten as fresh as possible.

225g/8oz/1¾ cups plain (all-purpose) flour
pinch of salt
1 tsp baking powder
150g/5oz/⅔ cup caster (superfine) sugar
100ml/3½fl oz/⅓ cup milk
2 free-range eggs
150g/5oz unsalted butter, melted
2 bananas, mashed
150g/5½oz/1 cup blueberries

1 Preheat the oven to 200°C/400°F/gas mark 6. Place 10 large paper cases in a deep muffin tin (pan).

2 Sift the flour, salt and baking powder into a mixing bowl, stir in the sugar and mix together. Make a well in the centre.

3 Put the milk, eggs and butter in a jug (pitcher) and whisk until combined. Add to the bowl with the bananas, stir just to combine, then fold in the blueberries. Spoon into the cases.

4 Bake for 20 minutes until risen. Cool on a wire rack.

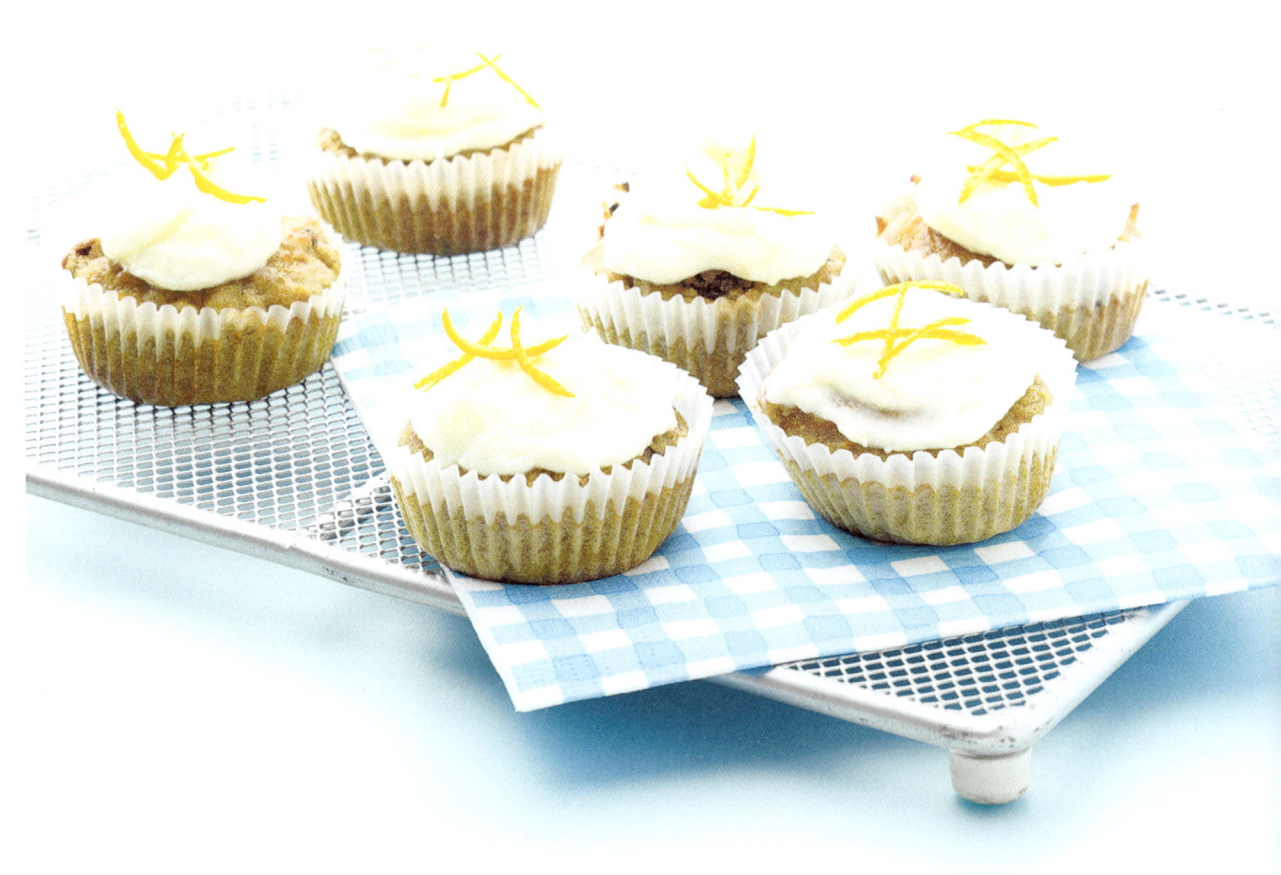

482 BUNNY BITES

MAKES 12

PREPARATION
15 minutes

COOKING
30 minutes

STORAGE
Keep the cakes without icing (frosting) for up to 2 weeks in an airtight container. Once iced, it is best to eat them within 3 days.

125ml/4fl oz/½ cup olive oil
115g/4oz/½ cup muscovado sugar
1 tsp ground cinnamon
½ tsp ground ginger
55g/2oz/scant ½ cup crushed walnuts
55g/2oz/⅓ cup sultanas (golden raisins)
225g/8oz carrot, peeled and grated
grated zest of 2 oranges
150g/5½oz/1½ cups self-raising flour
2 eggs
1 tsp vanilla extract
25g/1oz butter
115g/4oz cream cheese
85g/3oz/⅓ cup icing (confectioners') sugar
grated zest of 1 lemon
½ tbsp lemon juice

1. Preheat the oven to 200°C/400°F/gas mark 6. Put the oil, sugar, spices, walnuts, sultanas (golden raisins), carrot and half the orange zest into a bowl. Stir and then add and beat together the flour, eggs, and vanilla extract until smooth.

2. Pour the mixture into 12 cupcake cases, approximately 1 tablespoon in each. Bake in the oven for 30 minutes until lightly golden. Allow to cool for 30 minutes.

3. Meanwhile, to make the icing (frosting), put the remaining ingredients (reserving some of the zest) into a bowl and cream together. Spread 1 tbsp of icing (frosting) on each bunny bite, then decorate with the remaining orange zest.

483 CARROT CAKE

MAKES 15
PREPARATION 20 minutes
COOKING 50 minutes

STORAGE
Make in advance and keep in an airtight container for up to 1 week.

butter, for greasing
125g/4½oz/1 cup wholemeal self-raising flour
125g/4½oz/1 cup white self-raising flour
2 tsp ground mixed spice
250g/9oz/heaped 1 cup light soft brown sugar
250g/9oz carrots, grated
4 free-range eggs, lightly beaten
200ml/7fl oz/generous ¾ cup sunflower oil

ICING (FROSTING)
125g/4½oz/½ cup low-fat cream cheese
5 tbsp icing (confectioners') sugar
1 tsp vanilla extract

1. Preheat the oven to 180°C/350°F/gas mark 4. Grease the sides and line the base of a 20cm/8in square cake tin (pan).

2. Sift the flours into a mixing bowl, adding the bran left in the sieve. Stir in the spice, sugar and carrots and thoroughly combine.

3. Add the eggs and oil, then stir until all the ingredients are combined. Pour into the tin (pan) and smooth the top. Bake for 50 minutes until risen and golden. Leave in the tin (pan) for 10 minutes, then turn out onto a rack and leave to cool.

4. Beat the cream cheese and icing (confectioners') sugar in a mixing bowl until smooth and creamy. Stir in the vanilla extract. Chill for 10 minutes, then spread over the cake and smooth with a palette knife. Cut into 15 squares.

484 PARTY CAKE

SERVES 10
PREPARATION 15 minutes
COOKING 50 minutes

STORAGE
You can store the cake in the fridge for up to 3 weeks.

200g/7oz/1 2/3 cups self-raising flour
1 tsp ground cinnamon
1 tsp ground nutmeg
115g/4oz butter
55g/2oz/1/3 cup chopped walnuts
55g/2oz/1/2 cup raisins
2 apples, cored and grated
1 tbsp grated lemon zest
3 eggs
60ml/2fl oz/1/4 cup apple juice

1 Preheat the oven to 180°C/350°F/gas mark 4 and grease a 23cm/9in loaf tin (pan). Put the flour, cinnamon, nutmeg and butter in a bowl and mix well, rubbing between your fingers.

2 Stir in the walnuts, raisins and apple. Add the grated lemon zest, eggs and juice. Beat with a wooden spoon until combined. Pour the mixture into the baking tin (pan) and smooth the top flat. Place in the oven and bake for 40–50 minutes, or until the cake is well risen and lightly browned.

485 TAHINI CHOCOLATE FUDGE

MAKES 30-36
PREPARATION 15 minutes + 36 hours chilling

STORAGE
Store in the fridge up to 1 week or in the freezer up to 1 month.

40g/1½oz/1/4 cup sesame seeds
190g/6½oz/1 1/3 cups almonds
6 dates, chopped
1/2 tsp ground cinnamon
2 tbsp shredded coconut
1 tbsp ground flaxseeds
6 tbsp tahini (sesame paste)
6 tbsp honey or agave nectar
5oz dark chocolate, melted
olive oil, for greasing

1 Put the sesame seeds and almonds in a food processor and process until finely ground. Add the dates, cinnamon, coconut, and flax seeds and process to form a coarse paste. Transfer to a bowl.

2 Mix the tahini, honey, and chocolate until blended. Add to the almonds and stir well to form a sticky dough.

3 Lightly grease and line a 20x33cm/13 x8in pan with oil and press the mixture into the pan. Chill in the refrigerator for 2 to 3 hours until firm, then cut into 30 to 36 small pieces and serve.

486 BANANA AND MANGO CAKE

SERVES 8–10
PREPARATION
15 minutes
COOKING
40 minutes

STORAGE
Store in the fridge for up to 3 days.

125g/4½oz butter, melted, plus extra for greasing
75g/2½oz/1 cup dried mango, chopped
175g/6oz/1½ cups wholemeal self-raising flour
55g/2oz/½ cup desiccated (dried shredded) coconut
2 tsp baking powder
1 tsp ground cinnamon
3 bananas, mashed
2 eggs
55g/2oz/¼ cup caster (superfine) sugar
handful of dried banana chips

FILLING
250g/9oz cream cheese
1½ tbsp honey or agave nectar
½ mango, peeled, pitted and finely chopped

1. Preheat the oven to 180°C/350°F/gas mark 4 and grease a 20cm/8in cake tin (pan) with butter. Cover the dried mango with boiling water and soak for 10 minutes, then drain.

2. Mix the flour, coconut, baking powder and cinnamon in a bowl. Stir in the dried mango. Blend the

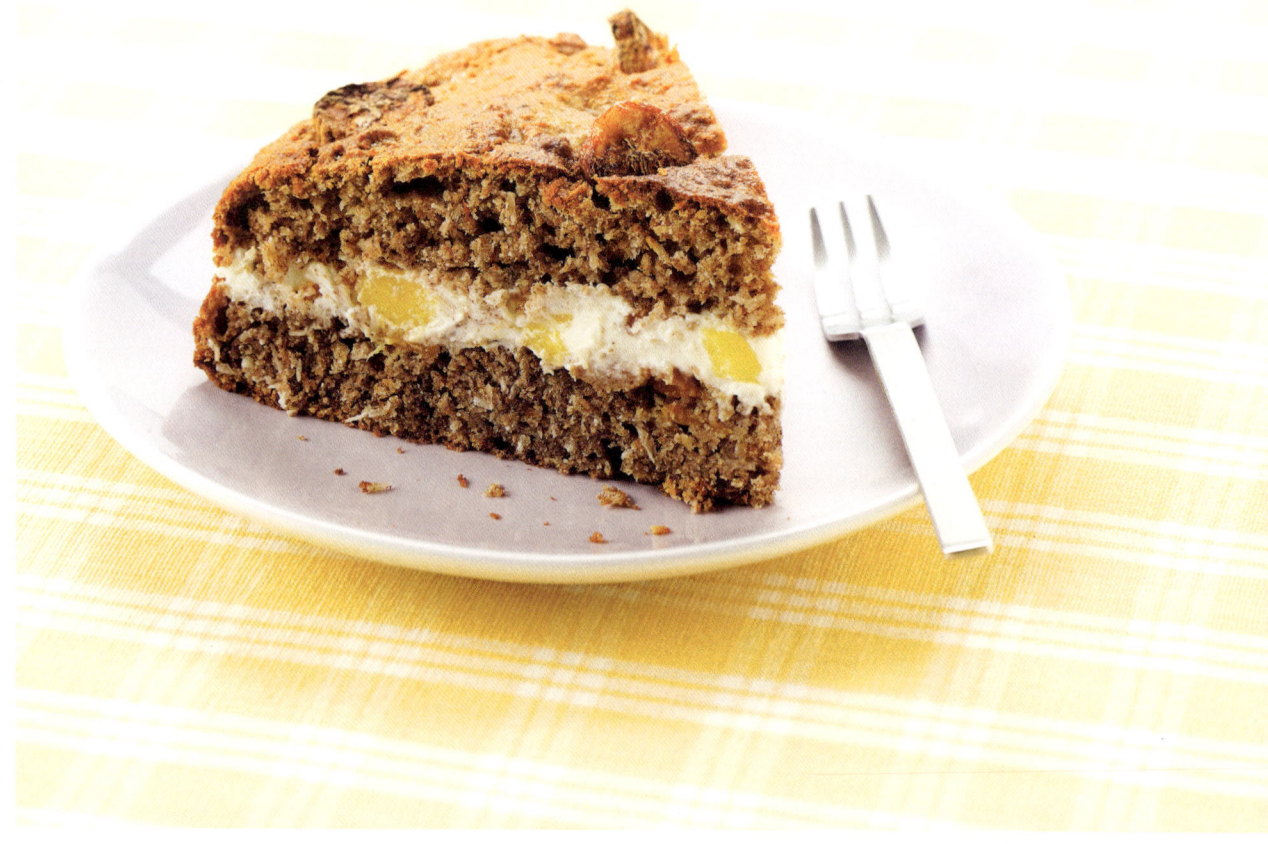

melted butter, bananas, eggs and sugar in a blender until smooth. Add to the flour and mix well. Spoon the mixture into the tin (pan) and top with the bananas chips. Bake for 30–40 minutes, or until firm and golden. Cool completely on a wire rack.

3 Beat the cream cheese and honey. Stir in the mango. Slice the cake in half horizontally, spread the filling in the centre and sandwich it back together, then serve.

487 SEEDED DOUGH BALLS

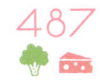

MAKES 20
PREPARATION
25 minutes +
proving
COOKING
20 minutes

350ml/12fl oz/1½ cups tepid water
2 tsp dried yeast
350g/12oz/3 cups strong white bread flour, plus extra for dusting
150g/5½oz/1¼ cups strong wholemeal bread flour
1½ tsp salt
5 tbsp toasted sunflower seeds
olive oil, for brushing

1 Pour 6 tablespoons of the water into a bowl. Sprinkle in the yeast, stir until dissolved and set aside for 5 minutes. Sift the flours and salt into a large bowl. Stir in the seeds.

2 Make a well in the centre of the flour and pour in the yeast mixture and 250ml/9fl oz/1 cup of the water. Gradually stir in the flour from the sides of the well. Stir in 3–4 tablespoons water, if necessary, to make a soft dough.

3 Turn the dough out on to a lightly floured work surface. Knead for 10 minutes until smooth and elastic. Put in a new bowl and cover with a dish towel. Leave for 1½–2 hours.

4 Preheat the oven to 220°C/425°F/gas mark 7. Press the dough with your knuckles, then divide into 20 pieces. Flatten each piece slightly, fold it over, then roll into a ball in your palm. Place on a floured baking sheet and leave for 10 minutes.

5 Brush the dough balls with olive oil and bake for 15–20 minutes until risen and golden. Cool on a wire rack.

488 CHEESE SCONES

MAKES 10
PREPARATION 10 minutes
COOKING 12 minutes

STORAGE Make in advance and keep in an airtight container for up to 3 days or freeze for up to 1 month.

150g/5½oz/1¼ cups self-raising flour
70g/2½oz/½ cup wholemeal self-raising flour
½ tsp baking powder
90g/3½oz Cheddar cheese, grated
2 tbsp extra-virgin olive oil
6–7 tbsp milk, plus for brushing
1 large free-range egg, beaten

1 Preheat the oven to 220°C/425°F/gas mark 7. Lightly dust a baking sheet with flour.

2 Sift both types of flour and the baking powder into a bowl. Stir in the Cheddar and make a well in the centre. Pour in the oil, milk and egg and mix to form a soft dough. Add a little extra milk if it seems dry. Transfer to a lightly floured work surface and knead until smooth.

3 Roll out the dough into a rectangle about 2.5cm/1in thick, then cut into 10. Arrange on the baking sheet and brush the tops with a little milk. Bake for 10–12 minutes until risen and golden.

489 CHEESE AND WALNUT BREAD

MAKES 1 LOAF
PREPARATION 20 minutes+ proving
COOKING 35 minutes

STORAGE Wrap and store in the fridge for up to 3 days or in the freezer for up to 1 month.

300g/10½oz/2¼ cups strong wholemeal bread flour
200g/7oz/1½ cups strong white flour, plus extra for kneading
15g/½ oz fast-acting dried yeast
1 tsp salt
75g/2½oz/½ cup walnuts, chopped
75g/2½oz Cheddar cheese, grated
1 tbsp olive oil, plus for greasing
milk, for brushing

1 Mix the flours, yeast and salt in a bowl with the walnuts and cheese. Make a well in the centre, add the oil and 300ml/10½fl oz/1¼ cups tepid water, then mix to a dough.

2 Turn the dough onto a lightly floured surface and knead for 10 minutes. Put in a bowl, cover with clingfilm (plastic wrap) and leave to rise for 1 hour until doubled in size.

3 Grease a baking sheet. Knead the dough briefly, shape it into a round loaf and put it on the baking sheet. Cover and leave to rise for 20 minutes, or until doubled in size.

4 Preheat the oven to 200°C/400°F/gas mark 6. Brush with milk and bake for 30–35 minutes until golden brown and hollow sounding when tapped underneath. Cool on a wire rack.

490 SEEDED RYE BREAD

MAKES 1 LOAF
PREPARATION
15 minutes+ proving
COOKING
35 minutes
STORAGE
Wrap and store in an airtight container for up to 2 days or in the freezer for up to 1 month.

350g/12oz/2¾ cups strong wholemeal bread flour, plus extra
150g/5½oz/1¼ cups rye flour
1 tsp salt
15g/½oz fast-acting dried yeast
50g/1¾oz/½ cup sunflower seeds
50g/1¾oz/½ cup pumpkin seeds
3 tbsp flaxseeds
5 tbsp sesame seeds
3 tbsp molasses
1 tbsp honey or agave nectar
olive oil, for greasing

1. Put the flours, salt, yeast and sunflower, pumpkin and flaxseeds in a large bowl. Mix in 2 tablespoons of the sesame seeds and make a well in the middle.

2. Mix the molasses and honey with 300ml/10½fl oz/1¼ cups warm water and add to the flour. Stir to form a stiff dough, then knead for 10 minutes on a floured surface. Put in a bowl, cover with clingfilm (plastic wrap) and leave to rise for 1 hour until doubled in size.

3. Grease a baking sheet with oil. Knead the dough briefly, shape into a round and put on the baking sheet. Score the top with a knife, brush with water and sprinkle with the remaining sesame seeds. Cover with clingfilm (plastic wrap) and leave to rise for 30 minutes. Preheat the oven to 200°C/400°F/gas mark 6.

4. Bake for 30–35 minutes until golden and hollow sounding when tapped underneath. Cool on a wire rack before serving.

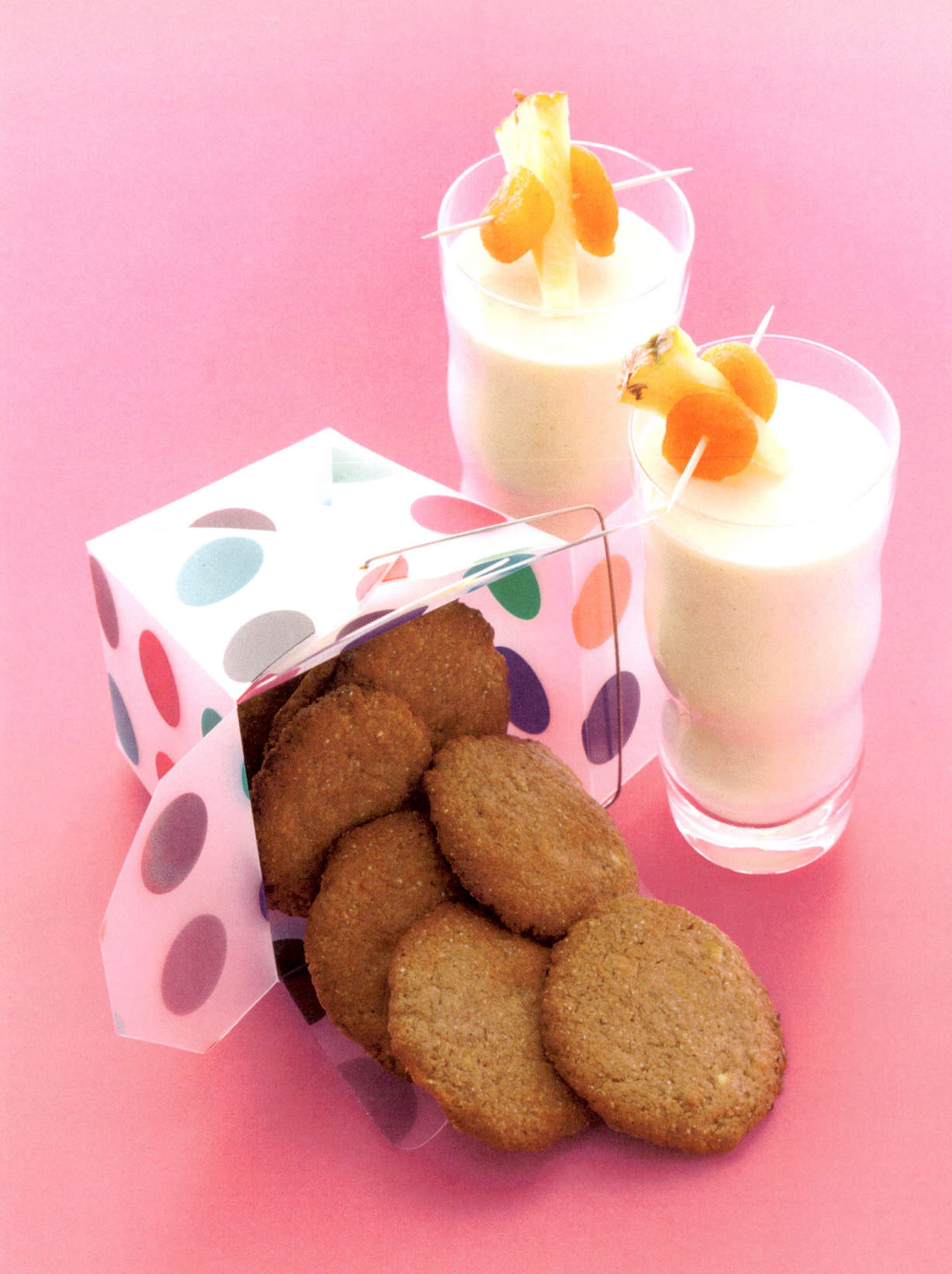

Drinks

Drinks aren't just for hydration – they also provide a good boost of essential vitamins and minerals in an easy-to-absorb form. In addition, making healthy drinks for your children reduces the amount of sugary, commercial drinks they are likely to request.

These smoothies and juices are ideal for getting extra fruit and vegetables into your family's diet. Serve the Tropical Explosion (see page 372) or Peach and Raspberry Shake (see page 374) for an exciting treat, or try the Spiced Apple Tea (see page 373) as a cooling, caffeine-free quencher on a summer's day.

491

CARIBBEAN COCKTAIL

SERVES 4
PREPARATION: 10 minutes
STORAGE: Best drunk fresh, but you can refrigerate for up to 12 hours.

1 pineapple
2 bananas
500ml/17fl oz/2 cups coconut milk
175g/6oz/¾ cup plain yogurt
seeds of ¼ vanilla pod
a little water, if required
4 dried apricots

1. Cut the top and skin off the pineapple. Cut the flesh into chunks, removing the core. Retain four chunks for garnish.

2. Peel the bananas, break into pieces and put into in a blender. Add the pineapple chunks, coconut milk, yogurt and vanilla seeds, and process until smooth. Add a little water if the consistency is too thick.

3. Pour the mixture into four glasses. Spear the apricots and reserved pineapple chunks onto cocktail sticks (toothpicks) and place on top of the glasses to serve.

492

TROPICAL EXPLOSION

SERVES 4
PREPARATION: 10 minutes
STORAGE: Best drunk fresh, but you can refrigerate for up to 12 hours.

6 oranges: 5 peeled and flesh chopped; 1 cut into slices
2 mangoes, peeled and chopped
2 passion fruit, deseeded and chopped
250ml/9 fl oz/1 cup apple juice
juice of 1 lime

1. Put the chopped orange flesh, mangoes and passion fruit into a blender. Add the apple and lime juices and process until smooth.

2. Remove any orange pips and serve in individual glasses, decorated with slices of orange.

493

CITRUS REFRESHER

SERVES 4
PREPARATION: 10 minutes + 4 hours chilling
COOKING: 5 minutes
STORAGE: Refrigerate for up to 24 hours.

8 lemons
2 limes
6 oranges
3 grapefruit
600ml/21fl oz/2½ cups water
225g/8oz/1 cup brown sugar
ice cubes

1. Grate the zest from a lemon, lime and orange. Place 1 tsp of each zest into a large saucepan. Squeeze the remaining fruit, removing as much juice as possible, and discard the skins.

2. Add the juice to the saucepan and then the water and sugar. Heat gently until the sugar dissolves and leave to simmer for 5 minutes.

3. Remove from the heat, allow to cool and then refrigerate for at least 4 hours before serving chilled with ice cubes.

494

SPICED APPLE TEA

SERVES 4
PREPARATION: 35 minutes
STORAGE: You can refrigerate for up to 3 days.

2 cinnamon sticks
1 lemon, sliced
4 spiced apple tea bags
1 litre/35fl oz/4 cups boiling water
1 apple, cored and sliced
115g/4oz/½ cup cranberries, frozen
ice cubes, optional

1. Place the cinnamon sticks, lemon slices and tea bags in a large measuring jug (pitcher).

2. Add the boiling water and allow to cool for 30 minutes. Place in the fridge overnight.

3. Just before serving, add the apple, frozen cranberries and ice cubes, if desired. Serve in individual glasses.

495

BLUEBERRY BRAINBOOSTER MILKSHAKE

SERVES 4
PREPARATION: 5 minutes
STORAGE: Best drunk immediately.

25g/1oz/¼ cup almonds, soaked in water overnight, then drained
250g/9oz/1¾ cups blueberries
1 small banana
150ml/5fl oz/scant ⅔ cup milk

1. Blend all the ingredients in a blender until smooth and creamy.

2. Divide the drink among four glasses and serve.

496

APRICOT AND TOFU BOOST

SERVES 4
PREPARATION: 5 minutes
STORAGE: Best drunk immediately, but it will keep for 3-4 hours in the fridge.

3 apricots, pitted
3 ready-to-eat dried apricots
1 small peach, pitted
150ml/5fl oz/scant 2/3 cup pineapple juice
250g/9oz silken tofu

1. Blend all the ingredients in a blender until smooth and creamy.

2. Divide the drink among four glasses and serve.

497

PINK ZINC HEAVEN

SERVES 4
PREPARATION: 5 minutes
STORAGE: Best drunk immediately, but it will keep for 3-4 hours in the fridge.

200g/7oz/2 cups strawberries
150g/5½oz/1 cup raspberries
2 passionfruit, flesh strained
1 banana
1 tbsp tahini (sesame paste)
1 tsp omega-blend oil or flaxseed oil
250ml/9fl oz/1 cup plain yogurt

1. Blend all the ingredients in a blender until smooth and creamy.

2. Divide the drink among four glasses and serve.

498

PEACH AND RASPBERRY SHAKE

SERVES 4
PREPARATION: 5 minutes
STORAGE: Best drunk immediately, but it will keep for 3-4 hours in the fridge.

2 peaches, pitted
25g/1oz/¼ cup mixed seeds (such as sunflower, sesame and pumpkin)
150g/5½oz/1 cup raspberries
2 tsp flaxseed oil
185ml/6fl oz/¾ cup plain yogurt
80ml/2½fl oz/⅓ cup milk

1. Blend all the ingredients in a blender until smooth and creamy.

2. Divide the drink among four glasses and serve.

499

REJUVENATING JUICE

SERVES 4
PREPARATION: 10 minutes
STORAGE: Refrigerate for up to 1 day. Stir before serving.

8 carrots
2 lemons
8 oranges
6 apples
12 celery stalks
4 celery tops

1. Peel the carrots, lemons and oranges. Squeeze the juice from the lemon.

2. Cut the apples in half, then remove the core, but leave the skin on.

3. Put all the fruit and celery stalks through a juicer, collecting the juice in a jug (pitcher). Add the lemon juice to the fruit and celery mixture and stir well. Serve in glasses with straws. Garnish with the celery tops.

500

SUPER FRUIT SMOOTHIE

SERVES 4
PREPARATION: 10 minutes
STORAGE: You can keep the smoothie in the fridge for up to 12 hours.

2 apples, cored and chopped
450g/1lb/3 cups frozen summer fruits
2 bananas, chopped
2 avocados, peeled, pitted and chopped
4 tbsp flaxseed oil
750ml/26 fl oz/3¼ cups unsweetened apple juice
4 tbsp ground almonds
juice of 1 lime
1 lime, cut into slices

1. Place the apple in a blender. Add all the other ingredients except the lime slices and blend until smooth.

2. Pour the smoothie mixture into glasses and decorate each glass with a slice of lime.

Index

almonds
   almond butter bites 63
   almond shortbread 357
   broccoli and almond soup 97
   carrot salad with almond dressing 136
   cranberry and almond quinoa 207
   soaked almonds 62
apples
   African curry 221
   apple, cherry and walnut crêpes 333
   apple coleslaw 122
   apple crumble 340
   apple flapjacks 74
   apple salad with cashew cream 313
   apple tart 344
   apricot and apple purée 308
   baked cinnamon apples 340
   blackberry and apple icicles 77
   blueberry and apple muffins 25
   cheese, apple and chutney bap 71
   cinnamon-spiced apple compote 328
   German salad 117
   great greens risotto 205
   mackerel, apple and potato salad 112–13
   millet and apple porridge 11
   pork with apples and pears 226
   spiced apple tea 373
   spiced apple volcanos 341
   toffee apple crisps 74
apricots
   apricot and apple purée 308
   apricot and cashew bars 352
   apricot and orange soufflés 334
   apricot and tofu boost 374
   apricot and tofu smoothie 21
   apricot cookies 356
   apricot muesli traybake 351
   Moroccan apricot parcels 281
   poached figs, apricots and cherries 22
   prune and apricot yogurt 20
artichokes, spaghetti with artichokes, beans and spinach 290
asparagus
   Asian asparagus 139
   asparagus egg scramble 31
   great greens risotto 205
   penne with asparagus and mushroom sauce 292
   salmon, mango and asparagus salad 110
aubergines
   aubergine and olive pâté 51
   aubergine farcie 230
   baba ganoush with avocado and fennel salad 52
   barbecued turkey and ratatouille kebabs 245
   lentil moussaka 283
   roasted aubergine dip 51
   spicy chickpeas with aubergine 278
avocados
   avocado and melon salad with creamy dressing 134
   avocado and seafood salad 116
   avocado with savoury crumbs 184
   baba ganoush with avocado and fennel salad 52
   bright bean salad 130
   creamed salmon rice cakes 29

INDEX

creamy guacamole 53
griddled chicken and guacamole baps 154
Italian flag salad 118
Mexican avocado soup 99
roast chicken and avocado focaccia 153
stuffed avocados 168
tropical salad 128

bacon
  bacon-baked Brussels 229
  braised Brussels sprouts 140
  Brazilian feijoa 220
  egg and bacon roll 149
  ham and barley broth 81
  wild mushroom, spinach and pancetta pizza 231
  winter vegetable soup 80
bananas
  April fool 325
  banana and blueberry muffins 361
  banana and buckwheat pancakes 26
  banana and coconut ice cream 316
  banana and mango cake 366-7
  date and walnut muffins 15
  nut butter and banana bagel 70
barley risotto 296
beans
  African-style broad beans 139
  baked bean melt 34
  bean & sausage hotpot 222
  bean cassoulet 301
  Brazilian feijoa 220
  bright bean salad 130
  crunchy country salad 130
  fighting fit fajitas 164
  giant baked beans on toasted rye 38
  Greek ragout 295
  ham, bean and pineapple salad 107
  Mexican bean tacos 193
  Mexican beanfeast 191
  Mexican casserole 216
  minestrone 98
  mixed bean salad 121
  prawn salad lunchbowl 115

quick and easy bean and ham salad 108
smashed bean and carrot spread 53
smoky butter bean soup 85
spaghetti with artichokes, beans and spinach 290
spiced bean and juniper casserole 299
spicy bean burgers 188
summer salad 131
super salad 120
beef
  beef tortillas with balsamic onions 211
  chow mein 210
  creamy beef korma 212
  oriental beef wrap 148
  steak ciabatta 147
  Tex-Mex burgers 213
beetroot
  baked chicory and beetroot 140
  beetroot cream soup 88
  bright bean salad 130
  crunchy country salad 130
  German salad 117
  Scandinavian beetroot burgers 284-5
  spicy beetroot soup 96
blackberries
  blackberry and apple icicles 77
  pear, blackberry and walnut crumble 339
blueberries
  banana and blueberry muffins 361
  blueberry and apple muffins 25
  blueberry brainbooster milkshake 373
  blueberry muffins 361
  blueberry salad 309
  blueberry yogo-pops 76
bread *see also* pizza; tortillas
  bread, butter and honey pudding 346
  cheese and walnut bread 368
  raisin French toast 16
  rigatoni with herb pangrattato 292
  seeded dough balls 367
  seeded rye bread 369
  socca Niçoise 69

summer berry pudding 322
summer puddings 336
broccoli
  broccoli and almond soup 97
  broccoli and Brazil nut stir 187
  broccoli and ginger stir-fry 274
  great greens risotto 205
  pesto pasta salad 127
  spaghetti with broccoli in yogurt and basil sauce 202
Brussels sprouts
  bacon-baked Brussels 229
  braised Brussels sprouts 140
bulgur wheat
  bulgur pilaf 182
  cool bulgur tabouleh 113
  spicy bulgur salad with nectarines 125
  tabouleh 125
  Turkish pilaf 244

cabbage
  apple coleslaw 122
  Caribbean casserole 268
  kimchi salad 129
  spring greens broth 93
cakes and bakes *see also* cookies; pies, pastries and tarts
  almond shortbread 357
  apricot and cashew bars 352
  apricot muesli traybake 351
  banana and blueberry muffins 361
  banana and mango cake 366-7
  blueberry muffins 361
  bunny bites 363
  carrot cake 364
  cheese scones 368
  chocolate and cranberry brownies 350
  date and pecan brownies 358
  flaxseed gingerbread men 355
  muesli crunchies 351
  party cake 365
calzone
  calzone 145
  pizza calzone 199
  tuna and cheese calzone 168
carrots
  braised Brussels sprouts 140
  bunny bites 363

carrot and courgette lentils 191
carrot and parsnip soup 93
carrot cake 364
carrot, date and pecan salad with ginger dressing 136
carrot, raisin and pinenut salad 122
carrot salad with almond dressing 136
carrot salad with sunflower seeds and parsley 137
curried carrot soup 94
Korean salad 128
smashed bean and carrot spread 53
spicy carrot and lentil soup 87
celeriac
   celeriac schnitzel 282
   sweet chestnut soup 95
celery
   celery smackers 60
   cheesy celery stalks 61
   crunchy country salad 130
   green giant soup 85
cheese *see also* pizza
   baked bean melt 34
   cheese and walnut bread 368
   cheese, apple and chutney bap 71
   cheese scones 368
   cheesy celery stalks 61
   cheesy potato and rocket pancakes 277
   Greek salad 123
   Italian flag salad 118
   Mediterranean melts 28
   melon and halloumi salad 123
   minted pea and cheese omelette 181
   mozzarella, cherry tomato and basil sticks 42
   mystery roll 174
   pasta with cheesy courgettes 204
   pesto pasta salad 127
   Popeye baked eggs 31
   roasted veg and halloumi pitta 177
   salami, cheese and pineapple sticks 43
   Spanish potato salad 131
   tuna and cheese calzone 168
   tuna melts 164
   tuna quesadilla 48

cherries
   apple, cherry and walnut crêpes 333
   hazelnut-cherry tart 332
   nut and cherry oat bars 21
   poached figs, apricots and cherries 22
   sweet cherry soup 310
chicken
   Caribbean chicken 235
   chicken & sweet potato casserole 242
   chicken and coconut curry 241
   chicken burgers 233
   chicken Caesar salad 109
   chicken dippers with peanut sauce 155
   chicken noodle nest 156
   chicken noodle soup 83
   chicken spring rolls 155
   chicken strips with satay dip 158
   chicken tikka naan 156
   curry with mango & coconut 238
   griddled chicken and guacamole baps 154
   Indian chicken korma 240
   Indonesian satay 246
   polenta gratin 237
   roast chicken and avocado focaccia 153
   Senegalese yassa 240
   sesame and honey goujons 234
   sesame-polenta chicken strips 234
   Spanish paella 238
   steamy soup 83
   sweet & sour 236
   sweet & sour buckwheat pasta 243
   tandoori chicken drumsticks 232
   Thai chicken salad 109
   Turkish pilaf 244
chickpeas
   bulgur pilaf 182
   chickpea veggie patties 284
   chunky Italian soup 86
   cool bulgur tabouleh 113
   corn pancakes with spicy peas 275
   falafel 176
   falafel and hummus lavash 197

hummus and seeded crackers 49
Mexican beanfeast 191
Moroccan apricot parcels 281
roasted red pepper hummus 45
spicy chickpeas with aubergine 278
spinach and chickpea soup 80
sweet potato scorchers 194
tomato and chickpea soup 89
chicory, baked chicory and beetroot 140
chocolate
   choco-nut ice cream 316
   chocolate and cranberry brownies 350
   chocolate fruit truffles 75
   date and pecan brownies 358
   fruity chocolate fondue 347
   orange and chocolate mousse 324
   tahini and chocolate fudge 75
   tahini chocolate fudge 365
coconut
   banana and coconut ice cream 316
   chicken and coconut curry 241
   coconut and clove rice 141
   curry with mango & coconut 238
   Hawaiian hulas 317
cod
   Caribbean casserole 268
   Cuban cod 263
   grilled cod with salsa 262
   spaghetti with Creole sauce 259
cookies
   apricot cookies 356
   gingerbread star cookies 355
   lemon oatmeal cookies 357
   oatmeal cookies 352
   peanut and oat cookies 353
   peanut butter cookies 353
   pumpkin cookies 356
courgettes
   barbecued turkey and ratatouille kebabs 245
   bright bean salad 130
   buckwheat noodles with spicy courgette sauce 278
   carrot and courgette lentils 191
   courgette and parmesan fritters 180

INDEX

pasta with cheesy courgettes 204
seafood tabouleh 117
Spanish omelette 173
tzatziki 56
couscous
  roast peppers 274–5
  royal couscous 119
  seafood tabouleh 117
  Turkish boreg 231
cream cheese and date bagel 71
cucumber
  Cajun salmon and cucumber roll 70
  gazpacho del campo 101
  Greek salad 123
  Korean salad 128
  Peruvian polenta cakes 54
  tabouleh 125
curries
  African curry 221
  chicken and coconut curry 241
  creamy beef korma 212
  curry with mango & coconut 238
  Indian chicken korma 240
  spring masala 256
  sweet potato and spinach curry 301

dates
  breakfast bars 20
  carrot, date and pecan salad with ginger dressing 136
  chewy date bars 73
  cream cheese and date bagel 71
  date and pecan brownies 358
  date and walnut muffins 15
duck, five-spice duck 251

eggs
  asparagus egg scramble 31
  Basque peppers with ham and eggs 151
  Beijing-style omelette 183
  breakfast kebabs 34
  Collioure salad 134
  egg and bacon roll 149
  egg and tomato cups 38
  fabulous frittata 181
  minted pea and cheese omelette 181
  mushroom omelettes 33

Niçoise wraps 172
omelette sandwich 150
pipérade pitta 29
Popeye baked eggs 31
pork and egg-fried rice 149
prawn omelette wraps 171
spaghetti frittata 180
Spanish omelette 173
tuna and onion tortilla 167
vegetable röstis with poached eggs 36

fennel
  baba ganoush with avocado and fennel salad 52
  fennel, monkfish and potato bake 267
  wild rice salad 135
figs, poached figs, apricots and cherries 22
fish *see also* seafood; *specific fish*
  creamy fish pie 258
  fish pâté 48
  Mediterranean fish parcels 252
  spicy fish tacos 253
fruit *see also specific fruit*
  baked fruit kebabs 343
  berry juicy yogurt 310
  berry muesli 10
  berry salad 15
  Caribbean cocktail 372
  chocolate fruit truffles 75
  citrus fruit salad 19
  citrus refresher 373
  dried fruit with fresh strawberries 16
  fruit and seed granola 11
  fruit brochettes 335
  fruit flowers 307
  fruit jellies 328
  fruit jelly 318
  fruit layer crisp 325
  fruit parfait 304
  fruity chocolate fondue 347
  fruity filo parcels 338
  fruity pancakes 24
  honey fruit salad 304
  hot waffles with fresh fruit 17
  jelly islands 317
  layered fruit and nut salad 18
  layered fruit salad 307

morning muesli 13
orchard harvest with custard 341
pink zinc heaven 374
rejuvenating juice 375
ruby-red salad 305
silky fruit salad 305
summer berry pudding 322
summer fruit salad 321
summer puddings 336
super fruit smoothie 375
tropical crème brûlée 326
tropical explosion 372
tropical fruit flambé 335
tropical fruit kebabs 326
tropical yogurt pots 18
winter fruit salad 336
winter sunshine salad 312

ham
  Basque peppers with ham and eggs 151
  carrot salad with almond dressing 136
  egg and tomato cups 38
  farfalle with chanterelle and thyme sauce 224
  ham and barley broth 81
  ham and egg pies 150
  ham, bean and pineapple salad 107
  ham roll-ups 43
  mushroom and ham pizza 230
  peach and prosciutto salad 106
  pear and ham bundles 46
  quick and easy bean and ham salad 108
  smoked ham and pepper pizza 144
herrings
  German salad 117
  herrings on rye 47
hummus
  celery smackers 60
  falafel and hummus lavash 197
  hummus and rye toasts 45
  hummus and seeded crackers 49
  hummus rice snacks 52
  pitta pockets 183
  roasted red pepper hummus 45
  spinach pancakes with hummus and wild mushrooms 276

ice cream
  banana and coconut 316
  choco-nut 316

kale
  caldo verde 81
  spicy chickpea pancakes 179
  spring green risotto 297

lamb
  chops with honey and thyme 214
  glazed lamb 213
  kofta pitta pockets 175
  lamb and pea samosas 148
  lamb Provençale 211
  mamma's meatballs 217
  Mexican casserole 216
  Moroccan lamb 215
  orange-roasted lamb chops 215
  oriental stir-fry 216

leeks
  brunch bonanza 39
  green giant soup 85
  leek and potato soup 102
  spring green risotto 297

lemons
  lemon oatmeal cookies 357
  lemon risotto with fresh basil 294
  Provençal lemon potatoes 141
  sesame-lemon turkey 248

lentils
  baked stuffed peppers 186
  carrot and courgette lentils 191
  creamy tomato and lentil soup 92
  lentil moussaka 283
  potato and lentil burgers 190
  spicy carrot and lentil soup 87
  Turkish pilaf 244
  winter vegetable soup 80

mackerel, apple and potato salad 112-13

mango
  banana and mango cake 366-7
  Caribbean chicken 235
  curry with mango & coconut 238
  mango and orange fool 319
  mango fool 324
  prawn and mango tarts 169
  salmon, mango and asparagus salad 110
  salmon with mango salsa 262
  tropical salad 128

melon
  avocado and melon salad with creamy dressing 134
  mellow melon 19
  melon and halloumi salad 123

millet and apple porridge 11

monkfish, fennel, monkfish and potato bake 267

mushrooms
  breakfast kebabs 34
  brunch bonanza 39
  Chinese soup with shiitake & noodles 104
  farfalle with chanterelle and thyme sauce 224
  mushroom and ham pizza 230
  mushroom and spinach quiche 286
  mushroom omelettes 33
  penne with asparagus and mushroom sauce 292
  pesto, spinach and mushroom pasta 273
  spinach pancakes with hummus and wild mushrooms 276
  stuffed mushrooms 287
  turkey escalopes in mushroom sauce 250
  wild mushroom pie 287
  wild mushroom, spinach and pancetta pizza 231

noodles
  buckwheat noodles with spicy courgette sauce 278
  chicken noodle nest 156
  chicken noodle soup 83
  Chinese five-spice noodles 264-5
  Chinese noodle salad 126
  Chinese soup with shiitake & noodles 104
  chow mein 210
  rice noodles with mangetout sauce 179
  rice paper rolls 153
  spring rolls 192
  tofu noodles 279
  turkey noodle soup 84

nuts
  berry muesli 10
  chocolate fruit truffles 75
  fruit and seed granola 11
  fruit layer crisp 325
  grilled peaches with macadamia cream 12
  layered fruit and nut salad 18
  morning muesli 13
  muesli crunchies 351
  nut and cherry oat bars 21
  soy-coated nuts and seeds 62
  tropical yogurt pots 18

oats & oatmeal
  apple flapjacks 74
  apricot muesli traybake 351
  berry muesli 10
  blueberry and apple muffins 25
  breakfast bars 20
  chewy date bars 73
  crunchy porridge 13
  fruit and seed granola 11
  fruit layer crisp 325
  lemon oatmeal cookies 357
  morning muesli 13
  muesli crunchies 351
  nut and cherry oat bars 21
  oatmeal cookies 352
  oatmeal pancakes with salmon 26
  peanut and oat cookies 353
  strawberry crunch pots 330

omelettes
  Beijing-style omelette 183
  eggless seaweed omelette 264
  eggless spring omelette 32
  eggless tofu and herb omelette 32
  minted pea and cheese omelette 181
  mushroom omelettes 33
  omelette sandwich 150
  prawn omelette wraps 171
  Spanish omelette 173

onions
  beef tortillas with balsamic onions 211
  pissaladière onion tart 187

tuna and onion tortilla 167
oranges
  apricot and orange soufflés 334
  braised Brussels sprouts 140
  citrus fruit salad 19
  creamy orange salad 312
  mango and orange fool 319
  mellow melon 19
  orange and chocolate mousse 324
  orange eskimo bowls 319
  orange-glazed sardines 256
  orange-roasted lamb chops 215
  pumpkin and orange crumble 339
  zesty citrus pancakes 23

pak choi, sesame Asian greens 137
pancakes
  apple, cherry and walnut crêpes 333
  banana and buckwheat pancakes 26
  buckwheat galettes with vegetables 28
  cheesy potato and rocket pancakes 277
  corn pancakes with spicy peas 275
  drop scones with fruit sauce 343
  eggless pancakes with spinach filling 35
  fruity pancakes 24
  Indian pancakes 178
  oatmeal pancakes with salmon 26
  Provençal pancakes 276
  spicy chickpea pancakes 179
  spinach pancakes with hummus and wild mushrooms 276
  zesty citrus pancakes 23
parsnips
  carrot and parsnip soup 93
  creamy parsnip soup 105
pasta *see also noodles*
  chunky Italian soup 86
  conchiglie with chunky sauce 203
  farfalle with chanterelle and thyme sauce 224
  fettuccine with walnut pesto 293

green tagliatelle with red hot pepper sauce 201
Lebanese macaroni salad 138
minestrone 98
pasta alla puttanesca 269
pasta and sun-dried tomato soup 99
pasta primavera 273
pasta with cheesy courgettes 204
pasta with goujons in a spinach sauce 250
pasta with sausage & tomato sauce 218
pasta with smoked trout and broccoli 259
pasta with vegetables and creamy mustard sauce 290
penne with asparagus and mushroom sauce 292
penne with Brazil nut sauce 200
penne with pesto and peas 202
penne with smoky pesto sauce 225
pesto pasta salad 127
pesto, spinach and mushroom pasta 273
prawn pasta salad 110
rigatoni with herb pangrattato 292
roasted tomato and basil pasta 288
seafood pasta 268
soupe au pistou 100
spaghetti bolognese 218
spaghetti frittata 180
spaghetti with artichokes, beans and spinach 290
spaghetti with broccoli in yogurt and basil sauce 202
spaghetti with Creole sauce 259
spaghettini with cool herbs and hot tomatoes 289
spinach fettuccine with fresh tomato sauce 203
sweet & sour pasta 243
vegetable lasagne 300
warm pasta salad 133
peaches
  grilled peaches with macadamia cream 12
  peach and almond rice pudding 334

peach and prosciutto salad 106
peach and raspberry shake 374
peanut butter
  breakfast bars 20
  chicken dippers with peanut sauce 155
  chicken strips with satay dip 158
  Indonesian satay 246
  peanut and oat cookies 353
  peanut butter cookies 353
  turkey satay 247
peanuts, nut butter and banana bagel 70
pears
  baked pears with honey and Brazil nuts 333
  hot pear soup 76
  pear and ham bundles 46
  pear, blackberry and walnut crumble 339
  pear tart 344
  pork with apples and pears 226
  sharon fruit with juicy pears 309
peas
  cool bulgur tabouleh 113
  corn pancakes with spicy peas 275
  eggless spring omelette 32
  green giant soup 85
  lamb and pea samosas 148
  minted pea and cheese omelette 181
  pea and mint soup with paninis 84
  pea and parmesan quinoa risotto 297
  penne with pesto and peas 202
  pesto pasta salad 127
  seafood tabouleh 117
pecans
  carrot, date and pecan salad with ginger dressing 136
  date and pecan brownies 358
  pecan pâté 56
peppers
  baked bean melt 34
  baked stuffed peppers 186
  barbecued turkey and ratatouille kebabs 245
  Basque peppers with ham and eggs 151

Brazilian feijoa 220
Collioure salad 134
gazpacho del campo 101
green tagliatelle with red hot pepper sauce 201
instant tortillas and pepper filling 195
Louisiana gumbo 221
Peruvian polenta cakes 54
pipérade pitta 29
polenta and pepper cakes with pesto 282
roast peppers 274–5
roasted red pepper hummus 45
Spanish omelette 173
pesto
  fettuccine with walnut pesto 293
  penne with pesto and peas 202
  penne with smoky pesto sauce 225
  pesto pasta salad 127
  pesto pizza 64
  pesto, spinach and mushroom pasta 273
  polenta and pepper cakes with pesto 282
  veg and pesto paninis 197
pies, pastries and tarts
  apple tart 344
  Catalan tart 263
  creamy fish pie 258
  custard tartlets 360
  fruity filo parcels 338
  half-moon pastries 69
  ham and egg pies 150
  hazelnut-cherry tart 332
  jammy heart tarts 360
  middle eastern puffs 184
  mini tarts 207
  Moroccan apricot parcels 281
  mushroom and spinach quiche 286
  pear tart 344
  pineapple pie 347
  pissaladière onion tart 187
  plum tart 346
  prawn and mango tarts 169
  Turkish boreg 231
  wild mushroom pie 287
  winter tapas tarts 260
pineapple

ham, bean and pineapple salad 107
Hawaiian hulas 317
pineapple and mint frozen yogurt 77
pineapple boats 308
pineapple cocktail 321
pineapple pie 347
salami, cheese and pineapple sticks 43
tuna kebabs with pineapple 270–1
wild rice salad 135
pizza
  calzone 145
  feisty fiesta pizza 198
  pepperoni pizza 144
  pizza calzone 199
  pizza grill 66
  pizza margherita 66
  pizza Napoletana 198
  simple mini pizzas 200
  smiley face pizza 146–7
  smoked ham and pepper pizza 144
  tomato and garlic pizza 64
  tuna and cheese calzone 168
plum tart 346
polenta
  Peruvian polenta cakes 54
  polenta and pepper cakes with pesto 282
  polenta gratin 237
popcorn
  cinnamon 72
  savoury spicy 63
pork
  African curry 221
  pork and egg-fried rice 149
  pork with apples and pears 226
  rice paper rolls 153
  spaghetti bolognese 218
  Turkish boreg 231
  Vietnamese pork 227
potatoes
  caldo verde 81
  cheesy potato and rocket pancakes 277
  chicken Caesar salad 109
  fennel, monkfish and potato bake 267
  German salad 117

Greek ragout 295
green giant soup 85
honey bangers and mash 229
leek and potato soup 102
mackerel, apple and potato salad 112–13
minted potatoes with hazelnuts 140–1
potato and lentil burgers 190
potato skin battalions 194
Provençal lemon potatoes 141
salmon and coriander fishcakes 162
salmon Niçoise salad 112
Scandinavian potato and sausage salad 107
Spanish potato salad 131
spicy chickpea pancakes 179
spinach bouillabaisse 299
tuna and onion tortilla 167
tuna Niçoise 115
prawns
  avocado and melon salad with creamy dressing 134
  brochettes with pili pili sauce 267
  Chinese five-spice noodles 264–5
  Hong Kong prawns 171
  prawn and mango tarts 169
  prawn omelette wraps 171
  prawn pasta salad 110
  prawn salad lunchbowl 115
  spring masala 256
prune and apricot yogurt 20
pumpkin
  Caribbean casserole 268
  hallowe'en soup 87
  Louisiana gumbo 221
  pumpkin and orange crumble 339
  pumpkin cookies 356
  pumpkin hotpot with roasted vegetables 189
  pumpkin soup 94
  sweet potato and pumpkin soup 98

quinoa
  cranberry and almond quinoa 207

INDEX

pea and parmesan quinoa risotto 297
sweet quinoa 12
rice
  barley risotto 296
  coconut and clove rice 141
  great greens risotto 205
  lemon risotto with fresh basil 294
  oriental rice salad 126
  peach and almond rice pudding 334
  pork and egg-fried rice 149
  seafood risotto 269
  Spanish paella 238
  spring green risotto 297
  sushi cones 161
  wild rice salad 135
rice paper rolls 153
rocket and trout salad 118

salmon
  Cajun salmon and cucumber roll 70
  cool bulgur tabouleh 113
  creamed salmon rice cakes 29
  creamy salmon and alfalfa pittas 163
  oatmeal pancakes with salmon 26
  salmon and coriander fishcakes 162
  salmon fish cakes 255
  salmon, mango and asparagus salad 110
  salmon Niçoise salad 112
  salmon with mango salsa 262
  smoked salmon pâté 160
  smoked salmon spirals 47
  sushi cones 161
  teriyaki salmon 254-5
  warm pasta salad 133
sardines
  orange-glazed sardines 256
  sardine bruschetta with herb dressing 166
  sardine soldiers 166
  sardines and tomato on brown 163
sausages
  aubergine farcie 230

bean & sausage hotpot 222
brunch bonanza 39
caldo verde 81
conchiglie with chunky sauce 203
cool dogs 151
honey bangers and mash 229
honey-sesame sausages 46
Louisiana gumbo 221
pasta with sausage & tomato sauce 218
sausage and barley salad 108
Scandinavian potato and sausage salad 107
seafood see also prawns
  avocado and seafood salad 116
  seafood kebabs 254
  seafood pasta 268
  seafood risotto 269
  seafood tabouleh 117
sharon fruit with juicy pears 309
spinach
  Caribbean casserole 268
  eggless pancakes with spinach filling 35
  half-moon pastries 69
  Japanese spinach soup 102
  Lebanese spinach 60
  mushroom and spinach quiche 286
  mystery roll 174
  pasta with goujons in a spinach sauce 250
  pepperoni pizza 144
  pesto pizza 64
  pesto, spinach and mushroom pasta 273
  Popeye baked eggs 31
  spaghetti with artichokes, beans and spinach 290
  spinach and chickpea soup 80
  spinach bouillabaisse 299
  spinach pancakes with hummus and wild mushrooms 276
  spring greens broth 93
  sweet potato and spinach curry 301
  wild mushroom, spinach and pancetta pizza 231
  wild rice salad 135
strawberries

dried fruit with fresh strawberries 16
minty strawberries 320
rhubarb and strawberry compote 331
strawberry cheesecake 315
strawberry crunch pots 330
sushi cones 161
sweet chestnut soup 95
sweet potatoes
  Brazilian feijoa 220
  brunch bonanza 39
  Caribbean casserole 268
  chicken & sweet potato casserole 242
  spicy sweet potatoes 127
  sweet potato and pumpkin soup 98
  sweet potato and spinach curry 301
  sweet potato scorchers 194
  sweet potato wedges 59

tarts see pies, pastries and tarts
tofu
  apricot and tofu boost 374
  apricot and tofu smoothie 21
  BBQ tofu baguette 174
  Chinese soup with shiitake & noodles 104
  choco-nut ice cream 316
  eggless tofu and herb omelette 32
  Japanese spinach soup 102
  miso and tofu broth 88
  smoked tofu salad 57
  summer kebabs 186
  tofu bites 175
  tofu noodles 279
tomatoes see also pizza
  aubergine and olive pâté 51
  Brazilian feijoa 220
  breakfast kebabs 34
  bright bean salad 130
  brunch bonanza 39
  creamy tomato and lentil soup 92
  crunchy country salad 130
  egg and tomato cups 38
  gazpacho del campo 101
  Greek salad 123

Italian flag salad 118
Louisiana gumbo 221
Mediterranean melts 28
minestrone 98
mozzarella, cherry tomato and basil sticks 42
mystery roll 174
pasta and sun-dried tomato soup 99
pasta with sausage & tomato sauce 218
pipérade pitta 29
quick tomato soup 68
roasted tomato and basil pasta 288
sardines and tomato on brown 163
spaghettini with cool herbs and hot tomatoes 289
spiced bean and juniper casserole 299
spinach fettuccine with fresh tomato sauce 203
stuffed tomato salad 133
summer tomato soup 91
tabouleh 125
tomato and chickpea soup 89
tomato soup with fresh coriander 91
tortilla dippers with tomato salsa 68
tuna quesadilla 48
tortilla (Spanish), tuna and onion 167
tortillas
  beef tortillas with balsamic onions 211
  fighting fit fajitas 164
  instant tortillas and pepper filling 195
  Moroccan turkey wraps 158
  Niçoise wraps 172
  tortilla dippers with tomato salsa 68
  tuna quesadilla 48
  veggie wrappers 192
trout
  pasta with smoked trout and broccoli 259
  rocket and trout salad 118

tuna
  fighting fit fajitas 164
  Niçoise wraps 172
  stuffed tomato salad 133
  tuna and cheese calzone 168
  tuna and onion tortilla 167
  tuna kebabs with pineapple 270-1
  tuna melts 164
  tuna Niçoise 115
  tuna patties 167
  tuna quesadilla 48
  tuna steak kebabs and sugar snaps 271
  winter tapas tarts 260
turkey
  barbecued turkey and ratatouille kebabs 245
  festive turkey balls 159
  Moroccan turkey wraps 158
  pan-fried turkey 246
  pasta with goujons in a spinach sauce 250
  sesame-lemon turkey 248
  towering turkey bagels 159
  turkey escalopes in mushroom sauce 250
  turkey meat balls in five-veg sauce 249
  turkey noodle soup 84
  turkey satay 247
  winter kebabs 244

vegetables *see also specific vegetables*
  autumn vegetable soup 105
  buckwheat galettes with vegetables 28
  chickpea veggie patties 284
  Chinese soup with shiitake & noodles 104
  chunky Italian soup 86
  conchiglie with chunky sauce 203
  Indonesian tempeh and vegetables 281
  minestrone 98
  pasta primavera 273
  pasta with vegetables and creamy mustard sauce 290
  pitta pockets 183
  Provençal pancakes 276
  pumpkin hotpot with roasted vegetables 189
  rejuvenating juice 375
  roasted veg and halloumi pitta 177
  soupe au pistou 100
  summer crudités 61
  summer kebabs 186
  summer salad 131
  super salad 120
  turkey meat balls in five-veg sauce 249
  veg and pesto paninis 197
  vegetable lasagne 300
  vegetable röstis with poached eggs 36
  vegetable samosas 172
  veggie dippers 59
  veggie wrappers 192
  warm pasta salad 133
  winter vegetable soup 80

waffles with fresh fruit 17
walnuts
  apple, cherry and walnut crêpes 333
  cheese and walnut bread 368
  date and walnut muffins 15
  fettuccine with walnut pesto 293
  middle eastern puffs 184
  pear, blackberry and walnut crumble 339
watermelon zest 313

yogurt
  April fool 325
  berry juicy yogurt 310
  blueberry yogo-pops 76
  fruit layer crisp 325
  Lebanese macaroni salad 138
  Lebanese spinach 60
  pineapple and mint frozen yogurt 77
  prune and apricot yogurt 20
  spaghetti with broccoli in yogurt and basil sauce 202
  strawberry crunch pots 330
  tropical crème brûlée 326
  tropical yogurt pots 18
  tzatziki 56